International and Cultural Psychology

Series Editor
Anthony J. Marsella, Alpharetta, GA, USA

Explores problems and challenges to mental health, psychosocial wellbeing, human growth and development, and human welfare that are emerging from our contemporary global context. It advances in psychological knowledge regarding the nature and consequences of the many social, cultural, economic, political, and environmental events and forces that affect individuals and communities throughout the world. The series covers areas like therapy, assessment, organizational psychology, community psychology, gender, child development, and specific disorders. In addition, it addresses major global challenges such as poverty, peace, urbanization, modernization, refugees, and migration. The series acknowledges the multidisciplinary, multisectoral, and multicultural nature of the global context of our lives, and publishes books that reflect this reality. Publish your next book in this series! Send your manuscript to Series Editor: Anthony J. Marsella, marsella@hawaii.edu.

More information about this series at http://link.springer.com/series/6089

Arthur W. Blume

Colonialism and the COVID-19 Pandemic

Perspectives from indigenous Psychology

Springer

Arthur W. Blume
Washington State University Vancouver
Ridgefield, WA, USA

ISSN 1571-5507 ISSN 2197-7984 (electronic)
International and Cultural Psychology
ISBN 978-3-030-92824-7 ISBN 978-3-030-92825-4 (eBook)
https://doi.org/10.1007/978-3-030-92825-4

This Springer imprint is published by the registered company Springer Nature Switzerland AG
The registered company address is: Gewerbestrasse 11, 6330 Cham, Switzerland

This book is dedicated to the memory of Dr. Jean Lau Chin and her husband Gene, who were early victims of the COVID-19 pandemic, as well as to all the other victims of color who have perished from the plague of colonialism and its consequential-isms. May you all rest in power. It is hoped that this book will help to close the colonial era and replace it with societies who are more aligned with the welfare of the whole rather the self-interests of the few—to end the pandemics of injustice once and for all.

Acknowledgments

I would like to acknowledge the ancestors who guided me throughout the writing of this book. The COVID-19 pandemic has reinstructed the lesson that we are nothing without those who went before us. I would also like to thank Dr. Karen Schmaling for reviewing and commenting upon yet another book for me. Your insightful comments as a gifted scholar of psychology were especially helpful to me during the extremely challenging task of writing a psychology text in real time as historical events unfolded. I would also like to thank the esteemed senior editor for the cultural and international psychology book series published by Springer Nature, Dr. Anthony Marsella, and the executive editor at Springer Nature, Sharon Panulla, for their consistent enthusiasm and support for the project from beginning to end, encouraging great optimism in the midst of writing about tragic circumstances. Many thanks to all—your spirits are reflected in this book.

Introduction

One cannot understate the irony that the progressive modern world in the early 2020s was about to be humbled by a relentless entity too small to be seen by the human eye. The COVID-19 pandemic would soon expose the significant vulnerabilities of modern human civilization. Beliefs of species superiority would not spare humanity from its collective vulnerability to one of nature's most miniscule members.

A couple of explanations are needed to introduce the content. First, this book was written during the pandemic and completed prior to its end, so it may contain an incomplete history of events. As discussed in Chapter 11, the story is not complete, so in some ways the text may try to anticipate a short-term future that has already passed, contributing to a potential overuse of past imperfect tenses. Second, I refer to the pandemic by discussing coronavirus, SARS-CoV-2, and COVID-19 sometimes interchangeably. Coronavirus describes the type of virus, and SARS-CoV-2 is the specific virus that causes a disease referred to as COVID-19.

Toward the end of 2019, there was an obscure story in a local newspaper about an unusual form of sickness with pneumonia that had emerged in Asia. The story caught my eye, as an Indigenous psychologist, because unknown sicknesses have killed millions of our people during the history of colonialism. When colonists arrived in the western hemisphere, they brought along several pathogens that had plagued Europe for centuries. The First People of the Americas were naïve to the viruses, meaning they were as vulnerable to those deadly diseases as the global population was to the novel SARS-CoV-2 virus. Repeated outbreaks, epidemics, and pandemics resulted in extreme loss of life as described in Chapter 1. Those extreme killing events remain on the mind of those who lost ancestors to those illnesses that decimated Indigenous American families and peoples, illnesses that left the Indigenous people of the Americans essentially defenseless to the colonizing armies that followed.

Five centuries of sickness have resulted in a wary and resilient people: A wary people primed to perceive the collective risk for sickness given current imbalances and a resilient people who have used the strengths of the cultural perspectives to survive and thrive despite five centuries of sickness. Radically different assumptions about human nature and humanity's place in the natural world primed the First People of the Americas to the risks of an unknown disease much earlier than European descendants, despite both having experienced significant sickness and death in their histories. Indigenous people, who assume interdependence with nature, would understand that humans could easily be humbled by a tiny little virus rippling throughout our interdependent planetary system.

Worldviews have certainly played a role in how to interpret and respond to epidemics and pandemics. Eurocentric cultural beliefs emerged with assumptions that individuals were the foundational unit of existence (e.g., Descartes, 1637). The hierarchical structures in European society likely reinforced those beliefs, suggesting that self and self-reliance were essential for survival in a hierarchical social order. Perhaps the era of plagues had played a role in the belief of the necessity to pursue self-interests in order to survive, and perhaps fear had an important role in the development of that trust in self-reliance. During the epidemics of the middle ages, when millions of Europeans were killed by diseases that were poorly understood, fear would have been a predominant feature of those societies.

Many Europeans in the middle ages would have understood diseases as caused by dark supernatural forces likely related to sin, and often spread through communities by miasma (putrid dark vapors) or poisoning by outsiders. Since darkness and evil forces were blamed for sicknesses, and since darkness and evil often were associated unfairly with non-Christian outsiders, outgroups such as Jews were blamed for the diseases (Getz, 1991; Glatter & Finkelman, 2020; Voigtländer & Voth, 2012; Winkler, 2005). Especially in hierarchical societies decimated by unknown illnesses, blaming others for these unknown tragic and disruptive events would have happened easily. Even with the advancement of science, the tendencies to blame others in those societies have persisted, readily observed during the COVID-19 pandemic. So, why did so many twenty-first century societies react to COVID-19 like medieval Europe?

Colonial Amnesia and Forgotten Horrors

Many colonial nations were slow to respond and surprised by the spread and ferocity of the SARS-CoV-19 virus, with very little historical recall of the risks and dangers of pathogens. Afterall, influenza continues to stalk humans and only 70 years has passed since polio was finally controlled with a vaccine (Conniff, 2020). I have known people who suffered the consequences of polio. I have a scar on my arm from the smallpox vaccines. Yet the collective memory about polio and smallpox seems to have been lost to the mainstream today.

Another largely forgotten pandemic was the so-called "Spanish Flu Pandemic" despite the fact it seems to have been first detected in the US in 1918 (Barry, 2018). Remember learning about the 1918 pandemic in American schools? Why wasn't the memory of masks and social distancing passed along to children and grandchildren so they would be prepared when history repeated itself? In Barry's book, *The Great Influenza* (2018), one reads an account that in many respects could have been mistaken as a book about the COVID-19 pandemic, suggesting the lessons of 100 years ago were not learned. How is it possible so many people would forget a pandemic that resulted in the deaths of probably more than 50 million (Barry, 2018; Champine & Marques, 2020; Conniff, 2020), or the lessons from those deaths?! Contrast that with the experience of Indigenous Americans. In 1918, American Indians and Alaska natives had significantly higher mortality rates for the Spanish Flu pandemic, and again in 2009, for the H1N1 pandemic, than other ethnic groups (Andrulis et al., 2012). Indigenous Americans have not had the luxury of forgetting pandemics that have continued to traumatize our communities routinely from the fifteenth to the twenty-first centuries.

Colonial nations conquered Indigenous people because they assumed that they were a superior people and entitled to dominate others. Colonial beliefs in superiority also help to explain pandemic amnesia before the COVID-19 pandemic. If one assumes the superiority of a people and a culture, one might also buy into the belief of a certain invulnerability of that particular people and culture. Some psychologists have noted an "unrealistic optimism bias" in which some believe they will not get sick during a pandemic (Taylor, 2019, p. 45), but such optimism would likely arise from beliefs of personal superiority to others. A belief in superiority might assume that past missteps are no longer possible since we are so much smarter now than our ancestors, or that technological progress has made us invulnerable. Wrong.

Even though societies have advanced in certain ways technologically speaking and science has advanced significantly since 1918, it did not help us avoid the pitfalls of COVID-19. Colonial superiority led to colonial complacency that left people vulnerably unprepared. Due to colonial amnesia of tragedies, many thought pandemics were left in the past to never disturb us again. Wrong again. The sad truth is that nearly everything discussed in this book was avoidable. Why were the lessons from 1918 not used to prepare for COVID-19? What is the common thread that contributes to continued vulnerability to pandemics despite certain advances in medicine and technology? What contributed to the divisiveness we saw in the pandemic response that prevented a coordinated and unified approach? What do we need to do to be better in order to be prepared for the next pandemic? What kind of mindset change will that require?

The answers to all of those questions are related to the history of colonialism. Colonialism has always been a killing proposition, so it should be no surprise that colonialism continues to kill today. The rest of this book is dedicated to sharing an Indigenous psychological perspective on how colonialism helped to create pandemic risks and severely hampered the response to COVID-19. The consequences of colonialism and their relationships to the COVID-19 pandemic will be examined and critiqued in great detail. Finally, the tenets of Indigenous psychology will be used to propose alternative and more humane methods to address future pandemics and retiring the colonial circumstances that make them more likely.

Without significant transformations, everything written about the next pandemic will likely have been avoidable, too, emphasizing that future pandemic preparation begins today. My hope is that we will prepare for a healthier future together by examining what must change.

—Arthur W. Blume, October 10, 2021

References

Andrulis, D. P., Siddiqui, N. J., Purtle, J., & Cooper, M. R. (2012). *H1N1 influenza pandemic and racially and ethnically diverse communities in the United States: Assessing the evidence and charting opportunities for advancing health equity*. US Department of Health and Human Services.

Barry, J. M. (2018). *The great influenza: The story of the deadliest pandemic in history*. Penguin Books.

Champine, R. D., & Marques, D. (2020). Flattening the curve in 1918. *National Geographic, 238*(3), 22-23.

Conniff, R. (2020). Stopping pandemics. *National Geographic, 238*(2), 40-73.

Descartes, R. (1637). *Discourse on the method*. Translated in 1983 by V. R. Miller and R. P. Miller (Springer-Verlag).

Getz, F. M. (1991). Black death and the silver lining: Meaning, continuity, and revolutionary change in histories of medieval plague. *Journal of the History of Biology, 24*(2), 265-289. https://www.jstor.org/stable/4331174

Glatter, K. A., & Finkelman, P. (2020). History of the plague: An ancient pandemic for the age of COVID-19. *The American Journal of Medicine, 134*(2), 176-181. https://doi.org/10.1016/j.amjmed.2020.08.019

Taylor, S. (2019). *The psychology of pandemics: Preparing for the next global outbreak of infectious disease*. Cambridge Scholars Publishing.

Voigtländer, N., & Voth, H-J. (2012). Persecution perpetuated the medieval origins of anti-Semitic violence in Nazi Germany. *The Quarterly Journal of Economics*. https://doi.org/10.1093/qje/qjs019

Winkler, A. (2005). The medieval holocaust: The approach of the plague and the destruction of Jews in Germany, 1348-1349. Faculty Publications. 1816. https://scholarsarchive.byu.edu/facpub/1816

Contents

Chapter 1
Colonialism and Pandemics

Abstract Modern colonialism was initiated by a series of European policies that indoctrinated the belief that European colonists exercised divinely sanctioned superiority over those they encountered and conquered. Assumptions of superiority entitled colonists to kill, enslave, and assimilate others, resulting in hierarchical societies that dehumanized whole groups of people and permitted widespread inherent inequities. Supremacy beliefs permitted conquest and subjugation by any means necessary, utilizing longstanding policies of deception to generate significant distrust and division. Epidemics played a critical role in colonization, weakening Indigenous resistance and killing millions through the Columbian Exchange. Colonial hierarchies fostered competition and conflict between self and others, promoting the self-interests of the privileged over the interests of others. Colonialism also has a decidedly material worldview focused the acquisition of property, resources, and wealth extracted from others—a worldview that conflicted significantly with that of Indigenous Americans. The legacy of colonial hierarchies, inequitable treatment, and sickness has been collective vulnerability and a colonial world order ill prepared to address the collective threats of COVID-19.

The reality of the European Middle Ages before the voyages of Columbus had been unkind. Europe endured war after war, fighting off invaders from inside and outside of Europe (e.g., Graham, 2015). Europe also endured several waves of epidemics of infectious diseases with high mortality rates, such as cholera, influenzas, bubonic and pneumonic plagues, and smallpox. The so-called Black Death may have resulted in the deaths of up to half of the population of the continent with more than 50 million lost (Conniff, 2020). Psychologically speaking, one can imagine how self-preservation might emerge as a central concern and where others might be perceived with distrust and as a threat due to the illnesses. Paranoia towards others might have appeared to be a functional response at the time without a rational framework to interpret the viral events. The circumstances of epidemics and pandemics may have contributed toward a particular view on the human condition and perhaps contributed to an adversarial mentality towards others that set the stage for colonial activities.

A. W. Blume, *Colonialism and the COVID-19 Pandemic*, International and Cultural Psychology, https://doi.org/10.1007/978-3-030-92825-4_1

Christianity provided religious interpretations of the mysterious and life-threatening events. The church became a consistent power in Europe during the periods of instability. The vast majority of Europeans were Christian and subject to the power and will of the church. There was no democracy at work in Europe and the ruling class was granted divinely sanctioned power by the church to lord over others so long as that ruling class remained defenders of the Christian faith. The underclass of Europe was instructed by the church to obey those divinely sanctioned rulers. Columbus and others who followed brought these values with them.

Some have argued that colonialism as it is experienced today may have begun with the Christian Crusades (Dunbar-Ortiz, 2014). The papal decrees directing the Crusades sanctioned not only the slaughter of other peoples but also the seizure of their lands and their possessions in the name of the church. Later, a papal edict by Pope Nicholas V known as the *Dum Diversas* (Pope Nicholas V, June 18, 1452) was used as the foundation of a doctrine that sanctioned the colonization of non-believers (as defined by the Roman church). The so-called *Doctrine of Discovery* of 1493 by Pope Alexander VI expanded upon *Dum Diversas* to create a blueprint for the conquest and division of the world. Included in the *Doctrine of Discovery* was papal permission to annihilate and control others, to seize and exploit the resources of others, and to enslave those who survived. Centuries thereafter, the *Doctrine of Discovery* was used as the legal precedent for supporting the methods and consequences of conquest and subjugation by colonial nations, including colonial policies carried out in the US (Davenport, 1917). Those policies and their consequences help us to understand current circumstances. Nearly every nation has been touched by the long arms of colonialism, negatively impacting the psychological wellness of the planet (Barber & Naepi, 2020; Blume, 2020).

Colonization has defined the assumptions under which much of the world lives under today, including assumptions concerning social structures and institutions (Blume, 2020). Hierarchy has been assumed as the natural state of affairs, such that inequities are tolerated and perpetuated even if disapproved by many. Many shrug-off the inequities as inevitable (natural) or unsolvable (entrenched), and apathetic resignation tends to perpetuate the inequitable status quo. Those inequities have played an important role with pandemics historically, including in the 2020s. The next section of this chapter describes how colonial assumptions have contributed to historic vulnerabilities to pandemics and their consequences.

Hierarchies and Dehumanization

When Columbus arrived in the western hemisphere, he and those who followed unwittingly brought the same pathogens that contributed to illnesses that depopulated Europe. The first known epidemic apparently involved a swine influenza in 1493 (Guerra, 1988; Thornton, 2002), likely a virus not unlike the one that contributed to 1918 pandemic. The Columbian Exchange of Pathogens exposed the Indigenous people of the western hemisphere to diseases for which there was no natural immunity. The Europeans were also exposed to novel diseases for which they had no natural immunity, but history has suggested that it was Indigenous people of the west who was most severely impacted by that exchange (Merbs, 1992). Waves of sickness swept through Indigenous communities, depopulating the western hemisphere--leaving empty lands and almost defenseless people. Millions were estimated to have died in what is now known as Mexico and Peru (Joralemon, 1982; Livi-Bacci, 2006).

The most virulent killers were diseases such as influenza, measles, smallpox, and typhus (Bianchine & Russo, 1992; Guerra, 1988; Snow & Lanphear, 1988). Estimates are that the Americas were depopulated by perhaps as much as 90% between the arrival of Columbus and 1650 and perhaps 95% by the year 1900 (Lewis & Maslin, 2015; Mann, 2006; Thornton, 1987). However, the depopulation of Indigenous people by epidemics through first contact with European colonists was not exclusive to just the western hemisphere (e.g., Barber & Naepi, 2020). Recent climate research has linked the tremendous depopulation of Indigenous people with climate change referred to as a Little Ice Age (Koch et al., 2019). As Indigenous people rapidly died, vegetation flourished, producing the appearance of wilderness.

Colonizers saw the impact of the illnesses on the Indigenous people as a potential opportunity to expand colonization (Milner, 1980). There were many early reports about severe illness and its consequences to Indigenous villages in what is now the northeastern and southeastern US, illnesses spread from the earliest English colonies at Jamestown and Plymouth (Beach, 1885; Milner, 1980; Mires, 1994; Snow & Lanphear, 1988). Unfortunately, epidemic losses reinforced original colonizing beliefs that the land and resources of the west were there for the taking--that the land was empty and abandoned. Some colonizers also saw the advantages of a weakened enemy who could be easily manipulated and conquered. Unscrupulous policy makers and military leaders saw the illnesses as potential weapons, resulting in tactics such as intentionally sharing smallpox infected blankets with Indigenous people in a crude act of biological warfare (Dunbar-Ortiz, 2014; Hawkins & Blume, 2002; Henderson et al., 1999). Using sickness as a method for enhancing colonization may have even involved the spread of tuberculosis into the late nineteenth century in the US (Rosenfeld, 2020).

These tactics toward the Indigenous people were rooted in the assumption that colonists represented a superior people with a superior culture (e.g., Bump et al., 2021), an essential tenet in colonialism that justified the conquest, killing, and subjugation of people deemed to be inferior (Blume, 2020). With Indigenous people assumed to be expendable and a nuisance to the goals of conquest and colonization, little concern was given for the health and well-being of Indigenous people. Today, those perspectives persist in the belief systems of modern colonialists. Former Senator Rick Santorum suggested in 2021, that America was a "blank slate" created "from nothing," and that "America culture" had not been significantly influenced by Indigenous Americans (Fitzsimons, 2021), illustrating both historic and contemporary colonial efforts to erase Indigenous peoples and their cultures.

Additionally, Indigenous people were further weakened by slavery, poverty, and hunger due to colonial exploitation. Archeological evidence suggests that Indigenous people were much healthier prior to the arrival of Columbus when compared with the post-Columbian era (Mann, 2006). Enslavement of indigenous people was evidence of how colonial hierarchical beliefs allowed for basic human rights to be denied to certain people considered to be inferior. However, the depopulation of Indigenous people by wave after wave of illness meant the slave labor force was diminished in the Americas and the Caribbean. Thus, in order to fill the emerging void in slave labor, West Africans became the next target for enslavement. They, too, were dehumanized in the process, killed and traumatized for centuries by the colonial entities that required their enslavement to prosper. As other racial and ethnic groups arrived in the US as immigrants, they were also treated as lesser people (McCorkle, 2018; Young, 2017). All was sanctioned through the perceived superiority of colonists and their cultures that viewed that the needs and rights of colonial immigrants superseded the needs and rights of others. The result has been generations of dehumanized and vulnerable people.

Dehumanization remains a serious problem in colonial societies today, as evidenced by the extreme inequities in these societies, the callous disregard with how certain people are regarded in those societies, and the ample evidence that these inequities have continued despite so-called "advances" of civilization. The huge gulf between the potential and the reality of human civilization has perhaps never been clearer than during COVID-19, as will be discussed throughout this book. Hierarchies inevitably contribute to assumptions concerning superiority and inferiority (Blume, 2020), and superiority-inferiority beliefs inevitably impact decisions about life and death. Historically in colonial societies, protection of life is typically reserved for a privileged few and the risk of death extended to many who are not privileged.

Colonial Hierarchies and Sanctioned Deception

Colonialism also has a history of deceiving others in order to achieve the goals of dominance, control, and exploitation. Deception was used during the very first moments when Columbus contacted the Indigenous people of Caribbean Islands. The deception of Christopher Columbus inspired Jamaican Reggae star *Burning Spear* (Winston Rodney) to release a song in which he repeatedly referred to Columbus as a "damn blasted liar" (Rodney, 1980). The goals of colonization were never about extending good will to the Indigenous people that were encountered in conquests, as made clear in the *Doctrine of Discovery*. Colonial deception was at work with the numerous treaties negotiated in poor faith that occurred between colonial powers and Indigenous people. From 1778 to 1871, 370 treaties were ratified between the US and various Indigenous tribes. Treaties were routinely broken and violated by the US, with the treaty era finally ending in 1871 when the US felt empowered enough to abandon the deception of wanting peace (Nies, 1996). Even when a treaty initially benefitted both parties, the treaty was often vacated when it was expedient for colonial self-interests to do so.

Many colonial policies were founded in deception. Deceptive historical policies have contributed to significant disadvantages as well as a significant distrust of colonial social systems such as criminal justice and health care. In fact, the protection of civil liberties and human rights within colonial societies has never been fully extended to ethnic outgroups and other disempowered groups (women, those sexually minoritized, and people with disabilities).

In another book on the topic of Indigenous Psychology (Blume, 2020), I discussed several colonial myths, including the myth of opportunity that also has been packaged as the myth of the American dream. Unfortunately, like many promises emanating from colonial societies, the myth of opportunity is fulfilled so rarely that it may do more damage than good. The myth of opportunity suggests meritocracy--that anyone may succeed if they will only work hard and assumes that the playing field for life is level in such a way that a person might be able to determine his or her own destiny from birth. However, the playing field was never meant to be level in these societies. The rules of these societies have been shaped and prescribed in such a way to benefit the status quo and severely restrict change that might threaten those in a state of privilege. Data concerning social class mobility and income and wealth inequity over the last 50 years suggest that very few people benefit from the myth of opportunity due to engrained intergenerational colonial hierarchies (Alvarado et al., 2018; Carr & Wiemers, 2016; Diamond, 2018; Song et al., 2020). Myths of opportunity, seductive as they are, are deceptive and not well-aligned to the realities of these societies.

The myth of opportunity served its purpose in attracting large numbers of colonizers that benefitted the needs and ambitions of the ruling classes of Europe. It may have benefitted those who came willingly, but those opportunities were accomplished on the backs of Indigenous people and African slaves—in other words, they were stolen opportunities. But when you look closely at the realities of colonial societies today, even many of the children and grandchildren of colonial immigrants do not seem to be living the dream, either. Deception has played a role in convincing people that the playing field and the dream is possible. A pandemic exposes the fallacies in that deception quickly, as seen in the 2020s. Colonial deception had a hand in the consequences of the pandemic and in the failed responses to address COVID-19.

Some may assume that alternative facts and fake news began with the term of former President Donald Trump (Ortutay, 2017; Wendling, 2018), but deception was a strategy to ensure conquest and control by colonial governments centuries before Donald Trump became the US president. The pattern of using smoke screens and making up facts has been used to misdirect outgroups for many years, although some government officials have been subtler in their approaches than the methods employed during the Trump administration. The history of using half-truths, obfuscation, and outright lies has a long history in colonial nations as a tool to disempower people deemed to be inferior and to engage in what I have referred to as colonial splitting (Blume, 2020; see Chap. 4)--strategies meant to drive wedges between different groups in order to get them fighting with one another rather than uniting against the colonial forces that are oppressing them. Although the use of deception had become more covert in the twenty-first century in some ways, there has been a reversal of that trend with the rise of colonial nationalism that mimics the overt deception tactics of yesteryear. Colonialism has sanctioned fudging on the facts in order to achieve its goals of superiority and control—it is not a new phenomenon.

A Vast Wilderness for the Taking and Taming

The *Doctrine of Discovery* justified acquisition of property and resources as booty from the conquests, with lands and its resources viewed as things to be exploited by European immigrants as they saw fit. Colonists arrived with a belief that ownership was a divinely-given right due to the *Doctrine of Discovery*, cultural beliefs in the pre-eminence of individuals and self-interests, and to hierarchical understandings that permitted dominance over others including the natural world (Blume, 2020). Ownership was a rather foreign idea to Indigenous people, who could not understand how nature could be owned by other creatures of the natural world. Indigenous people considered themselves equal participants in the natural world--they did not hold colonial hierarchical perspectives that could conceive of human creatures dominating the Earth Mother. When confronted with the material desires for possessing things of European immigrants, Indigenous people were baffled by cultural beliefs they did not share or understand. The clash of perspectives concerning resources could not have been more striking, with owning being of paramount importance to colonists and sharing being of paramount importance to the collective cultures of Indigenous people (Blume, 2020).

The widespread death that occurred as a result of the Columbian Exchange of pathogens depopulated the lands of the west, so they appeared to be empty spaces of wilderness to the European settlers (Mann, 2006). The first contact with these lands must have given an impression of a cornucopia of land and resources for the taking from a colonial perspective. One perhaps can understand why ownership would have seemed so important to both the ruling class and the underclasses of Europe. For the ruling classes, increased resources meant increased power, since material resources tended to support the expansion of power. For the underclasses, ownership would have been new, something to aspire to according to colonial cultural beliefs--a divinely sanctioned sign of material success (Blume, 2020). Going from having nothing to having something must have been very appealing in a culture in which superiority was a function of ownership. And a vastly empty wilderness would have been truly compelling to people from a materially-oriented culture that owned little. The cultural importance of self-interests would become engrained into colonialism in such a way that ownership would be used to define status and rank in society, beliefs that persist today.

More is Better

Accumulation of possessions was something to aspire to in colonial societies that defined individual success materially. This particular perspective has evolved from the colonial assumption that accumulation of the possessions of others was divinely sanctioned in the *Doctrine of Discovery*, therefore a tangible sign of divine favor. As a result of the cultural beliefs, colonial citizens learned to evaluate social progress from a material perspective, and for some, to hold accumulation of possessions and wealth as aspirational and a sign of righteous living.

An exaggerated belief in colonial materialism contributes to a more-is-better perspective, and consumerism has been the modern result. Accumulation of wealth has been easier for some than others due to the rules of colonial societies favoring the status quo of those groups perceived to be superior (Echo-Hawk, 2013). The net result has been a society that places importance upon economic winners and losers (Blume, 2020). In colonial societies, minoritized outgroups lost their resources to colonists and then were compelled to dwell under those exploitive social systems with their colonial laws and social rules (Echo-Hawk, 2013).

On the other hand, colonialism has greatly benefitted the privileged few that have been able to leverage the colonial system for significant personal gain. Some families of privilege have passed along wealth intergenerationally. However, for most members of colonial societies, more is better is simply not a reality and leaves them hoping or discouraged in a system stacked against them. Not only do colonial nations expect and sanction material hierarchies, they have used the rules of their societies to maintain those hierarchies over time and discourage progress for certain peoples determined to be inferior. Chap. 3 discusses economic inequities in the context of the COVID-19 pandemic more fully.

Boundaries, Fences, and Walls

Colonial ownership created the need to control possessions and resources and even defend those possessions and resources from others. Because of concerns to protect self-interests and ownership, boundaries, fences, and walls became an important colonial demarcation between what is owned (controlled) and what is not. In a hierarchical system such as seen in colonial nations, boundaries, fences, and walls became demarcations between what is mine or ours (considering national self-interest) versus what is theirs. Notice how the "othering" perspective of ownership and self-interests tends to place "me" and "us" into an adversarial position with "you" and "them." In colonialism, it is easy to justify the needs of me-us over others, a cultural perspective that profoundly hindered addressing COVID-19.

Psychologically speaking, the importance of borders, fences, and walls in colonial societies is to provide a sense of security that me and my things will be protected and defended from others. The difficulty with such a perspective is that many things in nature do not respect boundaries, fences, and walls--arbitrary human demarcations created by humans have little meaning when considering migrating animals or the air we breathe as two examples (Blume, 2020). Modern colonial nations became complacent, believing that their political power, technology, and demarcations would leave them isolated and safe. However, viruses do not respect boundaries, fences, or walls, and many colonial nations have stumbled greatly with complacent responses under their guise of the false senses of security of borders.

The Shortsightedness of Colonialism

Colonial cultures have often exhibited shortsightedness concerning the consequences of their behaviors (Blume, 2020). Colonial nations showed little evidence of insight or concern for how their resource and land grabs were impacting others, including future generations of their own progeny. The focus was very proximal (what can we get now and how), and that proximal orientation has tended to result in more impulsive or even reactive actions than planful. An out of sight out of mind mentality has persisted to modern times within these nations with an inability to connect the dots between colonial activities and their global impacts. An excellent example of this cultural shortsightedness is global climate change (Blume, 2020).

Europe experienced one of the largest pandemics in history but the progeny of European citizens seemed to have widely forgotten the lessons of their ancestors (Conniff, 2020). This amnesia seemed to occur despite multiple outbreaks of smallpox, influenza, cholera, and other deadly epidemics that occurred after the Black Death. Most recently, there have been the Spanish Flu and HIV pandemics (Barry, 2018; Conniff, 2020), which accounted for tens of millions of deaths. Yet the lessons of these pandemics were typically lost.

The focus on proximal outcomes perhaps has left colonial nations at a disadvantage for long-term planning to prevent pandemics. The proximal focus also seems to result in an impatience perhaps related to the problems with delayed gratification seen in colonial societies (Blume, 2020). Additionally, when the central focus of psychological concern is on self and self-interests, connectivity with others is easy to break down or be neglected, especially with regard to long-term intergenerational concerns. Sustained planning for the next pandemic does not match well to the proximal orientation of colonial culture. Readers will see ample evidence in this book that concern for proximal outcomes at the expense of distal outcomes significantly hindered preparation for and progress in addressing the COVID-19 pandemic. Important questions moving forward include how to maintain the historic memory of pandemics such that we are not starting from scratch repeatedly, and how to maintain the momentum of anticipating and addressing these events over time and across generations?

Table 1.1 briefly reviews how colonial assumptions informed colonial attitudes that contributed to colonial consequences for much of the world. The consequences of colonialism set the stage for vulnerabilities to COVID-19 when it appeared, and

Table 1.1 Colonial assumptions and their consequences on societies

Colonial assumption	Resulting attitudes	Consequences of attitudes
Divinely sanctioned	Special people, special privileges	Colonial activities justified
Centrality of the individual	Self vs. other	Self-orientation, self-interests, perceived independence and boundaries
Hierarchical world	Superiority-inferiority	Dehumanization and disrespect of others, deceit, exploitation, blame, manipulation, inequity, conflict
Emphasis on visible, observable	Materialism	Colonization, exploitation of nature, "ownership" and "more is better"
Proximal outcomes valued	Myopic vision of scope and duration of consequences	Unanticipated global and intergenerational problems, Historical amnesia

continue to contribute to vulnerabilities to future pandemics, as will be discussed throughout the book. The next section begins to assess the psychological vulnerabilities of colonialism through Indigenous lenses.

An Assessment of Psychological Vulnerabilities from an Indigenous Perspective

Indigenous ways of thinking contribute to a very different perspective of what constitutes psychological wellness, illness, and vulnerabilities to illness. To begin to understand the differences in interpreting psychological well-being and health, it may be helpful to briefly discuss the basic assumptions of an Indigenous American Psychological Paradigm (IAPP; Blume, 2020) as an example of Indigenous ways of thinking about psychology.

The worldview that constitutes the foundation of IAPP begins with the assumption that the whole is the foundational context for understanding human nature, existence, relationships, and behavior—and therefore foundational to understanding psychology. The "Creation" (essentially the universe—capitalized to demonstrate Indigenous respect) is assumed sacred, not in a religious way, but rather as a whole worthy of utmost respect and awe as that which has sustained us all. Psychological health and well-being in IAPP are defined by right relationships with Creation (the whole). The entities within Creation are assumed to be interdependent upon one another, and since they are interdependent, there is not a hierarchical understanding about the organization of Creation as there is in colonialism. Instead, entities that constitute an interdependent Creation by necessity must have egalitarian relationships in order to maintain healthy balances in Creation. When the entities work toward the goodness and wellness of the whole, they too exhibit sacred qualities—including humans when their relationships with others align with the health and well-being of the whole.

When viewed through the lenses of IAPP, many aspects of the colonial worldview are perceived to be psychologically unhealthy. For example, the assumption that one group is divinely ordained to have dominion and superiority over others has contributed to numerous wars and significant social problems, and civil unrest. Nothing in IAPP would suggest that others have a divine right to lord over others, given the assumption of egalitarianism. In fact, psychological health and well-being depends upon the healthy, equitable relationships with others, relationships that assume mutual respect and personal humility.

Indigenous people have also historically strayed from their own essential belief systems, walking in neither balance nor harmony. Under community slips into hierarchy, others were not treated with the egalitarian respect they deserved to the detriment of peace and community building. Indigenous Americans are subject to the temptations of self and self-interests just like other people, especially now in the context of larger hierarchical societies. Minoritized groups had little choice but to adapt to colonial ways, so some traditional values have been displaced by necessary adaptation to colonial methods. One example is the practice of ownership.

Hierarchies ignore the realities of interdependent egalitarian relationships in Creation, contributing to inequities that disturb psychological well-being and health, such as racism, sexism, ableism, homophobia, ageism, xenophobia, and all other -isms in social orders meant to put down certain groups of people (see Chap. 4). The differences between the Indigenous egalitarian worldview and the colonial hierarchical view would have been obvious at first contact. Indigenous Americans tended to be culturally tolerant and perhaps even curiously openminded about the practices of other cultures. Upon first contact with European colonists, Indigenous Americans were apparently receptive and curious rather than immediately belligerent toward colonists (Dunbar-Ortiz, 2014; Mann, 2006), likely because of the interdependent and egalitarian worldview that looks upon all entities as worthy of respect. When Indigenous Americans first met Europeans, they saw a different people but not instantly a threat. They were anything but xenophobic in their reaction. However, the colonists who arrived made it clear they were belligerent toward the inhabitants of the land and had arrived with goals to exploit and subdue. They had been socialized to believe in their superiority and therefore were oriented toward a more adversarial and xenophobic approach. When Europeans saw Indigenous Americans, they saw inferior people who represented a threat to achieving their interests. Indigenous people were not immediately belligerent but became so after being mistreated, exploited, and deceived by the European immigrants.

Over 50 years ago, the Kerner Commission identified White racism as the source of inequities and civil unrest in the US, but the report was quietly buried by White leaders (Kerner Commission, 1968). Hierarchies have contributed to education, health, income, and wealth disparities that have left significant portions of the people in colonial societies vulnerable to poor psychological health for generations (Blume, 2019, 2020; Diamond, 2018). Hierarchical beliefs that place the self-oriented needs of humans above the rest of Creation have contributed to environmental encroachment and degradation as resources have been exploited with little concern for others including subsequent generations. Colonial exploitation of the planet and how it related to the COVID-19 pandemic is discussed in Chap. 2.

The belief there should naturally be superior-inferior entities disrespects others. The IAPP would suggests that all are equals and should be treated as equals. Furthermore, the fallacies of a hierarchical worldview--of me versus you or us versus them--inaccurately assume from an IAPP perspective that self-interests supersede the interests of others and present the fallacious impression that managing the self-interests of 8 billion different humans is feasible on this small blue jewel of a planet. Emphasizing the needs of self above others would be considered irrational because it ignores the reality of an interconnected, interdependent world. Excessive pursuit of self-interests, including national self-interests, would be considered disrespectful of others and pathological due to disrupting balance and harmony of the whole. Such activities interfere with healthy relations, potentially resulting in a *narcissistic orientation* destructive to others or contributing to *relational psychopathology* that interferes with psychological health and happiness and contributes to psychological suffering (Blume, 2020).

Accumulation of material possessions results from an inordinate concern for self and self-interests. More is better is related to the winners-losers mentality, an assumption that hierarchical competition is good when in fact the results have been worsening inequities (Alvarado et al., 2018). These fallacious assumptions do not align with the realities of an interdependent planetary system that works well only when all are respected and treated as equals. Our psychological health is dependent upon the larger whole, and if that larger whole is psychologically unhealthy, then individual entities will be psychologically unhealthy as well. From an IAPP point of view, a system that weakens and disempowers certain people in the context of an interdependent Creation contributes to physical and psychological vulnerabilities for us all. Much of the book will be filled with examples of how shared vulnerability as a result of colonialism enhanced the health and mental health risks of the COVID-19 pandemic.

Colonialism has also contributed to highly suspicious and distrustful citizens. From the perspective of IAPP, this is not a surprise. After all, colonial cultural beliefs violate the IAPP assumptions of the necessary preconditions for collective psychological well-being and happiness (Blume, 2020). Despite the extraordinary evidence that Creation operates best when in balance and harmony in relationships with others, colonialism has operated on assumptions of a self-orientation, of superiority-inferiority, and of divinely ordained privilege and inequities. Colonialism has been an adversarial cultural model from its inception with goals to harm, dominate, and exploit others. In a system where deception is used to empower those of privilege and disempower everyone else, the great amount of animosity across groups is no surprise. Colonial societies have been unsafe for many of its citizens from their inceptions. Anger, fear, and distrust is a way of being for many people under those conditions, making those societies psychologically unwell at baseline. Beliefs that boundaries, fences, walls, or even implicit privilege would protect individuals from self-inflicted anger, distrust, and fear is irrational. An IAPP perspective holds that anger, distrust, and fear are inner struggles to be resolved spiritually. Externalizing one's anger, distrust, and fear onto others through blame or hostility only reverberates their psychologically toxic effects to the interdependent whole.

Finally, those engaged in colonial activities with proximal goals have been callously inconsiderate of the distal consequences of colonial assumptions on others. An IAPP perspective of time is very different than the linear time of colonialism that contributes to a proximal focus and, frankly, to impatience and problems with delaying gratification. For Indigenous Americans, time flows in cycles like the seasons, such that summers across time have connectivity of essential patterns even though they have different presentations each year. Past and future come together in the present moment such that there is connectivity of events across time. Time repeats patterns—it recycles—allowing multiple opportunities to learn from those patterns. Cyclical time with its repeating patterns is much more forgiving than linear time where the moment comes and goes, encouraging impatience. An IAPP conceptualization of time allows for the whole picture to be viewed—how past, present, and future can viewed holistically and distally, as well as proximally (Blume, 2020).

The large intergenerational problems that we face, such as climate change and intergenerational inequities, have been the result of not considering distal outcomes that have and will impact the health and mental health of Creation--to include the progeny of those who acted so thoughtlessly. Losing sight of distal outcomes has significantly impacted the response to COVID-19. Will the focus on proximal outcomes hinder the preparedness of colonial societies in future pandemics? Time will tell. From the perspective of IAPP, distal outcomes can be appropriately considered and addressed operating under the interdependent, egalitarian, and intergenerational psychological assumptions (Blume, 2020). Perhaps it is time to step outside the colonial box to address future pandemics (see Chapters 11 and 12).

It was under colonial psychological conditions that COVID-19 emerged--the virus capitalized greatly on the psychological weaknesses of colonial societies. Its stealth nature has made it a particularly formidable threat physically and psychologically. Diné (Navajo) spiritualists refer to COVID-19 as a ghost sickness that emerged as a result of thousands of animal deaths during the 2019 Australian bush fires (Quintero, 2021), an excellent illustration of an Indigenous perspective concerning the interdependent nature of collective wellness or illness. Psychologists and other health care professionals will be addressing the consequences of COVID-19 for years. Learning the lessons of this pandemic will benefit future generations the next pandemic (see Chap. 6 for discussion of COVID-19 symptoms and health consequences).

Colonialism and Intergenerational Consequences: An Indigenous Interpretation

Modern colonialism had its roots in the doctrines of *Dum Diversas* and *Discovery* that sanctioned colonists to conquer, enslave, accumulate, and exploit other people and their resources. Materialistic pursuits were foundational to colonialism and accumulated wealth was viewed as a sign of divine favor and superiority. Natural hierarchies were assumed in the colonial worldview, justifying colonists to treat others and their cultures as inferior and irrelevant. Colonial doctrine begins with the centrality of self, therefore justifying the perspective of self-orientation and its pursuit and defense of self-interests. In the context of hierarchy, the centrality of self-views others as a potential threat to self-interests, therefore prompting conquest, control, distrust, deception, and division. Human self-interests permit exploitation of nature with little regard for consequences. Colonial activities have contributed to inequities that leave societies vulnerable to collective threats such as viral pandemics.

Indigenous people offer a different worldview that begins with the whole rather than the self. Psychologically speaking, the wellbeing of the whole helps to ensure the well-being of the individual. Relationships rather than things are most important in an IAPP view of psychological health. An IAPP assumes interdependence of all entities, ensuring collective strength and collective vulnerability. In an interdependent world, egalitarianism rather than hierarchy is the reality of nature, hence assuming hierarchies are neither natural nor rational. Equity rather than inequity is assumed to be Indigenously normative. Healthy relationships rather than artificial walls or borders ensure the security of the whole. The collective Creation is considered sacred rather than something to be exploited or used for human self-interests. In other words, an Indigenous perspective offers a striking alternative interpretation of psychological well-being and health to a colonial worldview.

Cultural traditions often walk a fine line between connectivity to the past and hierarchical practices that reflect superiority. Colonial societies historically assumed superior methods because they were innately hierarchical. Colonial cultural traditions are infused and entrenched in many societies globally, traditions that were never allowed to be examined critically or challenged by other perspectives. However, the circumstances of COVID-19 offer ample evidence that colonial traditions centered in self, individualism, autonomy, self-interests, social hierarchy, and proximal outcomes have not worked well to address a collective problem such as a global pandemic. The post-pandemic world offers a rare opportunity to fully examine and challenge colonial traditions harming collective well-being and health. It is in our best interests to retire colonial societies in the face of overwhelming evidence they are inadequate for preparing the world for the next global crisis, pandemic or otherwise.

References

Alvarado, F., Chancel, L., Piketty, T., Saez, E., & Zucman, G. (2018). *World inequity report: Executive summary*. World Inequity Lab. https://wir2018.wid.world/files/download/wir2018-summary-english.pdf

Barber, S., & Naepi, S. (2020). Sociology in a crisis: Covid-19 and the colonial politics of knowledge production in Aotearoa New Zealand. *Journal of Sociology, 56*(4), 693–703. https://doi.org/10.1177/1440783320939679

Barry, J. M. (2018). *The great influenza: The story of the deadliest pandemic in history*. Penguin Books.

Beach, W. M. (1885). Contagions and epidemics in America. *JAMA, 4*(11), 281–285. https://doi.org/10.1001/jama.1885.02390860001001

Bianchine, P. J., & Russo, T. A. (1992). The role of epidemic infectious diseases in the discovery of America. *Allergy and Asthma Proceedings, 13*(5), 225–232. https://doi.org/10.2500/108854192778817040

Blume, A. W. (2019). Views from Indigenous Psychology: How people can make peace with the planet. *Psychology for a Better World: A Cross-cultural Journal on Emotional Intelligence*, 7, 45–58.

Blume, A. W. (2020). *A new psychology based on community, equality, and care of the earth: An indigenous American perspective*. ABC-CLIO/Praeger.

Bump, J. B., Baum, F., Sakornsin, M., Yates, R., & Hofman, K. (2021). Political economy of Covid-19: Extractive, regressive, competitive. *BMJ, 372*, n73. https://doi.org/10.1136/bmj.n73

Carr, M. D., & Wiemers, E. E. (2016, September 7). *The decline in lifetime earnings mobility in the U.S.: Evidence from survey-linked data*. Washington, DC: Washington Center for Equitable Growth. https://equitablegrowth.org/woring-papers/the-decline-in-lifetime-earnings-mobility-in-the-u-s-evidence-from-survey-linked-administrative-data/

Conniff, R. (2020). Stopping pandemics. *National Geographic, 238*(2), 40–73.

Davenport, F. G. (1917). *European treaties bearing on the history of the United States and its dependencies to 1648, volume 1*. Carnegie Institute.

Diamond, J. (2018). The global peril of inequality. *National Geographic, 234*(6), 17–20.

Dunbar-Ortiz, R. (2014). *An indigenous peoples' history of the United States*. Beacon Press.

Echo-Hawk, W. R. (2013). *In the light of justice: The rise of human rights in native America*. Fulcrum.

Fitzsimons, T. (2021, April 26). *Rick Santorum says 'there isn't much Native American culture in American culture.'* New York: NBC News. https://www.nbcnews.com/news/us-news/rick-santorum-says-there-isn-t-much-native-american-culture-n1265407

Graham, A. (2015). *Warfare (1450–1789)*. Mainz: Leibniz Institute of European History. http://ieg-ego.eu/en/threads/alliances-and-wars/warfare-1450-1789

Guerra, F. (1988). The earliest American epidemic: The influenza of 1493. *Social Science History, 12*(3), 305–325. https://doi.org/10.2307/1171451

Hawkins, E. H., & Blume, A. W. (2002). Loss of sacredness: A history of alcohol use and health services for American Indians in the United States. In P. D. Mail, S. Heurtin-Roberts, S. E. Martin, & J. Howard (Eds.), *Alcohol use among American Indians and Alaska natives: Multiple perspectives on a complex issue* (pp. 25–46). National Institute of Alcohol and Alcoholism Research Monograph Series, Research Monograph #37: United States Department of Health and Human Services.

Henderson, D. A., Inglesby, T. V., Bartlett, J. G., Ascher, M. S., Eitzen, E., Jahrling, P. B., Hauer, J., Layton, M., McDade, J., Osterholm, M. T., O'Toole, T., Parker, G., Perl, T., Russell, P. K., & Tonat, K. (1999). Smallpox as a biological weapon. *JAMA, 281*(22), 2127–2137. https://doi.org/10.1001/jama.281.22.2127

Joralemon, D. (1982). New world depopulation and the case of disease. *Journal of Anthropological Research, 38*(1), 108–127. https://doi.org/10.1086/jar.38.1.3629951

Kerner Commission. (1968). *Report of the National Advisory Commission on civil disorders*. Government Printing Office. https://www.ojp.gov/ncjrs/virtual-library/abstracts/national-advisory-commission-civil-disorders-report

Koch, A., Brierley, C., Maslin, M. M., & Lewis, S. L. (2019). Earth system impacts of the European arrival and great dying in the Americas after 1492. *Quaternary Science Reviews, 207*, 13–36. https://doi.org/10.1016/j.quascirev.2018.12.004

Lewis, S. L., & Maslin, M. A. (2015). Defining the Anthropocene. *Nature, 519*, 171–180. https://doi.org/10.1038/nature14258

Livi-Bacci, M. (2006). The depopulation of Hispanic America after the conquest. *Population and Development Review, 32*(2), 199–232. https://www.jstor.org/stable/20058872

Mann, C. C. (2006). *1491: New revelations of the America's before Columbus*. Vintage Books.

McCorkle, W. D. (2018). Using history to inform modern immigration debate in the United States. *Journal of International Social Studies, 8*(1), 149–167. http://www.iajiss.org/
Merbs, C. F. (1992). A new world of infectious disease. *Yearbook of Physical Anthropology, 35*, 3–42. https://doi.org/10.1002/ajpa.1330350603
Milner, G. R. (1980). Epidemic disease in the postcontact southeast: A reappraisal. *Midcontinental Journal of Archaeology, 5*(1), 39–56. https://www.jstor.org/stable/20707847
Mires, P. B. (1994). Contact and contagion: The Roanoke colony and influenza. *Historical Archaeology, 28*, 30–38. https://doi.org/10.1007/BF03374188
Nies, J. (1996). *Native American history: A chronology of a culture's vast achievements and their links to world events*. Ballantine Books.
Ortutay, B. (2017, January 23). *'Alternative facts' quip from trump adviser sparks mockery*. New York: Associated Press. https://apnews.com/article/1ddc3c4fcb944528a80a273e89cb6f5a
Quintero, D. (2021). The COVID-19 outbreak in the Navajo nation. *American Indian, 22*(2), 10–19.
Rodney, W. (1980). Columbus. In *Hail H.I.M.* Kingston, JA: Tuff Gong.
Rosenfeld, J. (2020). *How white people used tuberculosis to settle the southwest*. Teen Vogue. https://www.teenvogue.com/story/southwest-settlers-tuberculosis
Snow, D. R., & Lanphear, K. M. (1988). European contact and Indian depopulation in the northeast: The timing of the first epidemics. *Ethnohistory, 35*(1), 15–33. https://doi.org/10.2307/482431
Song, X., Massey, C. G., Rolf, K. A., Ferrie, J. P., Rothbaum, J. L., & Xie, Y. (2020). Long-term decline in intergenerational mobility in the United States since the 1850s. *PNAS, 117*(1), 251–258. https://doi.org/10.1073/pnas.1905094116
Thornton, R. (1987). *American Indian holocaust and survival: A population history since 1492*. University of Oklahoma Press.
Thornton, R. (2002). Health, disease, and demography. In P. J. Deloria & N. Salisbury (Eds.), *A companion to American Indian history* (pp. 68–84). Blackwell Publishers.
Wendling, M. (2018, January 22). *The (almost) complete history of 'fake news'*. London: BBC. https://www.bbc.com/news/blogs-trending-42724320
Young, J. G. (2017). Making America 1920 again? Nativism and US immigration, past and present. *Journal on Migration and Human Security, 5*(1), 217–235.

Chapter 2
The Colonial War with the Environment

Abstract Colonial supremacy has been applied broadly to justify human exploitation of the natural world, which has contributed to widespread environmental degradation to satisfy colonial self-interests. Environmental degradation has been profound, with global resources consumed at unsustainable rates, negative consequences of climate change impacting generations to come, and human exploitation causing the widespread Eocene Extinction of other species. Rapidly changing environmental conditions have significantly and negatively impacted human health—leaving humans vulnerable to opportunistic viruses and diseases. Environmental exploitation has contributed to vast encroachment of previously pristine areas of the natural world, increasing the likelihood of novel virus exposure and the possibility of pandemics as a result. Colonial materialistic values and shortsightedness concerning environmental impact have contributed to pandemic vulnerability and hindered pandemic preparedness to respond effectively. Restoration of an egalitarian and peaceful human relationship with the natural world—a relationship that interprets sustainability broadly across generations and species--represents an important first step to pandemic prevention and preparation. An Indigenous American Psychological Paradigm provides a blueprint for reconciling humans with the natural world in a sustainable relationship, viewing the health of the natural world as inextricably linked to the psychological well-being of human creatures.

The consequences of environmental degradation are readily apparent in the 2020s. Climate change has become a serious threat to life on the planet (Burke et al., 2018; Intergovernmental Panel on Climate Change, 2021; United States Global Change Research Program, 2017). Sea level rise threatens coastal communities as a result. The UN estimates there may be hundreds of millions of climate change refugees by the turn of the next century, creating significant challenges to support and place so many in need (Brown, 2008). Indigenous communities In Alaska, Louisiana, and Washington have already needed to relocate due to erosion and high sea levels (Davenport & Robertson, May 3, 2016; Mapes, August 10, 2021; United States Environmental Protection Agency, 2017).

Climate change also has impacted weather patterns where droughts become megadroughts, enhanced storms result in significant flood events, heat waves

A. W. Blume, *Colonialism and the COVID-19 Pandemic*, International and Cultural Psychology, https://doi.org/10.1007/978-3-030-92825-4_2

smashing records, and hurricanes rapidly intensify into monster storms (Ault et al., 2016; Coumou & Rahmstorf, 2012; Selsky, Selsky, 2021; Tippett, 2018). Two examples occurred during the historic delta variant surge of COVID-19, first when the west coast of India was struck by an unusually intense cyclone Tauktae, and second, when Louisiana was hit by category 4 Hurricane Ida –both complicating pandemic responses in different areas of the globe (Kumar & Allen, 2021; National Aeronautics and Space Administration [NASA], 2021). Desertification is accelerating Africa and the US (United Nations XE "United Nations" Convention to Combat Desertification, 2017). Shorter winters and hotter drier summers contributed to catastrophic fires in the Australia and North America (Lindsey, 2020; Smith, 2021). Fresh water is scarce in many places, placing human and non-human life at risk (United States Global Change Research Program, 2017).

The world is in the midst of a mass extinction event caused by human activities such as climate change and resource exploitation (Andermann et al., 2020; Ceballos et al., 2015; Radchuk et al., 2019; Rosenberg et al., 2019). Unsustainable renewable resource consumption *overshoots* the natural replacement rate significantly each year (Wackernagel et al., 2002). Global resource overshoot is the result primarily of consumption overuse by so-called advanced colonial societies (Global Footprint Network, 2021; Lin et al., 2018). Furthermore, resources are often wasted rather than recycled or used to their full potential. Resource consumption by a few privileged nations has created negative environmental consequences for the entire planet.

Climate change and other forms of environmental degradation negatively impact the health and mental health of human beings including children (Pierre-Louis, 2019). Health scientists are predicting that tropical diseases such as malaria, dengue fever, and other infectious viruses will be likely to migrate to currently temperate climates such as the US (Watts et al., 2021). Warmer climates are predicted to negatively impact immune systems and exacerbate seasonal allergies and asthma through longer growing seasons (D'Amato et al., 2015). Environmental degradation seems to increase the vulnerability of other species to viruses, creating enhanced opportunities for animal to human virus spread (Mackenzie, 2020). Climate change induced extreme weather events and food, health, and resource inequities have also hampered the response to the COVID-19 pandemic (Sala, 2020; Watts et al., 2021). Pollution and waste resulting from resource exploitation has also been found to be problematic for health outcomes, with air pollution in particular suspected to be a particular risk factor for COVID-19 mortality (Wu et al., 2020).

The smoke from larger fires and longer fire seasons will negatively impact cardiopulmonary health (Food and Agriculture Organization, 2012; Watts et al., 2021; Weinstein et al., 2018). Smoke particulates were positively associated with increased viral influenza the following flu season (Landguth et al., 2020). People all over the western US experienced the unhealthiness of prolonged exposure to forest fire smoke during the pandemic summer of 2020, threatening the health of US citizens with the worst air quality on the planet (Carlson et al., 2020; NASA, 2020). The smoke may have contributed to thousands of bird deaths in the western US (Higgins, 2020), and smoke particulates were associated with COVID-19 cases and deaths (Zhou et al., 2021).

Forest management in the era of climate change might benefit from a return to Indigenous methods for control of wildfire risks. Evidence suggests that Indigenous people in the Americas routinely used prescribed burns and brush clearing to reduce risks for catastrophic fires, efforts that were no longer feasible once the epidemics of the Colombian Exchange depopulated Indigenous civilizations (Mann, 2006; Warren, 2002). Indigenous Australians did likewise in Australia (Asmelash, 2020). For centuries, colonial societies in North America or Australia did not seek out Indigenous wisdom concerning fire control until recent megafires encouraged them to consider alternative perspectives.

There is also significant evidence that environmental degradation negatively impacts mental health. Environmental degradation and climate change have disrupted traditional cultural practices important to groups of people, such as creating scarcity in traditional plants, herbs, and foods, and contributing to the loss of sacred places and spaces (Norton-Smith et al., 2016; US Climate Resilience Toolkit, 2020). Climate change refugees are and will continue to experience the psychological consequences of loss, stress, and trauma (Brown, 2008: Swim et al., 2009). Research has suggested the importance of the natural environment to mental health, including the wilderness, despite colonial beliefs to the contrary (Koole & Van den Berg, 2005). The ongoing Eocene extinction period has and will see the loss of creatures and plants of great significance to certain groups of people, prompting genuine grief for those losses (Andermann et al., 2020; Cunsolo & Ellis, 2018). All of the environmental changes noted above will impact the mental health of humans in significant ways for centuries (Swim et al., 2009).

All of the aforementioned circumstances of environmental degradation (see Table 2.1) have placed people at risk for worsening health over time. The connectivity and interdependence of all entities in nature have provided shared strength but also shared vulnerability. The environmental consequences of colonial consumption patterns have set the stage for people to be more vulnerable to infections by

Table 2.1 Environmental degradation and pandemic risks

Human Activity	Environmental consequence	Pandemic risk
Climate change	Warming climate	Tropical disease risk
Climate change	Weakened species	Increased likelihood of novel virus vector
Climate change, pollution	Worsening human health, immune function	Premorbid health and mental health vulnerabilities to novel viruses
Climate change	Climate refugees	Economic vulnerabilities
Climate change	Extreme weather events	Premorbid health, mental health, and economic vulnerabilities
Climate change, pollution, resource overshoot	Cultural disruption	Premorbid mental health vulnerabilities
Climate change, pollution, resource overshoot	Species extinction	Decreased biodiversity may limit pharmaceutical development, mental health vulnerabilities

degrading overall health (Jowell & Barry, 2020; Sala, 2020; Schmeller et al., 2020; Weiss & McMichael, 2004). The rest of the chapter discusses how colonialism has contributed to environmental crises that are literally making us more vulnerable to viruses with the most recent example being COVID-19.

Environmental Degradation Compounds a Pandemic: A Case Study

Scientists had warned that data suggested that the polar vortex was weakening in such a way that it would become more mobile, increasing the risk of extreme winter weather outbreaks in the northern hemisphere (Zhang et al., 2016). The National Oceanic and Atmospheric Administration (NOAA) had predicted and warned the public at least three weeks in advance that a polar vortex outbreak would significantly impact the central US all the way to the gulf coast with extremely cold weather. Unfortunately, little preparation was done for the massive arctic event, resulting in tremendous human suffering and additional health risk superimposed upon the COVID-19 pandemic (Borenstein, 2021). In Texas, millions of people lost electricity for days in places in which the infrastructure was unprepared for arctic events and enhanced weather extremes (Weber & Bleed, 2021). Hospitals were not only challenged by COVID-19, but also faced water shortages as a result of the infrastructure failure (O'Kane, 2021). Residents faced days of subfreezing weather without heat or easy access to potable water, food shortages due to loss of refrigeration and disrupted supply chains (Gamboa & Siemaszko, 2021). Many were forced to seek warmth in crowded shelters that risked virus spread (Nix, 2021). The winter storms also slowed vaccination efforts nationally (Naishadham, 2021).

The winter weather event in Texas taught lessons concerning climate change and pandemics, but there were other lessons as well. The first lesson concerned colonial individualism and liberties, which were to blame for the crisis with the electric grid. In the 1930s, federal legislation was passed to regulate the national power grid and power industry, presumably in part to prevent disasters like the one that happened in 2021. Texas opted out of the national grid because it wanted to be independent and unregulated by the federal government, constructing its own grid. Texans got what they wanted—a grid and a power industry that was unregulated and therefore able to avoid the more expensive precautions and redundancies placed on the rest of the nation (Hampton, 2021). Even though updating power delivery was discussed to prepare Texas for potential crises such as the one in 2021, nothing was done because of a reluctance to regulate and upgrade (Koenig & Liedtke, 2021). Individual liberties and independence contributed to several miserable days for most of Texas in February, 2021—and over 100 deaths (Weber & Stengle, 2021).

The second additional lesson about colonialism concerned privilege. Many Texans did not have the resources to escape the consequences of the tremendous bungle by Texas state leaders and were left to endure the hardship. However, one high profile political leader of Texas, Senator Ted Cruz, decided to travel to Cancun, Mexico, to escape the circumstances of the loss of power and water, as well as the cold weather (Peoples & Bleiberg, 2021). Mr. Cruz was an active participant of a populist-nationalistic government, a government that favored the colonial principles of self and self-interests. Through the lenses of that particular worldview, he exercised his privilege to escape the tragic circumstances that many of his constituents could not--taking a recreational international trip in the midst of the COVID-19 pandemic against his own nation's travel advisories. During that same time, many of his constituents were warming up to the idea that their monthly unregulated utility bills could amount to thousands of dollars as a result of the individual, independent, and liberty-oriented decision made 80 years ago to have an unregulated power grid (Miranda, 2021).

The story of Texas in February, 2021, highlights the significant weaknesses of colonialism in the face of a changing climate, weaknesses that increase the likelihood of and compound the risks associated with global pandemics. Climate enhanced weather events are only likely to get worse and more frequent, meaning the risks to human health will persist and worsen (Daly & Knickmeyer, 2021). It is important to understand how we arrived at this place of environmental risk so we may do something about it. The colonial worldview has played a significant role in environmental degradation as will discussed subsequently.

Colonial Supremacy and Nature

As discussed in the previous chapter, colonialism assumes natural hierarchies that define relationships between various groups of people. Colonial cultures assume the superiority of their own positions, prioritizing the needs of those deemed superior to those deemed inferior. Those biases remain obvious today when examining inequities within the social orders. The rank ordering of entities in the natural world extends to the non-human world as well.

Indigenous scholar and spiritualist Vine Deloria (2003) noted that colonial cultures were heavily influenced by the cosmology of Christianity, including in their perceptions of the natural non-human world. He noted that in the Bible, creation is said to have fallen into a state of sin and evil, suggesting that creation in colonial cultures was considered to be essentially flawed. That cosmology re-emerges in other areas of the Judeo-Christian Bible with suggestions that humans are given dominion over the non-human natural world, implying the world exists for human use and benefit. In addition, the wilderness is portrayed negatively as dangerous and a place of temptation. In the *Doctrine of Discovery*, the intent was to seize and exploit the lands occupied by Indigenous people for the benefit of the conquering colonists from Europe.

The representation of nature as a potential threat would help to explain colonial beliefs that suggested the natural world was something to be conquered and tamed (Blume, 2019). In colonial America, there was an emphasis on taming the wilderness as immigrants colonized and settled the lands (de Tocqueville, 1945; Gómez-Pompa & Kaus, 1992). Viewing the non-human natural world as a potential threat would also make it likely that nature would be treated with lack of consideration for its well-being or even with hostility. Hence, one would predict that colonial societies would not have the best interests of the non-human natural world in mind. And hierarchical beliefs that would favor self-interests over the needs of or consequences to others would suggest that colonists had license to do whatever they wanted with their land and its resources without consideration for potential impact on neighbors and future generations (Blume, 2020), which is exactly what has happened historically in colonial nations.

Hierarchical beliefs would also justify exploitation of the natural world to benefit the privileged few (Bump et al., 2021), with an expectation that the privileged have priority for having their interests protected and needs met over others. Resources could be extracted from colonies to benefit the self-interests of colonizing nations. Colonial nations often coerced their colonies or other disempowered nations into providing resources to benefit colonizing nations, and in many instances those resource interests were protected by colonial armies and navies stationed nearby. Those practices continue today in more covert ways, such as stationing troops in or near the oil rich lands of the Middle East. In the US, forcing construction of the Dakota Access Pipeline against the wishes of the Cheyenne River and Standing Rock Nations is an excellent example of colonial disregard for both Indigenous people and the natural world.

The colonial assumptions concerning primacy of the self and of self-interests and the assumptions of hierarchies that consider nature subservient to the needs of a privileged few have left the planet in a tough place. The resource use of the planet is unsustainable. Climate change is rapidly (more rapidly than originally predicted by researchers) changing the planet. Extinction rates are out of control (Ceballos et al., 2015; Radchuk et al., 2019; Rosenberg et al., 2019). Hundreds of millions of people will be impacted in such a way they will become refugees. More catastrophic climate and weather events will occur. The resources of the planet will be challenged in ways they have not been previously. The colonial mindset is contributing to a non-sustainable existence and must be addressed to avoid significant global consequences that have already harmed human health for some, and eventually will harm human health for all, even those who are privileged.

Colonial exploitation has done something else—it has encouraged humans to encroach upon previously pristine areas where humans had not routinely trodden, exposing them to new viruses in the wild. They have encroached on the domain of wild animals where viruses percolate, and they have created opportunities for viruses that have been sequestered away in the wilderness for millennia awaiting opportunities for spread that are abundant in a modern world. Colonialism has forced humans to exploit resources in areas where human exposure had not occurred regularly, contributing to more frequent encounter with "novel viruses" previously unknown to humans--viruses for which there is no treatment, cure, or immunity. In an Indigenous understanding of the natural world, colonialism crossed a line and now the consequences of crossing that line are occurring (e.g., Nuwer, 2020). Have we forever crossed the line toward planetary sickness, or will we find ways to restore a healthy planet?

An Indigenous Understanding of Human Relationships with Nature

An IAPP perspective views right relationships with the natural world as essential to psychological well-being, a very different perspective than a colonial view that sees the natural world as something to exploit. Those differences began because of very different assumptions about reality. Indigenous people tend to view Creation as sacred and view the well-being of the whole as essential for the well-being of individuals. There is no sense that the natural world is flawed, fallen, or subservient to the needs of human creatures. Rather, the focus is how can human creatures coexist with other creatures in ways that promote balance and harmony throughout the whole of Creation. An IAPP perspective holds that exploitation of nature is an expression of *relational psychopathology*, a belief that unhealthy relationships contribute to sickness, suffering, and misery of the whole (Blume, 2020). Pandemics would be understood as one form of sickness that emerge from the relational psychopathology of exploiting nature.

Sacred Community The vision for peace with the planet is to see humans as equal participants contributing to a sacred community with the rest of Creation. Indigenous perspectives hold that each participant in the sacred Creation is a sacred entity worthy of respect. Our sacredness becomes apparent when we align our activities with advancing the welfare of the whole. When we stray from that vision and engage in self-interests that risk disharmony with others, we have not fully embraced their sacredness and therefore have not embraced our own sacredness. From an IAPP perspective, our daily activities require constant monitoring that we are advancing the interests of the whole rather than those of the self in order to prevent harm to others, including harm to our home the Earth.

The Myth of Apex Creatures: Size Does Not Matter Colonial perspectives include the belief that hierarchy is natural. Those beliefs allow for the perspective that there are *apex* creatures, those who sit atop the so-called food chain, who are considered to be powerful and cunning creatures that dominate others. Within the anthropocentric perspectives of colonial thinking, humans have been considered THE apex creatures of the planet, presumably because of higher intelligence and the rise of human civilization. However, if you were to review the results of human civilization from an Indigenous perspective, one might question whether human environmental degradation and the accompanying risks to human health and well-being really support assumptions concerning the primacy of human intelligence.

Indigenous people view healthy relationships as egalitarian rather than hierarchical as a necessity in an interdependent existence. Indigenous people as keen observers of the natural world understand that survival of communities depends upon living in peace with the environment (Blume, 2019). Indigenous people did not see apex creatures as invulnerable but rather observed how interdependence elevates the importance of respect and humility in relating to others. Sure, wolves may eat elk, but if they eat too many elk, then they starve when the elk are depopulated. There is nothing apex about the shared vulnerabilities of predator and prey. Both rely on balances to survive. Human creatures are no different.

Contrast that apex view of human supremacy with the reality of viruses. Viruses provide tough lessons as they humble human creatures, especially when they are novel viruses. Apex humans dread viruses but they also appear to have been important in our own evolutionary development as creatures (Quammen, 2021). "Apex" humans cannot see COVID-19 with their weak eyes, cannot hear the virus stalking them, and cannot detect the risks of the viruses through taste or smell until the viruses have already multiplied. Mighty COVID-19 has humbled humans, an infuriating reality that challenges human supremacy and anthropocentric thinking errors fostered by colonialism. Living as if we are apex creatures has increased pandemic risks.

Creation-Centrism Vs. Self-Ism Since the whole is foundational to understanding human psychology rather than the self, IAPP would suggest a Creation-centric perspective rather than an anthropocentric perspective in relating to the non-human natural world (Blume, 2020). Creation-centrism suggests that pursuit of health and wellness for the whole is the logical course of action to keep human beings healthy. Individuals are utterly dependent upon the health and well-being of the interdependent environmental in which they live. Destroying the environment around us inextricably destroys a part of ourselves. Humans can only be as healthy as the world in which they dwell. So, logically, exploitation of the natural world for human gain actually results in losses for humans (Cunsolo & Ellis, 2018), threatening psychological health and well-being and contributing to poorer collective health (Diamond, 2018). Colonial behaviors that have been spun as advancing and protecting self-interests are in reality contributing to a less safe and increasingly vulnerable world.

Overshoot as a Sign that Self-Interests Have Run Amok Indigenous people believe that psychological happiness is found in healthy relationships rather than in accumulating things. Global overshoot in the use of renewable resources is unsustainable and pathological from an IAPP perspective (Blume, 2020). Psychological research suggests that greater materialism tends to be associated with lesser concern for the natural environment (Hurst et al., 2013), not surprising when one considers the self-oriented goals of colonial materialism. Furthermore, unbridled consumerism has not been shown to increase psychological well-being or happiness (Kasser, 2002), creating circumstances that may destructive to the whole of Creation without being personally satisfying. Although one might understand how people in colonial nations might be tempted to stock up on goods for security purposes, true security comes from our relationships rather than our things (Blume, 2020). Unbridled consumerism does not protect human creatures from the consequences of a degraded world. Colonial materialism has contributed to imbalances so great that they threaten harm to all.

Waste Nothing Indigenous people often learned to value of using everything and wasting nothing as essential to community well-being. When hunting, Indigenous Americans use the whole animal out of respect to the animal that gave its life. Waste disrespectfully dishonors the sacredness of that which is sacrificed for the good of others. Global overshoot is considered to be profoundly disrespectful when the wasting of resources is so apparent.

Connectivity, Interdependence, and Shared Vulnerability Evidence from natural sciences actually refutes the myth of the independence of individuals in significant ways (Blume, 2020). From an Indigenous perspective, the echoes of our activities reverberate through the interdependent relationships of the planet. The connectivity that we have with an interdependent Creation shares the collective strength and vulnerable of the whole throughout the ecosphere (Blume, 2020). There are also so many things that we do not yet know about how that connectivity manifests itself in nature. For example, there is new evidence that trees in forests are connected to one another through webs of fungi, potentially sharing and exchanging nutrients through the web (Jabr, 2020). The consequences of colonialism also reverberate through the connectivity and interdependence of the natural world. As an example of the connectivity and interdependence of the natural world, an early 2021 study found that 40% of US deer sampled showed evidence of SARS-CoV-2 antibodies (Maron, 2021).

Victimization of the natural world places human needs above the needs of the whole. Such a perspective contributed to the deaths of 17 million mink in Denmark found to have a variant of the virus deemed a threat to humans (Kesslen, 2020). Perhaps it was an easy choice since the mink were to be sacrificed for their furs. Still, the heartbreaking story is a good example of prioritizing human need over the needs of others in the natural world.

Indigenous elders globally have been observing that the planet is attempting to restore balance and harmony by addressing the human threat to nature. They have known for some time that the world is out of balance and see the unhealthiness of humans as a direct result of human generated disharmony and imbalances in the natural world (Nuwer, 2020). The pandemic has been interpreted as the planet is attempting to restore balance. Humans have crowded nature with population growth and resource exploitation (Mackenzie, 2020). Others noted that human encroachment on the natural world is "practically an invitation for animal viruses to infect humans" that might be interpreted as "nature's revenge" (Zakaria, 2020, p. 17). A backlash against human creatures is one way to interpret COVID-19, but an Indigenous perspective would interpret it as self-inflicted harm due to reckless exploitation of nature.

The real wealth of the world is in our relationships with others that help us access the collective strengths of Creation. One solution to reducing the vulnerability of human creatures to the risks of pandemics and other poor health and mental health outcomes is to rethink our relationships with the environment. Reducing environmental exploitation and working collectively toward a sustainable Creation would go far in reducing the encroachment across the lines of nature that risk exposure to novel viruses. The UN warned during the COVID-19 pandemic that too little pandemic recovery money had been used to control climate change as a contributor to virus exposure and its spread (Borenstein & Knickmeyer, 2021).

Climate scientists express serious concerns about the lack of coordinated attempts to reduce environmental degradation that is contributing to rapid and serious climate changes. Policymakers may not be taking seriously the idea that there may be serious "tipping points" where the consequences of environmental might severely impact climate with catastrophic warming in a way that will be difficult to reverse (Lenton et al., 2019). Catastrophic warming will seriously and negatively impact health and mental health. An Indigenous perspective challenges the climate roulette being played out through under responses and inaction--unconscionable behavior by the current generation to fail to protect future generations of life.

An Indigenous Interpretation: Disrespecting the Natural World Disrespects Ourselves

One of the great failings of colonialism has been the exploitation of the natural world. Colonial superiority has contributed to a sense of invulnerability--an anthropocentric arrogance that suggests humans are above and independent from the rest of the natural world. Assumptions of colonial superiority have contributed to disrespect toward other human beings AND toward the natural world. Environmental degradation has occurred because some have viewed the planet as nothing more than a supermarket for the human race. Colonial privilege has allowed some countries and individuals to use more resources than can be replaced. Encroachment on nature has expanded significantly due to increased demand for consumables, with resources being used at a rate at which they are not easily recycled or replaced.

Climate change will impact generations of human and non-human life. The activities of humans are contributing directly to a large extinction event with consequences for us all. The loss of biodiversity will harm humans practically speaking, but a greater loss may be the grief of slowly losing our home one entity at a time. The collective trauma of environmental degradation will impact the psychological well-being of the planet for centuries. Exposure to viruses due to encroachment and physical vulnerabilities from the unhealthiness of environmental degradation will compound the misery and grief.

An IAPP perspective suggests that environmental degradation in an interdependent natural order is self-defeating to all. Disrespecting the sacredness of Creation means disrespecting ourselves. We are increasing collective vulnerability to sickness in doing so, including to our progeny. Restoration requires that we restore a healthy relationship with the rest of the planet now and across time in order to embrace our own sacredness and acknowledge the sacredness of others. We do not have the moral right to do otherwise.

For a Moment Nature Rejoiced One interesting example of the re-emergence of the natural world during the COVID-19 pandemic was the visit by a snowy owl to New York City's Central Park, the first sighting in more than 120 years (CBS New York Team, 2021). Owls are majestic creatures bestowed with great spiritual powers highly respected by indigenous peoples. Owls are also symbolic forebearers of death in some Indigenous cultures. The visit by the owl represented a rebirth of nature at a time of death for humans. However, deadly pandemics due to environmental encroachment are not necessarily inevitable--humans do not need to war with the rest of the environment—it is a selfish choice to do so.

Some scientists have suggested that addressing the COVID-19 may be a dress-rehearsal for addressing environmental degradation such as climate change (Salas, 2020). With its respectful focus on the whole of Creation, IAPP is well-positioned to be a tool for addressing the broad and intergenerational challenges of climate change (Blume, 2020) and therefore potentially useful for reducing the climate risk that promotes the pandemics of the future.

The initial shutdown and shelter in place orders of 2020 shocked the economy (discussed more fully in Chap. 3), but nature rebounded. For example, air, noise, and water pollution all declined in 2020 (National Geographic Society, 2021). Global daily CO_2 emissions fell during the lockdown by about 17% in April, 2020 (Le Quéré et al., 2020). Estimates were that tens of thousands of people were saved from COVID-19 mortality due to the lower air pollution rates (Chossière et al., 2021). However, when many economies reopened later in the year, emissions climbed (Tollefson, 2021). Despite the rebound of emissions late in the year, the shutdown showed that it was indeed possible to bring global emissions under control, good news for the planet and its creatures, including humans. Two competing truths became much more obvious in the pandemic. First, a carbon-based energy economy and the health and well-being of the natural world were incompatible, and second, the natural world thrived when the human world was shutdown. During the spring of 2020, nature seemed to rejoice at its liberation from exploitation. The shutdown provided evidence that we can choose to reduce environmental degradation, good news for the whole of Creation. Human creatures must value that which keeps us alive, rather than war with it. Every loss that humans deal to the environment results in a greater loss to our health, and ultimately to our humanity.

References

Andermann, T., Faurby, S., Turvey, S. T., Antonelli, A., & Silvestro, D. (2020). The past and future human impact on mammalian diversity. *Science Advances, 6*(eabb2313), 1–17. http://advances.sciencemag.org/

Asmelash, L. (2020, January 12). Australia's indigenous people have a solution for the country's bushfires. *And it's been around for 50,000 years*. New York: CNN. https://www.cnn.com/2020/01/12/world/aboriginal-australia-fire-trnd/index.html

Ault, T. R., Mankin, J. S., Cook, B. I., & Smerdon, J. E. (2016). Relative impacts of mitigation, temperature, and precipitation on 21st-Century megadrought risk in the American southwest. *Science Advances, 2*(10), e1600873. https://advances.sciencemag.org/content/2/10/e1600873

Blume, A. W. (2019). Views from indigenous psychology: How people can make peace with the planet. *Psychology for a Better World: A Cross-Cultural Journal on Emotional Intelligence, 7*, 45–58.

Blume, A. W. (2020). *A new psychology based on community, equality, and care of the earth: An indigenous American perspective*. ABC-CLIO/Praeger.

Borenstein, S. (2021, February 20). *Weather experts: Lack of planning caused cold catastrophe*. New York: Associated Press. https://apnews.com/article/weather-texas-2a309531 1cf760fb9f 1a6d2e835e5bc0

Borenstein, S., & Knickmeyer, E. (2021, March 10). *UN: Too little of recovery spending fights climate change*. New York: Associated Press. https://apnews.com/article/environment-climate-climate-change-untied-nations-b523cc54d5e3fc8c0256d0c77be1329e

Brown, O. (2008). *Migration and climate change (Geneva: International Organization for Migration)*. https://www.ipcc.ch/apps/njlite/srex/njlite_download.php?id=5866.

Bump, J. B., Baum, F., Sakornsin, M., Yates, R., & Hofman, K. (2021). Political economy of Covid-19: Extractive, regressive, competitive. *BMJ, 372*, n73. https://doi.org/10.1136/bmj.n73

Burke, K. D., Williams, J. W., Chandler, M. A., Haywood, A. M., Lunt, D. J., & Otto-Bliesner, B. L. (2018). Pliocene and Eocene provide best analogs for near-future climates. *PNAS, 115*(52), 13288–13293. https://www.pnas.org/content/115/52/13288

Carlson, A., McMinn, S., & Eng, J. (2020, September 23). *1 in 7 Americans have experienced dangerous air quality due to wildfires this year*. Washington, DC: National Public Radio. https://www.nrp.org/2020/09/23/915723316/1-in-7-americans-have-experienced-dangeous-air-quality-due-to-wildfires-this-year

CBS New York Team. (2021, January 29). *Snowy owl spotted in Central Park for first time in more than a century, experts say*. https://newyork.cbslocal.com/2021/01/29/snowy-owl-central-park/

Ceballos, G., Ehrlich, P. R., Barnosky, A. D., García, A., Pringle, R. M., & Palmer, T. M. (2015). Accelerated modern human-induced species losses: Entering a sixth mass extinction. *Science Advances, 1*(e1400253), 1–5. https://doi.org/10.1126/sciadv.1400253

Chossière, G. P., Xu, H., Dixit, Y., Isaacs, S., Eastham, S. D., Allroggen, F., Speth, R. L., & Barrett, S. R. H. (2021). Air pollution impacts of COVID-19–related containment measures. *Science. Advances, 7*(21), eabe1178. https://doi.org/10.1126/sciadv.abe1178

Coumou, D., & Rahmstorf, S. (2012). A decade of weather extremes. *Nature Climate Change, 2*, 491–496. https://doi.org/10.1038/nclimate1452

Cunsolo, A., & Ellis, N. R. (2018). Ecological grief as a mental health response to climate change-related loss. *Nature. Climate Change, 8*, 275–281. https://www.nature.com/articles/s41558-018-0092-2.pdf

D'Amato, G., Holgate, S. T., Pawankar, R., Ledford, D. K., Cecchi, L., Al-Ahmad, M., Al-Enezi, F., Al-Muhsen, S., & Annesi-Maesano, I. (2015). Meteorological conditions, climate change, new emerging factors, and asthma and related allergic disorders. A statement of the world allergy organization. *World Allergy Organization Journal, 8*(25), 1–52. https://doi.org/10.1186/s40413-015-0073-0

Daly, M., & Knickmeyer, E. (2021, February 18). *US needs to brace itself for more deadly storms, experts say*. New York: Associated Press. https://apnews.com/article/us-deadly-winter-storms-2021-df7d37d12ef13633bb5666e1151bcf9e

Davenport, C. & Robertson, C. (2016, May 3). *Resettling the first American 'climate refugees'. The New York times*. Retrieved from https://www.nytimes.com/2016/05/03/us/resettling-the-first-american-climate-refugees.html

de Tocqueville, A. (1945). In P. Bradley (Ed.), *Democracy in America* (Vol. 2). Alfred A. Knopf.

Deloria, V. (2003). *God is red: A native view of religion*. Fulcrum Publishing.

Diamond, J. (2018). The global peril of inequality. *National Geographic, 234*(6), 17–20.

Food and Agriculture Organization. (2012). *State of the World's forests*. UN.

Gamboa, S., Siemaszko, C. (2021, February 24). *3 million Texans boil water amid 'plumbing catastrophe,' food shortages after devasting storm*. New York: NBC News. https://www.nbcnews.com/news/us-news/8-million-texans-boiling-water-after-wintry-blast-n1258648

Global Footprint Network. (2021). *Country overshoot day*. Author. https://www.overshootday.org/newsroom/country-overshoot-days/

Gómez-Pompa, A., & Kaus, A. (1992). Taming the wilderness myth. *Bioscience, 42*(4), 271–279. https://www.jstor.org/stable/1311675

Hampton, D. J. (2021, February 19). *Texas set the stage for its energy crisis more than 80 years ago*. New York: NBC News. https://www.nbcnews.com/news/us-news/texas-set-stage-its-energy-crisis-more-80-years-ago-n1258341

Higgins, D. (2020, November 10). *Researchers still don't know why so many birds died this fall*. Oakland, CA: Sierra Club. https://www.sierraclub.org/sierra/researchers-still-don-t-know-why-so-many-birds-died-fall

Hurst, M., Dittmar, H., Bond, R., & Kasser, T. (2013). The relationship between materialistic values and environmental attitudes and behaviors: A meta-analysis. *Journal of Environmental Psychology, 36*, 257–269. https://doi.org/10.1016/j.jenvp.2013.09.003

Intergovernmental Panel on Climate Change. (2021). *Climate change 2021: The physical science basis*. University Press. https://www.ipcc.ch/report/ar6/wg1/#SPM

Jabr, F. (2020, December 5). *The social life of forests*. New York: New York Times Magazine. https://www.nytimes.com/interactive/2020/12/02/magazine/tree-communication-mycorrhiza.html

Jowell, A., & Barry, M. (2020). COVID-19: A matter of planetary, not only national health. *Journal of Tropical Medicine and Hygiene, 103*(1), 31–32. https://doi.org/10.4269/ajtmh.20-0419

Kasser, T. (2002). *The high price of materialism*. MIT Press.

Kesslen, B. (2020, December 1). *Here's why Denmark culled 17 million minks and now plans to dig up their buried bodies*. The Covid mink crisis explained. New York: NBC News. https://www.nbcnews.com/animal-news/here-s-why-denmark-culled-17-million-minks-now-plans-n1249610

Koenig, D., & Liedtke, M. (2021, February 17). *EXPLAINER: Why the power grid failed in Texas and beyond*. New York: Associated Press. New York: Associated press. https://apnews.com/article/why-texas-power-grid-failed-2eaa659d2ac29ff87eb9220875f23b34

Koole, S. L., & Van den Berg, A. E. (2005). Lost in the wilderness: Terror management, action orientation, and nature evaluation. *Journal of Personality and Social Psychology, 88*(6), 1014–1028. https://doi.org/10.1037/0022-3514.88.6.1014

Kumar, D. K., & Allen, J. (2021, August 30). *Hurricane Ida lashes Louisiana, knocking out power in New Orleans* London: Reuters. https://www.reuters.com/world/us/louisiana-braces-powerful-hurricane-covid-19-taxes-hospitals-2021-08-29/

Landguth, E. L., Holden, Z. A., Graham, J., Stark, B., Mokhtari, E. B., Kaleczyc, E., Anderson, S., Urbanski, S., Jolly, M., Semmens, E. O., Warren, D. A., Swanson, A., Stone, E., & Noonan, C. (2020). The delayed effect of wildfire seasons particulate matter on subsequent influenza season in a mountain west region of the USA. *Environment International, 139*, 105668. https://doi.org/10.1016/j.envint.2020.105668

Le Quéré, C., Jackson, R. B., Jones, M. W., Smith, A. J. P., Abernethy, S., Andrew, R. M., De-Gol, A. J., Willis, D. R., Shan, Y., Canadell, J. G., Friedlingstein, P., Creutzig, F., & Peters,

G. P. (2020). Temporary reduction in CO_2 emissions during the COVID-19 forced confinement. *Nature Climate Change, 10*, 647–653. https://doi.org/10.1038/s41558-020-0797-x

Lenton, T. M., Rockström, J., Gaffney, O., Rahmstorf, S., Richardson, K., Steffen, W., & Schellnhuber, H. J. (2019). Climate tipping points—Too risky to bet against. *Nature, 575*, 592–595. https://doi.org/10.1038/d41586-019-03595-0

Lin, D., Hanscom, L., Murthy, A., Galli, A., Evans, M., Neill, E., Mancini, M. S., Martindill, J., Medouar, F.-Z., Huang, S., & Wackernagel, M. (2018). Ecological footprint accounting for countries: Updates and results of the national footprint accounts, 2012-2018. *Resources, 7*, 58. https://www.mdpi.com/2079-9276/7/3/58/pdf

Lindsey, R. (2020, January 3). *Catastrophic wildfires in southeastern Australia in 2019–2020.* Silver Springs, MD: National Oceanic and Atmospheric Administration. https://www.climate.gov/news-features/event-tracker/catastrophic-wildfires-southeastern-australia-2019-20

Mackenzie, D. (2020). *COVID-19: The pandemic that never should have happened and how to stop the next one*. Hachette Books.

Mann, C. C. (2006). *1491: New revelations of the Americas before Columbus*. Vintage Books.

Mapes, L. V. (2021, August 10). *This tribe has lived on the coast of Washington for thousands of years. Now climate change is forcing it uphill.* Seattle, WA: Seattle Times. https://www.seattletimes.com/seattle-news/environment/this-tribe-has-lived-on-the-coast-of-washington-for-thousands-of-years-now-climate-change-is-forcing-it-uphill/?amp=1

Maron, D. F. (2021, August 2). *Wild U.S. deer found with coronavirus antibodies*. Washington, DC: National Geographic. https://www.nationalgeographic.com/animals/article/wild-us-deer-found-with-coronavirus-antibodies

Miranda, L. (2021, February 19). *As Texas deep freeze subsides, some households now face electricity bills as high as $10,000*. New York: NBC News. https://www.nbcnews.com/business/business-news/deep-freeze-subsides-texans-now-face-electricity-bills-10-000-n1258362

Naishadham, S. (2021, February 17). *Crippling weather hampers vaccine deliveries, distribution*. New York: Associated Press. https://apnews.com/article/weather-hampers-vaccine-distribution-7a8e8908a0d68da784d1335b3bd6ead8

NASA. (2020, September 9). *A wall of smoke on the U.S. west coast*. Greenbelt, MD: Author. https://earthobservatory.nasa.gov/images/147261/a-wall-of-smoke-on-the-us-west-coast

NASA. (2021, May 17). *Cyclone Tauktae strikes India*. Greenbelt, MD: Author. https://earthobservatory.nasa.gov/images/148325/cyclone-tauktae-strikes-india

National Geographic Society. (2021). The year that hope endured. *National Geographic, 239*(1), 121.

Nix, M. (2021, February 15). *North Texas counties, cities, others open warming shelters for residents without power*. Dallas, TX: Dallas Morning News. https://www.dallasnews.com/news/weather/2021/02/16/north-texas-counties-cities-others-open-warming-shelters-for-residents-without-power/

Norton-Smith, K., Lynn, K., Chief, K., Cozzetto, K., Donatato, J., Redsteer, M. H., Kruger, L. E., Maldonado, J., Viles, C., & Whyte, K. P. (2016). *Climate change and indigenous peoples: A synthesis of current impacts and experiences*. General technical report PNW-GTR-944. Washington, DC; United States Department of Agriculture. https://www.cakex.org/sites/default/files/documents/pnw_gtr944.pdf

Nuwer, R. (2020, May 4). For hundreds of years, indigenous groups have warned that destroying the environment leads to disease and adversely affects lives and culture. Is the world ready to listen? London: BBC. https://www.bbc.com/travel/story/20200503-the-indigenous-communities-that-predicted-covid-19

O'Kane, C. (2021, February 18). *Texas hospitals suffer from water issues amid widespread power outages*. New York: CBS News. https://www.cbsnews.com/news/texas-power-outage-hospitals-water/

Peoples, S., & Bleiberg, J. (2021, February 19). *'Obviously a mistake': Cruz returns from Cancun after uproar*. New York: Associated Press. https://apnews.com/article/ted-cruz-mexico-vacation-amid-storm-b0cdc326db95bf25d93de9e877e05862

Pierre-Louis, K. (2019, November 13). *Climate change poses threats to children's health worldwide*. New York: New York Times. https://www.nytimes.com/2019/11/13/climate/climate-change-child-health.html

Quammen, D. (2021). How viruses shape our world. *National Geographic, 239*(2), 41–67.

Radchuk, V., Reed, T., Teplitsky, C., van de Pol, M., Charmantier, A., & Hassall, C.…Karmer-Schadt, S. (2019). Adaptive responses of animals to climate change are most likely insufficient. *Nature Communications, 10*, 3109. https://doi.org/10.1038/s41467-019-10924-4

Rosenberg, K. V., Dokter, A. M., Blancher, P. J., Sauer, J. R., Smith, A. C., Smith, P. A., Stanton, J. C., Panjabi, A., & Marra, P. P. (2019). Decline of the north American avifauna. *Science*. https://doi.org/10.1126/science.aaw1313

Sala, E. (2020). The cost of harming nature. *National Geographic, 238*(3), 15–18.

Salas, R. N. (2020, April 23). Lessons from the covid-19 pandemic provide a blueprint for the climate emergency. *BMJ Opinion.*. https://blogs.bmj.com/bmj/2020/04/23/renee-n-salas-lessons-from-the-covid-19-pandemic-as-a-blueprint-for-the-climate-crisis/

Schmeller, D. S., Courchamp, F., & Killeen, G. (2020). Biodiversity loss, emerging pathogens and human health. *Biodiversity and Conservation, 29*, 3095–3102. https://doi.org/10.1007/s10531-020-02021-6

Selsky, A. (2021, July 1). *Hundreds believed dead in heat wave despite efforts to help*. New York: Associated Press. https://apnews.com/article/canada-heat-waves-science-health-government-and-politics-ea770a153d84b8774190a96affe2c2e3

Smith, A. B. (2021, January 8). *2020 U.S. billion-dollar weather and climate disasters in historical context*. Silver Springs, MD: National Oceanic and Atmospheric Administration. https://www.climate.gov/news-features/blogs/beyond-data/2020-us-billion-dollar-weather-a

Swim, J., Clayton, S., Doherty, T., Gifford, R., Howard, G., Reser, J., Stern, P., & Weber, E. (2009). *Psychology & global climate change*. Washington. *DC: American Psychological Association.*. https://www.apa.org/science/about/publications/climate-change.aspx

Tippett, M. K. (2018). Extreme weather and climate. *Climate and Atmospheric Science, 1*, 45. https://doi.org/10.1038/s41612-018-0057-1

Tollefson, J. (2021). COVID curbed 2020 carbon emissions—But not by much. *Nature, 589*, 343. https://www.nature.com/articles/d41586-021-00090-3

United Nations Convention to Combat Desertification. (2017). *The global land outlook, 1st Edition* (Bonn: Author, 2017). https://www.unccd.int/sites/default/files/documents/2017-09/GLO_Full_Report_low_res.pdf

United States Climate Resilience Toolkit. (2020). *Tribal nations*. National Oceanic and Atmospheric Administration. https://toolkit.climate.gov/topics/tribal-nations

United States Environmental Protection Agency. (2017). *Climate impacts in Alaska*. Retrieved from https://www.epa.gov/climate-impacts/climate-impacts-alaska

United States Global Change Research Program. (2017). *Climate science special report: Fourth national climate assessment, volume I*. U.S. Global Change Research Program. https://science2017.globalchange.gov/downloads/CSSR2017_FullReport.pdf

Wackernagel, M., Schulz, N. B., Deumling, D., Linares, A. C., Jenkins, M., Kapos, V., Monfreda, C., Loh, J., Myers, N., Norgaard, R., & Randers, J. (2002). Tracking the ecological overshoot of the human economy. *PNAS, 99*(14), 9266–9271. https://doi.org/10.1073/pnas.142033699

Warren, L. S. (2002). The nature of conquest: Indians, Americans, and environmental history. In P. J. Deloria & N. Salisbury (Eds.), *A companion to American Indian history* (pp. 287–306). Blackwell Publishers.

Watts, N., Amann, M., Arnell, N., Ayeb-Karlsson, S., Beagley, J., Belesova, K., Boykoff, M., Byass, P., Cai, W., Campbell-Lendrum, D., Capstick, S., Chambers, J., Coleman, S., Dalin, C., Daly, M., Dasandi, N., Dasgupta, S., Davies, M., Napoli, D., & C.,…Costello, A. (2021). The 2020 report of the *lancet* countdown on health and climate change: Responding to converging crises. *Lancet, 397*, 129–170. https://doi.org/10.1016/50140-6736(20)32290-X

Weber, P. J., & Bleed, J. (2021, February 19). *Some electricity restored in Texas, but water woes grow*. New York: Associated Press. https://apnews.com/article/texas-power-outages-icy-weather-186cf801eade2d221f001a99b3aaa936

Weber, P. J., & Stengle, J. (2021, March 26). *Texas death toll from February storm, outages surpasses 100*. New York: Associated Press. https://apnews.com/article/hypothermia-health-storms-power-outages-texas-ffeb5d49e1b43032ffdc93ea9d7cfa5f

Weinstein, Z. S., Hoshiko, S., Fahima, J., Harrison, R. J., Cascio, W. E., & Rappold, A. G. (2018). Cardiovascular and cerebrovascular emergency department visits associated with wildfire smoke exposure in California in 2015. *Journal of the American Heart Association, 7*(e007492), 1–15. https://doi.org/10.1161/JAHA.117.007492

Weiss, R. A., & McMichael, A. J. (2004). Social and environmental risk factors in the emergence of infectious diseases. *Nature Medicine, 10*(12), S70–S76.

Wu, X., Nethery, R. C., Sabath, M. B., Braun, D., & Dominici, F. (2020). Air pollution and COVID-19 mortality in the United States: Strengths and limitations of an ecological regression analysis. *Science. Advances, 6*(45), eabd4049. https://doi.org/10.1126/sciadv.abd4049

Zakaria, F. (2020). *Ten lessons for a post-pandemic world*. W. W. Norton.

Zhang, J., Tian, W., Chipperfield, M. P., Xie, F., & Huang, J. (2016). Persistent shift of the Arctic polar vortex towards the Eurasian continent in recent decades. *Nature Climate Change, 6*, 1094–1100. https://doi.org/10.1038/NCLIMATE3136

Zhou, X., Josey, K., Kamareddine, L., Caine, M. C., Liu, T., Mickley, L. J., Cooper, M., & Dominici, F. (2021). Excess of COVID-19 cases and deaths due to fine particulate matter exposure during the 2020 wildfires in the United States. *Science. Advances, 7*, eabi8789. https://doi.org/10.1126/sciadv.abi8789

Chapter 3
Colonial Economics and COVID-19

Abstract Materialism has been central to colonialism from its inception and remains as a fundamental value in contemporary colonial societies. Social hierarchy permits widespread economic inequities that favor the privileged and harm the disfavored. The pandemic highlighted the weaknesses of an economic system that has benefitted the privileged while contributing to intergeneration income and wealth inequities. Centuries of inequitable policies have contributed to economically vulnerable societies, compounding pandemic preparation and response. Wealth building during COVID-19 pandemic highlighted how colonial economic systems perpetuate and advance privilege. Colonial economics rather than human need have historically defined public health policies. During COVID-19, economically driven responses created innumerable barriers to controlling virus spread and protecting the vulnerable. When addressing a pandemic, placing economic considerations first was consistently harmful to the common good and particularly deadly in results. Effectively preparing for future pandemics requires a vision for collective wellness. Advancing psychological well-being demands policies that promote collective well-being and health. Colonial materialism, self-interests, and economic hierarchy must be transformed to promote a more balanced humanitarian response to future global crises including pandemics.

Economics are very important to understanding colonialism. As discussed earlier in the book, the *Doctrine of Discovery* granted the spoils of conquest to colonizers and their ruling classes. Colonialism from its inception was about building wealth and exploiting resources for self-gain (Bump et al., 2021), hence the importance of economics in colonial nations even today. Contrast the model of economics for material self-gain with the barter economies for community survival that Indigenous Americans had before conquest illustrates the remarkable differences that worldviews can have on economics. Colonialism has a decidedly material perspective when it comes to understanding health, well-being, and happiness (Blume, 2020), and therefore economics have been highly influential on the trajectory of the pandemic.

Economic power in colonial nations has always been centralized into the hands of very few privileged citizens, beginning with the ruling class in Europe, morphing

A. W. Blume, *Colonialism and the COVID-19 Pandemic*, International and Cultural Psychology, https://doi.org/10.1007/978-3-030-92825-4_3

into the entrepreneurial tycoons, and eventually into the uber wealthy of the present. The privilege of accumulating wealth has been a protected liberty within colonial societies--viewed as a visible sign of success, power, and even mystique, and the wealthy are often revered. Original colonial perspectives that resource accumulation was divinely sanctioned contributed to the modern colonial myths such as the American dream that suggests anyone can share in that wealth (Blume, 2020). However, the uber wealthy also may be socialized to protect their wealth intergenerationally, at least in the US (Disney, 2021), suggesting they may not want to share too much. Evidence of class migration within these societies is not encouraging, especially in the US (Carr & Wiemers, 2016; Song et al., 2020). In fact, intergenerational poverty is perhaps a more likely outcome than class migration, especially for outgroups (Chetty et al., 2018; Smeeding, 2016). In 2021, the situation was so obviously bleak that Jamie Dimon, CEO of JP Morgan Chase, suggested the American dream was "fraying" (La Monica, 2021), a harsh assessment from a high-profile proponent of colonial economics.

Colonial economic systems were never meant to be equitable. In Europe, the ruling class was rewarded with material spoils without needing to be physically present during the conquest—it was expected that the ruling class would receive such tributes. In the US, only property owners were allowed to vote in the original US constitution, with many people unable to own property in the beginning of the republic. Certain demographic groups were forbidden to share in the accumulation of wealth, and for slaves, indentured servants, and Indigenous peoples, their wealth was seized by others. The result was an economic system that privileged some and slighted many. Many minoritized groups started their association with colonial economies impoverished and have found it difficult to climb out of that poverty with unequal access to education, health care, and vocational opportunities (ISSC, 2016; Smeeding, 2016). Colonial societies have never been shy about prioritizing economics ahead of people, especially people from outgroups. Using the analogy of a car, colonial economies were fueled by gasoline siphoned from others, and then the car was never allowed to operate with all eight cylinders functioning smoothly due to the inequities imposed on many groups in those economies. Such were the circumstances of many colonial economies when the COVID-19 pandemic emerged.

Colonial Shortsightedness in Preparing for Pandemics

Colonialism has been centered on achieving proximal goals but experiences difficulty with long-term planning (Blume, 2020). Colonization historically has been focused on self-gratification through material acquisition of land and possessions, executed through immediate actions to achieve those proximal goals. Colonization featured material aspirations, such as *Manifest Destiny* in the US that dreamt of controlling North America from sea to shining sea, and then later colonial conquests beyond North America (Kluger, 2007). However, colonial dreamers did not consider the negative consequences of pursuing those dreams, such as the victims who were either harmed by the dreams or excluded from them. Psychologically speaking, the activities of colonialism were not well-considered with regard to the long-term consequences of how colonial acts would impact others, including subsequent generations of their own progeny (Blume, 2020). We continue to see those societies principally focused on "now is all that matters" orientations, emphasizing self-gratification of the moment without considering the consequences over the long-term to others. Many examples follow of how these activities prevented a strong and compassionate pandemic response.

One economic result of proximal ways of thinking is that many colonial societies have emphasized efficiency over sufficiency. The first apparent casualty of efficiency over sufficiency during the Trump administration that impacted COVID-19 pandemic response was the 2018 elimination of a National Security Council unit charged with global health security and biothreats, greatly reducing the ability to carry out global surveillance to detect and mitigate biological threats before they became national security threats to the US (Morrison, 2018; Riechmann, 2020). The decision appeared to be made in the context of economic efficiency but unwittingly contributed to a deficient pandemic response early in the pandemic, a consequence predicted shortly after the decision (Morrison, 2018).

Efficiency rather than sufficiency also left societies without enough personal protective equipment (PPE) on hand to address a pandemic (Ranney et al., 2020). Global supply chains were developed to be cost effective--economically efficient—to save businesses and governments money. The manufacture of many products was outsourced to other areas of the world in order to benefit the profit margin of corporations but creating vulnerable supply chains. In an example of both colonial shortsightedness and arrogance related to the perception of colonial superiority and invulnerability, governments did not stockpile sufficient PPE or other essential goods for a global emergency. The pandemic disrupted globally "efficient" supply chains since "sufficiency" had not thoughtfully considered.

Concerns were immediately voiced by US hospitals and other health care entities that did not stockpile sufficient PPE. Safety was palpably compromised, contributing to significant psychological stress and consequences such as anxiety, depression, and psychological distress due to lack of protections for human services workers (Grover et al., 2020; Spoorthy et al., 2020). Disruptions in the global supply chain contributed to health-threatening shortages on important medications (Schondelmeyer et al., 2020). In other words, hospitals had prepared for only short-term proximal needs just like their colonial governments--unprepared for a prolonged crisis response that had more distal consequences.

The US was forced to turn to the strategic reserve to access PPE and other health care equipment such as ventilators early in the pandemic. The strategic national stockpile in the US is designed to hold essential items in reserve to be available in the case of a national emergency or disaster. Unfortunately, the strategic national stockpile was only envisioned to be used as a stop-gap solution and was never conceived as a long-term solution to a prolonged interruption to the supply chain of

PPE, medical equipment, or other disaster response items (Fitzpatrick, 2020). Sadly, the assumptions of the strategic national stockpile match perfectly the proximal tenets of a colonial society to fulfill short-term rather than long-term needs of a global crisis like the COVID-19 pandemic. Supply problems of some items persisted throughout the pandemic, exacerbated by individualized and independent national policy barriers (International Chamber of Shipping, 2021). Despite beliefs of economic efficiency, the proximal biases of colonial societies left many nations resource insufficient during COVID-19 and even more vulnerable to addressing pandemics of the future.

Hoarding As a Consumer Response to Emotional Insecurity and Self-Interests Another economic consequence was the phenomenon of consumer hoarding that occurred partly due to concerns about the supply chain. Consumers were restricted from purchasing lifesaving PPE online, such as n-95 masks and hand sanitizer, due to tremendous shortages for health care institutions and professionals. As is typical with impending emergencies in material societies, there were runs on stores for certain supplies in anticipation of long lock-down orders and supply chain problems. Shelves were emptied in retail stores with some items difficult to locate.

Hoarding behaviors are often a response to extreme emotions, such as the anger, anxiety, fear, and sadness experienced during the COVID-19 pandemic (Baddeley, 2020; Shaw et al., 2015). Hoarding behavior further aggravated the difficulties in the supply chain associated with the colonial model of economic efficiency over sufficiency. Cohen-Louck and Levy (2021) compared the fears related to the unseen and pervasive threat of the coronavirus (or any other pandemic) to the generalized fear of threats some perceive related to terrorism. Addressing anxiety and fear would have been helpful early in the pandemic, but unfortunately many colonial governments were more interested in using blame to encourage externalized anxiety and fear directed toward others. The populist-nationalist governments in power during the COVID-19 pandemic were masters of division and externalizing threats to stoke fear and anxiety (as well as anger), so citizens of those countries were primed to be at risk for hoarding. In addition to the link of hoarding to extreme emotions, a study of adolescent early in the pandemic found an association with hoarding grocery items and values of self-interest and social responsibility. Higher self-interested values were associated with greater self-report of hoarding and higher social responsibility values with lesser hoarding behaviors (Oosterhoff & Palmer, 2020), suggesting that the colonial values of self-interests over social responsibility may have been associated with COVID-19 hoarding, at least among adolescents. The perception of externalized threats from others also likely prompts competition to stockpile personal consumables before hypothetical others get to them first. Externalized anxiety and fear appeared to hinder a willingness to share at a time when concern for others was most needed.

Colonial Deception and Pandemic Economics

Many colonial nations acted as if they were economically invulnerable pre-pandemic to a significant breakdown in the global system. The resulting colonial arrogance contributed to poor pandemic preparation that profoundly disrespected those who were needed the most: health care workers. But they were not been alone. Colonial arrogance contributed to acts that significantly placed many others at risk through decisions made to protect the economy without sufficient methods to protect the workers. In the early stages of the pandemic, many colonial nations used *a laissez faire* approach toward COVID-19, slow walking responses to the pandemic and downplaying risks through deception. As discussed in Chap. 1, deception has been a historically common tactic by colonial nations, and so it is no surprise that deception was used during COVID-19 to manipulate the citizens of those societies.

One of the most striking examples of deception was perpetrated by the US government. The administration of former President Trump made a conscious decision to downplay the risks associated with the pandemic to minimize economic concerns before the 2020 election (Woodward, 2020). The Trump administration deceived by statements that the virus was a hoax or would simply disappear (Wolfe & Dale, 2020), and other times suggested the virus was essentially harmless and the risk had been overstated by public health professionals (Levin, 2020; Subramaniam et al., 2020; Woodward, 2020). Trump officials even attempted to tamper with CDC documents to downplay pandemic severity and its extent (Stracqualursi & Holmes, 2021). Deceptive practices significantly hindered mitigation efforts. When asked about the discrepancies between messages of science versus the colonial acts of deception in the Trump administration, Dr. Anthony Fauci, longtime Director of the National Institute on Allergies and Infectious Disease (NIAID), said in exasperation, "I can't jump in front of the microphone and push him down" (Azad, 2020).

Pre-Pandemic Tax Policies Created Greater Vulnerability for Many People

Even though colonial economies appeared superficially healthy immediately before the shutdowns of 2020 to some, many were not well. One of the most remarkable developments of early 2020 was how quickly economies collapsed--like houses of cards--suggesting the perceived strengths were masking the overwhelming vulnerabilities of income and wealth inequities (Alvarado et al., 2018; ISSC, 2016). And without significant stimulus efforts by many nations, the global economy might have collapsed even further. Projections have been that the overall impact of COVID-19 through 2030 on global economies would results in tremendous losses to the global gross domestic product, perhaps many trillions of US dollars (Yeyati & Filippini, 2021), having consequences for global health and mental health over time.

One pre-existing vulnerability to the US economy came in the form of a new tax code that was passed in late 2017. The tax code changes have resulted in significantly increased wealth for the upper class and corporations while simultaneously increasing the US budget deficit over time (Beyer, 2019; Leonhardt, 2021). The tax was portrayed as a mechanism to help stimulate the economy, but empirical evidence suggests there was little economic benefit resulting from the changes (Gravelle & Marples, 2019). This is not a surprising outcome since researchers have found little support for the notion that tax reductions on the upper class stimulate the economy. Instead, the policy appears to increase income inequality (Hope & Limberg, 2020; Zidar, 2019). Despite no evidence tax cuts would stimulate the economy or help those who are suffering economically, the Trump administration considered additional tax cuts to benefit the upper class and corporations again--against the advice of economic scientists (Hope & Limberg, December 29, 2020). The tax cut proposal was an excellent example of how political decisions that benefit the privileged few are often packaged in deceptive populist messages assuring benefits to all. The tax cuts favoring the privileged would have left the vulnerable even more vulnerable to the health and mental consequences of the pandemic.

Open for Business

One policy that profoundly impacted the health and well-being during the COVID-19 pandemic was the inordinate effort to keep countries open for business despite unaddressed health risks. Efforts to keep businesses open, damn the consequences, often occurred under the guidance of populist governments with nationalist agendas—in other words, the most regressive of colonial governments (see also Chap. 4). Within the US with its splintered political system, there were significant policy differences to opening businesses safely across different states and municipalities. The efforts to keep the US economy open were happening in the context of PPE shortages, often hampering safe reopening of businesses. The expensive results of the largely uncontrolled spread were not economically efficient (Bartsch et al., 2020).

Colonial nations, especially the US, entered the pandemic with an air of colonial arrogance regarding the health of the economy. Perhaps the best example of this arrogance was a statement made by American Airlines CEO Doug Parker in early 2018, when he suggested that his company would never lose money again due to efficiencies to the industry (Kuehner-Hebert, 2018). Psychologists often see the use of the word "never" as sign than one is engaged in a thinking error that needs to be challenged. The errors of Mr. Parker's thinking became clear when airlines required financial bailouts to survive in 2020. In addition, the comment by Mr. Parker is an excellent example of the shortsighted colonial worldview and its inability to anticipate distal outcomes. The level of arrogance helps to understand the irrational thinking processes of colonial leaders that hindered lifesaving pandemic responses.

Unfortunately, airlines also highlighted the risks of the open economy amidst the pandemic in very dramatic ways. For example, the difficulty with social distancing on flights made safety an ongoing problem. The CDC provided evidence that exposure to COVID-19 on flights was likely widespread due to the inability to socially distance, despite numerous precautions provided by the airlines (CDC, 2020; Muntean et al., 2020). The CDC later in the pandemic found evidence that risks to passengers were significantly decreased by blocking middle seats in coach, but airliners often filled those seats anyway for financial reasons (Dietrich et al., 2021). Compliance with flight crew instructions on masking were spotty and difficult to enforce (Laris, 2021), despite the fact that at least two people died of COVID-19 in flight (Duncan, 2020; Sampson, 2020). Airline passenger misbehavior (e.g., fighting, refusing to mask and follow flight attendants' instructions) was so common as to constitute a threat to flight safety (Federal Aviation Administration, 2021). The travel industry suffered greatly. Many became unemployed due to the difficulties with traveling safely (Rugaber, 2021), suffering psychological stress from economic uncertainty and insecurity.

The problem has not been with keeping businesses open, but rather how to keep businesses open safely. Different businesses had different challenges related to their abilities to protect employees and customers while ensuring a reasonable cashflow to remain open. It became increasingly clear that businesses with crowds and poor ventilation were risky for both employees and customers. For example, bars and restaurants, fitness centers, and hotels/motels were identified as risky places for COVID-19 spread without protections in place (Chang et al., 2020). Limiting indoor capacity for businesses was recommended to reduce social spread as a result of the study (Carey, 2020). Later in the pandemic, modeling research called into question whether the six-foot social distancing rule routinely suggested was enough given poor indoor ventilation in many buildings (Bazant & Bush, 2021).

Unfortunately, many businesses have not been well-supported when pushed to reopen by governmental entities. Many suffered mightily as a result (e.g., Hartmans, 2020). Plus, similar to airlines, many citizens have refused to comply with safety guidelines, risking health and mental health consequences to others. Interestingly, collective societies seemed to have done better with social compliance as might be expected, and therefore experienced significantly fewer pandemic problems. New Zealand did very well in controlling COVID-19 and its consequences--likely no accident since the culture of New Zealand is heavily influenced by Indigenous values with 16.7% of its population being Maori (Stats, 2020). South Korea was also another country that did well in controlling COVID-19 with a much larger population (Dyer, 2021). Both South Korea and New Zealand had strong collectivistic cultural influences at work that promoted collective health and protection rather than self-interests.

Privilege and Pandemic "Wealth Building"

There are periodic reminders that health care in colonial nations is essentially defined by economics. Those reminders have occurred frequently with COVID-19. Health care in colonial nations reflects the material assumptions of colonial cultures. Economics have tended to define important aspects of health care such as accessibility and quality of care. In societies where colonial inequities contribute to wide variations in accessibility and quality of care, economic decisions tend to benefit the privileged in society, often at the expense of outgroups. US health care mostly operates under a business rather than public health model, meaning that economics drive health care delivery, rather than health care need driving the economics.

One example of economics driving the agenda on health care could be seen in which hospitals did well during the pandemic and which did not. Safety net hospitals care for the most vulnerable in society. During the pandemic, safety net hospitals suffered significant financial distress, whereas many hospitals serving more affluent patients generated significant financial gains (Sullivan & Jingnan, 2021)--the haves of the health care world prospering significantly at a time when the have-nots struggled mightily. Another victim of pandemic economics was rural America. Rural hospitals were at a significant disadvantage pre-pandemic because of their small sizes, lack of resources, and because many serve older populations with fixed incomes or those with lower SES (Mason, 2017). Rural communities also have limited access to mental health care, especially during the COVID-19 pandemic (Renner, 2020). The pandemic left an already challenged rural hospital system struggling for financial survival (Tribble, 2020), especially those serving Black rural communities (Goldhill, 2021). Rural hospitals are often owned by for-profit hospital systems whose decisions with an eye to the profit motive may not have helped prepare them for a pandemic. For-profit hospital systems closed unprofitable rural hospitals, leaving broad geographical areas as hospital deserts (Morgenson et al., 2020), yet another example of how economics driving health care hindered the COVID-19 response.

Another example of the economics driving health care occurred on November 9, 2020, when Pfizer announced that preliminary findings for their COVID-19 vaccine were very positive, suggesting that the vaccine might be more than 90% effective (Pfizer, 2020a). The announcement occurred 11 days prior to those data being submitted to the Federal Drug Administration (FDA) on November 20 (Pfizer, 2020b). Meanwhile, a regularly scheduled sell-off of Pfizer stock was carried out on behalf of Pfizer CEO Albert Bourla that amounted to approximately 5.6 million dollars and for the executive vice president of Pfizer, Sally Susman, that netted Ms. Susman approximately 1.8 million dollars (Mohamed, 2020). Pfizer suggested that since the stock sell-off had been pre-scheduled, there was no impropriety involved. Bourla and presumably Susman reportedly learned the preliminary findings of the phase 3 clinical trial the day before the sell-off, a Sunday when the markets would have been closed. Pfizer officials were not alone with stock sell-offs after positive press releases, with Moderna executives doing likewise (Nagarajan, 2020).

The optics of these sell-offs were obviously not good and reflect a certain economic insensitivity present in colonial business decisions that often favor self- and organizational interests at the expense of others (Blume, 2020). The stock sell-offs were a reminder that the profit motive is a major driver of health care delivery, especially in the US. And even though the sell-off was pre-arranged, the timing of the announcement of the preliminary results of the clinical trial was not necessarily pre-set and could have been made the day after the sell-off rather than the morning before the sell-off. Colonial health care has historically reflected the material assumptions its culture, with variations in accessibility and quality of care driven by economic decisions that benefit those who are the privileged in society.

Regardless of how one feels about lucrative stock sell-offs, they represent an excellent example of what has been referred to as *wealth building*. Accumulation of material wealth has been an important aspect of colonial culture consistently though history. Modern wealth building strategies are merely an extension of that tradition. Wealth building during the pandemic was highly visible and produced extreme results in the middle of an economic collapse that required governmental interventions to keep economies afloat. As an aside, it is worth noting that the federal government has been used to prop up the fragile American economy innumerable times over its history (Davis, 2021). One wonders why it is necessary to bail out what some view as a premier economic system over and over again. History provides evidence of inherent flaws that challenge the viability of the American economy without periodic governmental stimulus. Ironical to some, government stimulus has fueled some of the pandemic wealth building, affirming its misuse to protect existing privilege.

Many US citizens have found it extremely difficult to understand how the stock markets could reach historical highs in the context of lock downs, significant unemployment and widespread sickness and death. At first, the reaction of stock markets to the pandemic is what one would have expected--a significant loss as the uncertainty of the pandemic provoked fear. Individual COVID-19 stimulus checks and unemployment benefits prevented millions from sinking into poverty (Alonso-Zaldivar, 2021). But as stimulus was provided to keep the economy afloat, a record comeback was staged by the stock market, at a time when underclasses were suffering mightily (Rugaber, 2020; Tensley, 2020). Stock markets seemed to exist in another reality, oblivious to the suffering of many people.

One result was unprecedented wealth building for the privileged few of society at the expense of the rest of the population. Wealth inequity has exploded in the US, some brought on by the pre-existing inequities to the pandemic that placed outgroups at risk but the balance was a historic example of how privilege enhances privilege (Rugaber, 2020; Tensley, 2020). For example, the privileged have been able to social distance and maintain their incomes (Blow, 2020), and have also been able to leverage pandemic circumstances for building more wealth (Rugaber, 2020). The COVID-19 pandemic was a most striking recent exhibit of how economic privilege works. Those with pre-existing privilege were able to enhance that privilege easily and naturally within social orders designed to maintain and defend privilege. The same era that has created unprecedented wealth building will be followed by a wave of serious mental health issues that will be with us for years, a totally predictable outcome given the level of relational psychopathology that has benefitted the few and risked the many (Blow, 2020; Blume, 2020).

There are many more examples of the privileged benefitting from the pandemic and the traditionally disposed and oppressed of society being victimized. One example involved who benefitted from the stimulus packages, and it was not necessarily those who needed it most. Some mistakes appeared to be innocent. For example, some of the stimulus checks from the CARES Act were sent to non-citizens overseas (Pfeiffer, 2020). However, other misuses of the stimulus money appeared to be better explained by colonial self-interests. For example, minoritized businesses were turned down repeatedly by the CARES Act Paycheck Protection Program (PPP) and only considered after others had received benefits (Shalvey, 2021). Contrast that experience with the benefits provided to companies much earlier in the program that clearly did not need the protections—large corporations and businesses with tremendous financial reserves (Sherman, April 24, 2020). Businesses owned by Trump family members received significant benefits from the CARES Act PPP (Popken & Lehren, 2020). Companies debarred (prevented) from receiving federal funds for past violations also received PPP funds (Lehren & Siegel, 2021). The uneven distribution of stimulus resources is another example of how the colonial values of hierarchical injustice and protection of privilege complicated efforts to address the pandemic. Small businesses owned by people of color were disproportionately harmed (US Chamber of Commerce, 2020), exacerbating post-pandemic economic challenges to those communities. In reality, the 2020 US business stimulus initiatives proved to be primarily a safety net for the privileged.

The Gig: Essential Yet Disposable

The realities of COVID-19 redefined who is an essential worker—those who had little choice but to work in harm's way of the virus. Essential workers were often subject to prolonged virus exposure. Many essential workers suffered from a lack of PPE to prevent exposure and worried not only for their own welfare but also for the welfare of family members who might become sick from them. Some essential workers are compensated well but many were not, with those working in food and agricultural jobs having median wages of $13.12 an hour—not much to compensate for keeping the US fed (McNicholas & Poudock, 2020). Approximately 43% of essential workers were from minoritized groups, and among food and agricultural workers, approximately 50% (McNicholas & Poudock, 2020). As a result, ethnic-racial disparities of COVID-19 at US workplace outbreaks early in the pandemic were not uncommon (Bui et al., 2020). From an IAPP perspective, essential workers should be greatly honored for their courage and for the importance of their service to others. However, in colonial societies, many essential workers were not compensated or treated well, and often worked under conditions deemed undesirable from the perspective of the privileged.

Research findings confirm the risks that essential workers faced when interfacing with others. In general, researchers found that less mobile people during the pandemic were less likely to be infected (Chang et al., 2020). Those who had occupations that offered the possibility of teleworking from home were significantly less likely become infected (Fisher et al., 2020). Social distancing in the workplace was strongly recommended by health policy professionals. However, social distancing was difficult for essential workers, many from low SES circumstances and afflicted with health-related risk factors (Weill et al., 2020).

Health care providers understood the risks of their professions, but they probably never counted on the persistent level of risks they would face during the pandemic. Those risks were compounded by the lack of PPE upon which lives depended; therefore, many improvised with their own forms of protection--reusing supposedly disposable items, enhancing substandard equipment, or creating their own means of protection. Those fears were warranted—researchers found that front-line health care professionals were significantly more likely to become ill with COVID-19 than others in their communities (Nguyen et al., 2020). By summer of 2020, hundreds had passed away from COVID-19, with analyses findings mortality disparities for Asian American and Black American health care workers (Hughes et al., 2020).

The long-term exposure to these psychological stressors, traumatic events, anxiety, and worry, as well as the despairing circumstances contributing to depression, have taken a serious toll on the health and mental health of care providers globally (Grover et al., 2020; Lin et al., 2020; Spoorthy et al., 2020; Trougakos et al., 2020). Many health and mental health care providers of color had workplace stress and trauma compounded by acts of bias and discrimination (Miu & Moore, 2021). A majority of health care workers and psychologists in the US are female (American Psychological Association [APA], 2016; McNicholas & Poudock, 2020), another historically disempowered group in colonial societies (Blume, 2020).

Health care was not the only risky profession related to essential services. As an example, firefighters combatting the wild and forest fires associated with a warming climate were sometimes not provided PPE or encouraged to practice pandemic safety measures (Lozano, 2021). In another example, those who worked in food processing plants endured superspreader events early in the pandemic due to unsafe practices including insufficient PPE but were designated as essential workers to coerce staying on the job despite the risks. One such example was a Tyson Food plant in Iowa where spread was so common that managers set up a betting pool to guess the total number of employees who would get infected (Ali, 2020). When asked, a manager indicated that the betting pool was meant to increase the morale of the office (Foley, 2020b). There are several issues to psychologically unpack about this particular incident. First, the callousness toward the worker-victims by their managers demonstrates a clear hierarchical perspective common to colonial cultures. Second, since a significant number of workers getting ill were likely Latinx given the demographics of the area (Foley, 2020a), minoritized hierarchical bias likely entered into the callousness. Finally, one wonders how pandemic stress might have impacted the managers' judgement in this incident. From an IAPP perspective, relational psychopathology was clearly at work (Blume, 2020). Regardless, essential workers were putting their health on the line for their families and country and yet were being disrespected and dehumanized by their "superiors."

The Vulnerability of the Pre-Pandemic Gig Economy As many as 150 million workers in the North America and Europe and perhaps 24% of all Americans aged 18 or older participated in what is known as the gig economy (Edison Research, 2018; Petriglieri et al., 2018). Gig jobs often include a patchwork of part-time positions dependent upon consumer demand, potentially allowing a flexible schedule for the entrepreneur. Gig jobs tend to be more temporary and perhaps more vulnerable to changing economic circumstances than regular employment. Workers aged 18–34 have gig work necessary due to economic factors disfavoring their age group. Over half reporting gig work as a primary source of income--larger than any other age group (Edison Research, 2018). The gig job market rapidly expanded post-Great Recession, perhaps to fill the void of permanently lost positions (Frazer, 2019). The sheer number of people employed in gig jobs post-Great Recession suggests that economic growth was oriented towards unstable jobs, which also suggests a vulnerable economy pre-pandemic—a house of cards as suggested earlier.

Although some gigs are meant to either supplement income from other employment, many gig workers depend on gig jobs as the primary source of income, especially true for Black and Latinx Americans (Edison Research, 2018). When the COVID-19 pandemic emerged, many gig workers lost significant sources of income due to the vulnerability of those jobs (Lavietes & McCoy, 2020). Young adults in particular fared poorly in the COVID-19 economy (Sherman, 16 October, 2020). The fragile gig economy represented an economic vulnerability of many colonial nations pre-pandemic. Gig workers with their economic uncertainties and inherent risks of exposure to COVID-19 also experienced significant psychological stress during the pandemic. Long-term consequences of chronic job insecurity have been associated with negative outcomes to psychological health and well-being (Wu et al., 2020).

Income and Wealth Inequities and COVID-19

One of the greatest economic risks entering into the COVID-19 pandemic were pre-existing income and wealth disparities that enhanced vulnerability to sickness. Income and wealth inequities are important contributors to intergenerational poverty and poor health and mental health, depriving people of access to appropriate health and mental health services (Blundell et al., 2020; Chetty et al., 2018; ISSC, 2016; United Nations, 2020). In the US, income and wealth disparities were increasing immediately before the COVID-19 pandemic (Horowitz et al., 2020), and those trends accelerated during the pandemic. Mean US salaries remained equivalent to pre-pandemic levels, even with millions of newly unemployed earning nothing (Rugaber, 2021). Global billionaires saw their wealth expand greatly during the pandemic when many others experienced high unemployment and lost income (Ziady, 2020). Contrast that pandemic windfall with the projections that Africa will see an increase of perhaps 100 million people entering into severe poverty (World Bank, 2020).

Economic inequities contributed to increased risk for mortality from COVID-19 mortality in Mexico (Gutierrez & Bertozzi, 2020), another nation with a populist-nationalist president (Andrés Manuel López Obrador). As discussed earlier in the chapter, populist-nationalistic responses to the pandemic have contributed to significant health consequences to benefit a few at the expense of many. Using Mexico as an example, the likely death toll by the spring of 2021 rivaled both the US and Brazil (Reuters, 2021). Economic inequity erodes trust in societies, and certainly colonialism has contributed to that distrust. In a study of 84 countries, societies with greater economic inequity experienced greater social distrust and higher mortality from COVID-19 (Elgar et al., 2020). Perceived economic hardship during the pandemic was also associated with elevated depressive symptoms and anxiety, with workers in socially devalued professions perhaps most vulnerable to elevated mental health symptoms (Witteveen & Velthorst, 2020). Economic instability in the US contributed tremendous stress and uncertainty for many. US Black and Latinx people reported greater worries about employment, rent and mortgage, childcare, and repaying student loans during the pandemic than White Americans (American Staffing Association, 2020). People traditionally disempowered by colonial hierarchies would be the most likely to suffer from the risks of economic hardships and perceptions of lower prestige (Blume, 2020), another example of how colonial values perpetuate mental health risks.

Intergenerational poverty and unemployment contributed to hunger and long food lines in the US during COVID-19. Pandemic unemployment and closures contributed to widespread food insecurity in the US (Feeding America, 2020), exacerbated pre-pandemic food insecurity that impacted 25% of Indigenous American families, 20% of Black families, and 17% of Latinx families (Spratling, 2021). One pandemic oddity was the use of autos to socially distance, such as by drive-through COVID testing centers, vaccination sites, and social services. Miles long lines of autos quickly became a common sight at emergency food distribution sites (Alonso & Cullinane, 2020). Racial economic inequities contributed to worsening food insecurity among Black Americans as a consequence of COVID-19 (Hardy & Logan, 2020).

The threat of homelessness followed the economic challenges of the pandemic. Political indecision sometimes compounded the consequences of income and wealth inequities, contributing to increased poverty and homelessness (Dougherty, 2020; Sherman, October 15, 2020). In the US, tens of millions of Americans fell months behind in their rent and faced eviction (Benfer et al., 2020). In December of 2020, it was estimated that between 7–14 million American households were at risk of eviction with an estimated shortfall of 10–20 billion dollars in rent (Stout Risius Ross LLC, 2020). Rental housing has been stressed since the Great Recession and vulnerable pre-pandemic. Stimulus initiatives provided rental relief for some, but the rules concerning amount available varied by states and favored White and rural Americans (Ruiz-Goiriena & Bajak, 2021). Homelessness has significantly increased as a result of the evictions, even with a periodic moratorium on foreclosures in place (Dougherty, 2020). Another wave of increased homelessness was anticipated when the US Supreme Court rejected an extension of the federal moratorium (BBC, 2021). Minoritized individuals have been particularly vulnerable to foreclosures, exacerbating social tensions already enhanced by policing shootings (e.g., Vera & Toropin, 2020).

The COVID-19 pandemic pushed the capacity of homeless shelters to the brink, with social distancing restricting capacity and evictions increasing numbers. Homeless citizens were at risk if they sought shelter due to the virus, and at risk from weather exposure if they did not, especially during winter (Silva, 2020). With large numbers of first time homeless, there was great concern about their well-being during the winter of 2020–21. No one seemed to be tracking US mortality rates for people who were homeless during the pandemic, but the numbers must have been great (McFarling, 2021). A study from New York City through October, 2020, found mortality rates to be about 75% higher than the norm for the city (Coalition for the Homeless, 2020). People who were homeless were caught between the usual survival challenges and the novel risks of COVID-19 without resources for personal protection.

Worsening inequities will have serious post-pandemic consequences for health and mental health. The pandemic has exposed the weaknesses of social safety nets (Bump et al., 2021), wreaking havoc on personal finances and ability to access health care. Worsening inequities ensure that disempowered groups in colonial societies will remain economically disadvantaged for the foreseeable future. As an example of pandemic specific financial consequences, the amount of retirement savings available to people of color diminished greatly due to economic stressors, exacerbating an existing disparity (Reinicke, 2020).

Global stimulus packages during the COVID-19 pandemic were historic, rapidly escalating deficits of many nations (Horowitz, 2021; Woodward, 2021). Without stimulus, human suffering would have been compounded, so enacting stimulus was an appropriate short-term (proximal) solution to economic problems of the COVID-19 pandemic. However, there are serious concerns concerning the long-term (distal) economic consequences to using such extreme measures to keep the economies afloat (Horowitz, 2021).

How Colonial Beliefs Slowed the Response: An Indigenous Interpretation

A distal, more holistic view common to Indigenous thinking would view colonial economies as systemically flawed. The economic policies of colonial nations have been the source of tremendous relational psychopathology that contributes to the psychological wounding of billions of people (see Table 3.1). An IAPP psychological perspective would interpret current circumstances as evidence that the social

Table 3.1 Colonial economics and pandemic risk

Colonial barriers to pandemic response	Alternatives for a psychologically well society
Assuming inequities are normative	Pursing an egalitarian model
Disposable approach to economics	Sustainable approach to economics
Economics driving policies	Policies driving economics
Emphasizing efficiency	Pursuing sufficiency
Emphasizing proximal material goals	Seeking intergenerational equity-sustainability
Privilege drives necessity	Collective Well-being drives necessity
Pursuing self-interests	Pursuing collective planetary interests
Wealth building drives economics	Relationship building drives economics

system requires transformation to reduce victimization in need of economic bandaging to moderate future global catastrophes.

Why were people so divided in deciding how to balance opening the economy with controlling SARS-CoV-2 spread in colonial nations? From an IAPP perspective, it likely was related to the high value placed on economic prosperity in their societies. Colonial societies from their inception have linked self-esteem and happiness closely with material well-being and wealth and acquisition as evidence of individual success in hierarchical societies (Blume, 2020).

Psychological assumptions concerning the importance of self and autonomy in colonial societies suggest that economic success or failure is in the hands of the individual, which has never been true. Due to the nature of the material rules of those societies, competing self-interests divide people, pitting them against each other. Colonial methods to maintain the status quo of privilege exacerbate those divisions. People feel naturally insecure, often using material means to ward off those perceived insecurities. Anger, anxiety, and fear of others is ever-present with the inequities of colonial social orders--chronic psychological stressors externalized onto others who are blamed for the inherent insecurities of colonial societies. An IAPP perspective assumes that externalized anger, anxiety, and fear harm relationships—fuel for relational psychopathology if the person does not view the anger, anxiety, and fear as an internal growth opportunity for growth rather than an external threat (Blume, 2020).

Societies appear to do best when the have a common vision and purpose—a collective vision of their social contracts. From an IAPP perspective, social orders that operate on individual assumptions would not foster the cohesiveness needed to work collaboratively. Such a society would likely splinter, especially in the face of an overwhelming crisis such as a pandemic. A foundational tenet of colonial social contract was the acquisition and accumulation of material wealth for a privileged few. Today, a basic belief that individual pursuit of material well-being underlies the social contract of colonial societies—that happiness and well-being may be found in the pursuit of the materially driven dream to have and to own (Blume, 2020). However, from its inception, those societies have excluded many within the borders of those countries from that social contract. The reality is that the foundational assumption concerning the individual pursuit of material well-being has divided nations rather than united them. Colonial societies were splintered by their self-orientations and self-interests pre-pandemic, making a collectively healthy economic response to the pandemic difficult to impossible. The splintered self-interests of colonial citizens contributed to inadequately addressing both economy and health well. The impact of colonial splintering on health care, mental health care, and governance is elaborated upon in subsequent chapters.

Colonialism was founded as an economic enterprise that derived its resources and wealth from others. Economic opportunities to the privileged of colonial societies were not extended to everyone dwelling in those nations. As hierarchical societies, colonial nations have assumed and accepted inequities as an economic reality, often wielding political power to ensure those inequities. Widespread income and wealth disparities as well as intergenerational poverty among minoritized groups have been the result. The health and mental health consequences to those societies as a result of economic inequities were profound pre-pandemic, and will be even more profound in the post-pandemic world.

Privilege highlights the schizoid nature of colonial economics. The pandemic offered a tremendous opportunity for wealth building for those with privilege when millions of others lost their jobs. The non-privileged often worked in the presence of the virus whereas those with privilege were able to work remotely. As a result, those without privilege were more likely to become ill. Non-privileged families were often left with physical and mental health consequences they could not afford in the context of worsening family economies. The trajectory of the pandemic was driven by economics defined by privilege and inequity. Success of future pandemic responses relies on whether societies have the courage and wisdom to eliminate economic inequities. Addressing COVID-19 has been extremely costly in human capital and economic resources. It is an open question as to whether even the richest of colonial nations can withstand more of these economic shocks over the long-term.

Dr. Martin Luther King, Jr., (1956) once said, "we need leaders not in love with money, but in love with justice." Colonial proponents would like us to believe that economic systems are valuable because they provide material opportunities for individuals, but the unspoken reality is that the inequities that they have created and perpetuated threaten us all. Pandemic preparedness requires a transformation from a self-oriented economic mindset to an economic approach that benefits and protects the whole. Such an approach would go a long-ways toward improving the psychological well-being and happiness of the planet.

References

Ali, S. S. (2020, December 16). *Tyson fires 7 after probe into managers betting if workers would get COVID-19 at Iowa plant*. New York: NBC News. https://www.nbcnews.com/news/us-news/tyson-fires-7-after-probe-managers-betting-if-workers-would-n1251487

Alonso, M., & Cullinane, S. (2020, November 16). *Thousands of cars form lines to collect food in Texas*. New York: CNN. https://www.cnn.com/2020/11/15/us/dallas-texas-food-bank-coronavirus/index.html

Alonso-Zaldivar, R. (2021, September 14). *Census: Relief programs staved off hardship in COVID crash*. New York: Associated Press. https://apnews.com/article/business-health-coronavirus-pandemic-poverty-covid-19-pandemic-a1ba01f49c641ce1da8b21cc54d8b1ff

Alvarado, F., Chancel, L., Piketty, T., Saez, E., & Zucman, G. (2018). *World inequity report: Executive summary*. Paris: World Inequity Lab. https://wir2018.wid.world/files/download/wir2018-summary-english.pdf.

American Staffing Association. (2020). *2020 workforce monitor. Pandemic worries vary by race, job sector, and more*. Washington, DC: Author. https://americanstaffing.net/asa-workforce-monitor/worries-vary/

APA. (2016). *Frequently asked questions about psychology workforce: Demographics*. Washington, DC: Author. https://www.apa.org/workforce/about/faq.

Azad, A. (2020, March 23). *Fauci on Trump: 'I can't jump in front of the microphone and push him down.'* : CNN. https://www.cnn.com/2020/03/23/politics/fauci-trump-science-interview/index.html

Baddeley, M. (2020). Hoarding in the age of COVID-19. *Journal of behavioral economics for. Policy, 4*(S), 69–75.

Bartsch, S. M., Ferguson, M. C., McKinnell, J. A., O'Shea, K. J., Wedlock, P. T., Siegmund, S. S., & Lee, B. Y. (2020). The potential health care costs and resource use associated with COVID-19 in the United States. *Health Affairs, 39*(6), 927–935. https://doi.org/10.1377/hlthaff.2020.00426

Bazant, M. Z., & Bush, J. W. M. (2021). A guideline to limit indoor airborne transmission of COVID-19. *PNAS, 118*(17), e2018995118. https://doi.org/10.1073/pnas.2018995118

BBC. (2021, 27 August). *Supreme court: Biden eviction moratorium shot down by supreme court*. : Author. https://www.bbc.com/news/world-us-canada-58351798

Benfer, E., Robinson, D. B., Butler, S., Edmonds, L., Gilman, S., McKay, K. L., Owens, L., Steinkamp, N., Yentel, D., & Neumann, Z. (2020, August 7). *The COVID-19 eviction crisis: An estimated 30–40 million people in America are at risk*. Washington, DC: Aspen Institute. https://www.aspeninstitute.org/blog-posts/the-covid-19-eviction-crisis-an-estimated-30-40-million-people-in-america-are-at-risk/

Beyer, D. (2019). *Two years of evidence show 2017 tax cuts failed to deliver promised economic boost*. Joint Economic Committee of the US Congress.

Blow, C. M. (2020, April 5). *Social distancing is a privilege*. New York: New York Times. https://www.nytimes.com/2020/04/05/opinion/coronavirus-social-distancing-html

Blume, A. W. (2020). *A new psychology based on community, equality, and care of the earth: An indigenous American perspective*. ABC-CLIO/Praeger.

Blundell, R., Costa Dias, M., Joyce, R., & Xu, X. (2020). *Fiscal studies, 41*(2), 291-319. https://doi.org/10.1111/1475-5890.12232.

Bui, D. P., McCaffrey, K., Friedrichs, M., LaCross, N., Lewis, N. M., Sage, K., Barbeau, B., Vilven, D., Rose, C., Braby, S., Willardson, S., Carter, A., Smoot, C., Winquist, A., & Dunn, A. (2020, August 21). Racial and ethnic disparities among COVID-19 cases in workplace outbreaks by industry sector—Utah, march 6-June 5, 2020. *MMWR, 69*(33), 1133–1138. https://doi.org/10.15585/mmwr.mm6933e3

Bump, J. B., Baum, F., Sakornsin, M., Yates, R., & Hofman, K. (2021). Political economy of Covid-19: Extractive, regressive, competitive. *BMJ, 372*, 73. https://doi.org/10.1136/bmj.n73

Carey, B. (2020, November 10). *Limiting indoor capacity can reduce coronavirus infections, study shows*. New York: The New York Times. https://nyti.ms/32wXR6e

Carr, M. D., & Wiemers, E. E. (2016, September 7). *The decline in lifetime earnings mobility in the U.S.: Evidence from survey-linked data*. Washington, DC: Washington Center for Equitable Growth. https://equitablegrowth.org/woring-papers/the-decline-in-lifetime-earnings-mobility-in-the-u-s-evidence-from-survey-linked-administrative-data/

CDC. (2020, December 2). *Domestic travel during COVID-19*. Atlanta: Author. https://www.cdc.gov/coronavirus/2019-ncov/travelers/travel-during-covid19.html

Chang, S., Pierson, E., Koh, P. W., Gerardin, J., Redbird, B., Grusky, D., & Leskovec, J. (2020, 10 November). Mobility network models of COVID-19 explain inequities and inform reopening. *Nature* https://doi.org/10.1038/s41586-020-2923-3

Chetty, R., Hendren, N., Jones, M. R., & Porter, S. R. (2018). *Race and economic opportunity in the United States: An intergenerational perspective*. Harvard University. http://www.equality--of-opportunity.org/assets/documents/race_paper.pdf

Coalition for the Homeless. (2020). *Age-adjusted mortality rate for sheltered homeless new Yorkers*. : Coalition for the Homeless. https://www.coalitionforthehomeless.org/age-adjusted-mortality-rate-for-sheltered-homeless-new-yorkers/

Cohen-Louck, K., & Levy, I. (2021). Viruism: The need for a new term describing COVID-19 impact in context of viral victimization. *Psychological Trauma: Theory, Research, Practice, and Policy, 13*(1), 1–8. https://doi.org/10.1037/tra0000945

Davis, M. (2021, January 24). *US government financial bailouts*. New York: Investopedia. https://www.investopedia.com/articles/economics/08/government-financial-bailout.asp

Dietrich, W. L., Bennett, J. S., Jones, B. W., & Hosni, M. H. (2021). *Laboratory modeling of SARS-CoV-2 exposure reduction through physically distanced seating in aircraft cabins using bacteriophage aerosol—November 2020*. MMWR, 70. https://www.cdc.gov/mmwr/volumes/70/wr/pdfs/mm7016e1-H.pdf

Disney, A. (2021, June 17). *I was taught from a young age to protect my dynastic wealth*. New York: The Atlantic. https://www.theatlantic.com/ideas/archive/2021/06/abigail-disney-rich-protect-dynastic-wealth-propublica-tax/619212/

Dougherty, C. (2020, August 7). *Millions of evictions are a sharper threat as government support ends*. New York: New York times. https://nyti.ms/31sBugU

Duncan, I. (2020, October 31). *A woman died of coronavirus on a plane. Her passengers were never notified*. Washington DC: Washington Post. https://www.washingtonpost.com/local/trafficandcommuting/woman-diescoronavirus-plane/2020/10/31/2d824dc-1878-11eb-82db-60b15c874105_story.html

Dyer, P. (2021, June 15). *Policy and institutional responses to COVID-19: South Korea*. Washington, DC: Brookings Institute. https://www.brookings.edu/research/policy-and-institutional-responses-to-covid-19-south-korea/

Edison Research. (2018). *The gig economy*. Author. https://www.edisonresearch.com/americans-and-the-gig-economy/

Elgar, F. J., Stefaniak, A., & Wohl, M. J. A. (2020). The trouble with trust: Time-series analysis of social capital, income inequality, and COVID-19 deaths in 84 questions. *Social Science & Medicine, 263*, 113365. https://doi.org/10.1016/j.socscimed.2020.113365

Federal Aviation Administration. (2021, August 30). *Unruly passengers*. Washington, DC: Author. https://www.faa.gov/data_research/passengers_cargo/unruly_passengers/

Feeding America. (2020, April 22). *The impact of the coronavirus on food insecurity*. Washington, DC: Author. https://www.feedingamerica.org/research/coronavirus-hunger-research#:~:text=The%20Impact%20of%20the%20Coronavirus%20on%20Food%20INSECURITY%20IN%202020&text=Combining%20analyses%20at%20the%20nationalmillion%2C%20including%2017%20million%20children

Fisher, K. A., Olson, S. M., Tenforde, M. W., Feldstein, L. R., Lindsell, C. J., Shapiro, N. I., Files, D. C., Gibbs, K. W., Erickson, H. L., Prekker, M. E., Steingrub, J. S., Exline, M. C., Henning, D. J., Wilson, J. G., Brown, S. M., Peltran, I. D., Rice, T. W., Hager, D. N., & Ginde, A. A. (2020). CDC COVID-19 Response Team. Telework before illness onset among symptomatic adults aged ≥ 18 years with or without COVID-19 in 11 outpatient health care facilities— United States, July 2020. *MMWR, 69*(44), 1648–1653. https://doi.org/10.15585/mmwr.mm6944a4

Fitzpatrick, S. (2020, March 28). *Why the strategic National Stockpile isn't meant to solve a crisis like coronavirus: The country's largest repository of drugs and medical equipment is designed to be used as a stopgap—Not a solution—During emergencies*. New York: NBC News. https://www.nbcnews.com/health/health-care/why-strategic-national-stockpile-isn-t-meant-solve-crisis-coronavirus-n1170376

Foley, R. J. (2020a, May 5). *Nearly 1,400 Tyson workers at 3 Iowa plants get coronavirus*. New York: Associated Press. https://apnews.com/article/c8286cc4dd670e88850ad33e977866a4
Foley, R. J. (2020b, December 28). *Fired Tyson boss says COVID office pool was a 'morale boost.'* New York: Associated Press. https://apnews.com/article/iowa-waterloo-lawsuits-iowa-city-coronavirus-pandemic15fe07ecd7799f91f6d9dd5b6972c38d#:~:text=IOWA%20CITY%2C%20Iowa%20(AP),and%20intended%20to%20boost%20morale
Frazer, J. (2019, February 15). *How the gig economy is reshaping careers for the next generation*. Jersey City, NJ: Forbes. https://www.forbes.com/sites/johnfrazer1/2019/02/15/how-the-gig-economy-is-reshaping-careers-for-the-next-generation/
Goldhill, O. (2021, May 26). *Shuttered hospitals, soaring Covid-19 deaths: Rural black communities lose a lifeline in the century's worst health crisis*. Boston: STAT News. https://www.statnews.com/2021/05/26/shuttered-hospitals-soaring-covid19-deaths-rural-black-communities-lose-lifeline-in-pandemic/
Gravelle, J. G., & Marples, D. J. (2019, May 22). *The economic effects of the 2017 tax revisions: Preliminary conclusions*. Congressional Research Services.
Grover, S., Dua, D., Sahoo, S., Mehra, A., & Nehra, R. (2020). Why all COVID-19hospitials should have mental health professionals: The importance of mental health in a worldwide crisis. *Asian Journal of Psychiatry, 51*, 102147. https://doi.org/10.1016/j.ajp.2020.102147
Gutierrez, J. P., & Bertozzi, S. M. (2020). Non-communicable diseases and inequities increase risk of death among COVID-19 patients in Mexico. *PLoS One, 15*(10), e0240394. https://doi.org/10.1371/journl.pone.0240394
Hardy, B. L., & Logan, T. D. (2020, August 13). *Racial economic inequality amid the COVID-19 crisis*. Washington, DC: Brookings Institute, the Hamilton Project. https://www.hamiltonproject.org/papers/racial_economic_inequality_amid_the_covid_19_crisis
Hartmans, A. (2020, December 7). *Roughly 17% of US restaurants have permanently shut down since the start of the pandemic as industry leaders warn of an 'unprecedented economic decline.'* New York: Business Insider. https://www.businessinsider.com/thousands-us-restaurants-closed-coronavirus-pandemic-2020-12
Hope, D., & Limberg, J. (2020). *The economic consequences of major tax cuts for the rich. International inequalities institute, working paper 55*. The London School of Economics and Political science. https://eprints.lse.ac.uk/107919/1/Hope_economic_consequences_of_major_tax_cuts_published.pdf
Hope, D., & Limberg, J. (2020, December 29). *Trump and republicans prefer covid tax cuts to hikes. Our research proves they're wrong*. New York: NBC News. https://www.nbcnews.com/think/opinion/trump-republicans-prefer-covid-tax-cuts-hikes-our-research-proves-ncna1252242
Horowitz, J. (2021, March 11). *The world went on a debt binge last year. There could be a nasty hangover*. New York: CNN. https://www.cnn.com/2021/03/11/investing/government-debt-bond-yields-interest-rates/index.html
Horowitz, J. M., Igielnik, R., & Kochhar, R. (2020, January 9). *Trends in come and wealth inequality*. Washington, DC: Pew Research Center. https://www.pewsocialtrends.org/2020/01/09/trends-in-income-and-wealth-inequality/
Hughes, M. M., Groenewold, M. R., Lessem, S. E., Xu, K., Ussery, E. N., Wiegan, R. E., Qin, X., Do, T., Thomas, D., Tsai, S., Davidson, A., Latash, J., Eckel, S., Collins, J., Ojo, M., McHugh, L., Li, W., Chen, J., Chan, J., & Stickey, M. J. (2020). Update: Characteristics of health care personnel with COVID-19—United States, February 12-July 16, 2020. *MMWR, 69*(38), 1364–1368. https://doi.org/10.15585/mmwr.mm6938a3
International Chamber of Shipping. (2021, September 29). *Joint open letter-transport heads call on world leaders to secure global supply chains*. London: Author. https://www.ics-shipping.org/press-release/joint-open-letter-transport-heads-call-on-world-leaders-to-secure-global-supply-chains/
ISSC, Institute of Development Studies, & United Nations Educational, Scientific and Cultural Organization. (2016). *World social science report*. Author. https://en.unesco.org/wssr2016

King, M. L., Jr. (1956, August 11). *The birth of a new age*. Buffalo, NY: Alpha Phi Alpha. https://kinginstitute.stanford.edu/king-papers/documents/birth-new-age-address-delivered-11-august-1956-fiftieth-anniversary-alpha-phi

Kluger, R. (2007). *Seizing destiny: The relentless expansion of American territory*. Viking Press.

Kuehner-Hebert, K. (2018, February 20). *American Airlines will never lose money again, says CEO Doug Parker*. https://chiefexecutive.net/american-airlines-will-never-lose-money-says-ceo-doug-parker/

La Monica, P. R. (2021, April 15). *Jamie Dimon says 'American dream is fraying.'* New York: CNN. https://www.cnn.com/2021/04/15/investing/jamie-dimon-david-axelrod/index.html

Laris, M. (2021, January 1). Sneezed on, cussed at, *Ignored: Airline workers battle mask resistance with scant government backup*. Washington, DC: Washington Post. https://www.washingtonpost.com/local/trafficandcommuting/coronavirus-mask-airplanes/2020/12/3109c12d52-4565-11eb-975c-d17b8815a66d_story.html

Lavietes, M., & McCoy, M. (2020, October 19). *Waiting for work: Pandemic leaves U.S. gig workers clamoring for jobs*. London: Reuters. https://www.reuters.com/article/us-biggerpicture-health-coronavirus-gigw-idUSKBN2741DM

Lehren, A. W., & Siegel, E. R. (January 16, 2021). *Derelict, dangerous and debarred: Millions in PPP funds given to banned companies*. New York: NBC News. https://www.nbcnews.com/business/business-news/ppp-funds-given-debarred-companies-n1254437

Leonhardt, D. (2021, April 8). *Good morning. What's the reason taxes on the very wealthy have declined? The fall in corporate taxes*. New York: New York Times The Morning. https://messaging-custom-newsletters.nytimes.com/template/oakv2?campaign_id=9&emc=edit_nn_20210408&instance_id=28991&nl=themorning&productCode=NN&regi_id=100564608&segment_id=55179&te=1&uri=nyt%3A%2F%2Fnewsletter%2Fb34f53b6-3d74-5beb-ad39-62b17b4e86b5&user_id=13a05c9d7e7662b4a38a1af96eeabb61

Levin, B. (2020, February 11). *Trump claims coronavirus will "miraculously" go away by April*. New York: Vanity Fair. https://www.vanityfair.com/news/2020/02/donald-trump-coronavirus-warm-weather

Lin, K., Yang, B. X., Luo, D., Liu, Q., Ma, S., Huang, R., Lu, W., Majeed, A., Lee, Y., Lui, L. M. W., Mansur R. B., Nasri, F., Subramaniapillai, M., Rosenblat, J. D., Liu, Z., & McIntyre, R. S. (2020). 74 The mental health effects of COVID-19 on health care providers in China. *Psychiatry Online*. https://doi.org/10.1176/appi.ajp.2020.20040374

Lozano, A. V. (2021, March 13). *'They left us out to dry': Wildland firefighter says he was 'blacklisted' for speaking against lack of Covid safety*. New York: NBC News. https://www.nbcnews.com/news/us-news/they-left-us-out-to-dry-wildland-firefighter-says-he-was-n-n1260302

Mason, D. J. (2017). Rethinking rural hospitals. *JAMA, 318*(2), 114–115. https://doi.org/10.1001/jama.2017.7535

McFarling, U. L. (2021, March 11). *The uncounted: People who are homeless are invisible victims of Covid-19*. Boston: STAT News. https://www.statnews.com/2021/03/11/the-uncounted-people-who-are-homeless-are-invisible-victims-of-covid-19/

McNicholas, C., & Poudock, M. (2020, May 19). *Who are essential workers? A comprehensive look at their wages, demographics, and unionization rates*. Washington, DC: Economic Policy Institute. https://www.epi.org/who-are-essential-workers-a-comprehensive-look-at-their-wages-demographics-and-unionization-rates/

Miu, A. S., & Moore, J. R. (2021). Behind the masks: Experiences of mental health practitioners of color during the COVID-19 pandemic. *Academic Psychiatry*. https://doi.org/10.1007/s40596-021-01427-w

Mohamed, T. (2020, November 12). *Pfizer's CEO cashed out $5.6 million of stock after trumpeting its COVID-19 vaccine. That's 30% of his total compensation last year*. New York: Business Insider. https://markets.businessinsider.com/news/stocks/pfizer-ceo-sold-stock-6-million-30-percent-compensation-vaccine-2020-11-1029798146

Morgenson, G., Nguyen, V., Ferguson, C., & Enright, M. (2020, December 12). *Already struggling, the nation's rural hospitals face another challenge: For-profit own-*

ers. New York: NBC News. https://www.nbcnews.com/health/health-care/already-struggling-nation-s-rural-hospitals-face-another-challenge-profit-n1250912

Morrison, J. S. (2018, June 28). *Health security downgraded at the white house*. Washington, DC: Center for Strategic and International Studies. https://www.csis.org/analysis/health-security-downgraded-white-house

Muntean, P., Gumbrecht, J., & Wallace, G. (2020, September 23). *Thousands of passengers on commercial flights may have been exposed to coronavirus in 2020, CDC says*. New York: CNN. https://www.cnn.com/world/live-news/coronavirus-pandemic-09-23-20-int/h_7cd28b4c3d78cab443440db75afc2c2d

Nagarajan, S. (2020, November 23). *Moderna's CEO sold nearly $2 million of his stock ahead of the company's emergency use vaccine filing. He's now worth $3 billion*. New York: Business Insider. https://markets.businessinsider.com/news/stocks/moderna-ceo-sold-million-stock-company-emergency-use-vaccine-filing-2020-11-1029830266

Nguyen, L. H., Drew, D. A., Graham, M. S., Joshi, A. D., Guo, C.-G., Ma, W., Mehta, R. S., Warner, E. T., Sikavi, D. R., Lo, C.-H., Kwon, S., Song, M., Mucci, L. A., Stamfer, M. J., Willett, W. C., Eliassen, A. H., Hart, J. E., Chavarro, J. E., Rich-Edwards, J. W., & Chan, A. T. (2020). Risk of COVID-19 among front-line health-care workers and the general community: A prospective cohort study. *The Lancet Public Health, 5*, e475–e483. https://doi.org/10.1016/S2468-2667(20)30164-X

Oosterhoff, B., & Palmer, C. A. (2020). Attitudes and psychological factors associated with news monitoring, social distancing, disinfecting, and hoarding behaviors among US adolescents during the coronavirus disease 2019 pandemic. *JAMA Pediatrics, 174*(12), 1184–1190. https://doi.org/10.1001/jamapediatrics.2020.1876

Petriglieri, G., Ashford, S. J., & Wrzesniewski, A. (2018, March-April). Thriving in the gig economy. *Harvard Business Review.*. https://hbr.org/2018/03/thriving-in-the-gig-economy

Pfeiffer, S. (2020, November 30). *IRS says its own error sent $1,200 stimulus checks to non-Americans oversees*. Washington, DC: National Public Radio. https://www.npr.org/2020/11/30/938902523/irs-says-its-own-error-sent-1-200-stimulus-checks-to-non-americans-overseas

Pfizer. (2020a, November 9). *Pfizer and Biontech announce vaccine candidate against COVID-19 achieved success in first interim analysis from phase 3 study*. New York: Author. https://www.pfizer.com/news/press-release/press-release-detail/pfizer-and-biontech-announce-vaccine-candidate-against

Pfizer. (2020b, November 20). *Pfizer and Biontech to submit emergency use authorization request today to the U.S. FDA for COVID-19 vaccine*. New York: Author. https://www.pfizer.com/news/press-release/press-release-detail/pfizer-and-biontech-submit-emergency-use-authorization

Popken, B., & Lehren, A. W. (2020, December 1). *Release of PPP loan recipients' data reveals troubling patterns*. New York: NBC News. https://www.nbcnews.com/business/business-news/release-ppp-loan-recipients-data-reveals-troubling-patterns-n1249629

Ranney, M. L., Griffeth, V., & Jha, A. K. (2020). Critical supply shortages-the need for ventilators and personal protective equipment during the Covid-19 pandemic. *New England Journal of Medicine, 382*(18), e41. https://doi.org/10.1056/NEJMp2006141

Reinicke, C. (2020, November 15). *The pandemic has made the racial retirement gap worse. Here's how individuals can close it*. New York: NBC News. https://www.nbcnews.com/news/nbcblk/pandemic-has-made-racial-retirement-gap-worse-here-s-how-n1247771

Renner, R. (2020, December 30). *COVID-19 is taking heavy toll in America's mental health-care deserts*. Washington, DC: National Geographic. https://www.nationalgeographic.com/science/2020/12/coronavirus-is-taking-heavy-toll-america-mental-health-care-deserts/

Reuters. (2021, March 28). *Mexico says COVID-19 deaths likely 60% higher than confirmed toll*. London: Reuters. https://www.reuters.com/article/us-health-coronavirus-mexico-toll-idUSKBN2BK0EY

Riechmann, D. (2020, March 14). *Trump disbanded NSC pandemic unit that experts had praised.* New York: Associated Press. https://apnews.com/article/donald-trump-ap-top-news-virus-outbreak-barack-obama-public-health-ce014d94b64e98b7203b873e56f80e9a

Rugaber, C. (2020, September 21). *Soaring wealth during pandemic highlights rising inequality.* New York: Associated Press. https://apnews.com/article/virus-outbreak-stock-prices-financial-markets-stock-markets-archive-28a44dd1a025d9b9af5a8d4ff8c5a033

Rugaber, C. (2021, February 12). *Sign of inequality: US salaries recover even as jobs haven't.* New York: Associated Press. https://apnews.com/article/inequality-us-salaries-recover-jobs-02ce81649c9e6518d6bd2c6c96f5ead8

Ruiz-Goiriena, R., & Bajak, A. (2021, February 11). *How much rent relief will I get? You're more likely to get help if you're white and live in rural America.* Tysons Corner, VA: USA Today. https://www.usatoday.com/story/news/nation/2021/02/10/covid-rent-relief-emergency-rental-assistance-not-big-states/4413471001

Sampson, H. (2020, December 22,). *Man who died following medical emergency on united flight had coronavirus, coroner says.* Washington, DC: Washington Post. https://www.washingtonpost.com/travel/2020/12/22/united-flight-death-covid/

Schondelmeyer, S. W., Seifert, J., Margraf, D. J., Mueller, M., Williamson, I., Dickson, C., Dasararaju, D., Caschetta, C., Senne, N., & Osterholm, M. T. (2020, October 21). *COVID-19: The CIDRAP viewpoint. Part 6: Ensuring a resilient US prescription drug supply.* Minneapolis: University of Minnesota. https://www.cidrap.umn.edu/covid-19/covid-19-cidrap-viewpoint

Shalvey, K. (2021, January 3). *Struggling minority-owned businesses were kept waiting until the last minute for PPP loans.* New York: Business Insider. https://www.businessinsider.com/minority-owned-businesses-kept-waiting-for-months-ppp-loans-2021-1

Shaw, A. M., Timpano, K. R., Steketee, G., Tolin, D. F., & Frost, R. O. (2015). Hoarding and emotional reactivity: The link between negative emotional reactions and hoarding symptomatology. *Journal of Psychiatric Research, 63*, 84–90. https://doi.org/10.1016/jpsychires.2015.02.009

Sherman, E. (2020, April 24). *Many public companies that got PPP loans had lots in the bank.* Jersey City, NJ: Forbes. https://www.forbes.com/sites/eriksherman/2020/04/24/public-companies-ppp-loans-money/

Sherman, N. (2020, October 15). *Coronavirus: US poverty rises as aid winds down.* London: BBC. https://www.bbc.com/news/business-54559008

Sherman, N. (2020, October 16). *US election 2020: The young people struggling in the 2020 economy.* London: BBC. https://www.bbc.com/news/election-us-2020-54471388

Silva, D. (2020, December 6). *With winter approaching, homeless shelters face big challenges against coronavirus.* New York: NBC News. https://www.nbcnews.com//news/us-news/winter-approaching-homeless-shelters-face-big-challenges-against-coronavirus-n1249906

Smeeding, T. M. (2016). Multiple barriers to economic opportunity for the "truly" disadvantaged and vulnerable. *RSF, 2*(2), 98–122. https://doi.org/10.7758/RSF.2016.2.2.04

Song, X., Massey, C. G., Rolf, K. A., Ferrie, J. P., Rothbaum, J. L., & Xie, Y. (2020). Long-term decline in intergenerational mobility in the United States since the 1850s. *PNAS, 117*(1), 251–258. https://doi.org/10.1073/pnas.1905094116

Spoorthy, M. S., Pratapa, S. K., & Mahant, S. (2020). Mental health problems faced by healthcare workers due to the COVID-19 pandemic—A review. *Asian Journal of Psychiatry, 51*, 102119. https://doi.org/10.1016/j.ajp.2020.102119

Spratling, C. (2021). America's hunger crisis. *National Geographic, 240*(2), 86–109.

Stats NZ. (2020). *Māori population estimates ay 30 June, 2020.* https://www.stats.govt.nz/information-releases/maori-population-estimates-at-30-june-2020

Stout Risius Ross, LLC. (2020). *Estimation of households experiencing rental shortfall and potentially facing eviction.* Author. https://app.powerbi.com/view?r=eyJrIjoiNzRhYjg2NzAtMGE1MC00NmNjLTllOTMtYjM2NjFmOTA4ZjMyIiwidCI6Ijc5MGJmNjk2LTE 3NDYtNGE4OS1hZjI0LTc4ZGE5Y2RhZGE2MSIsImMiOjN9

Stracqualursi, V., & Holmes, K. (2021, July 27). *New evidence shows trump appointees' political interference with CDC weekly Covid data reports, house subcommittee says*. New York: CNN. https://www.cnn.com/2021/07/27/politics/house-covid-committee-trump-administration-cdc-data-reports/index.html

Subramaniam, T., Lybrand, H., Hickey, C., & Fleischer, V. (2020, April 5). *A timeline of trump promises and predictions on coronavirus—And how they stack up to the facts*. New York: CNN. https://www.cnn.com/2020/04/05/politics/timeline-trump-promises-coronavirus/index.html

Sullivan, L. & Jingnan, H. (2021, May 18). *Hospitals serving the poor struggled during COVID. Wealthy hospitals made millions*. Washington, DC: National Public Radio. https://www.npr.org/2021/05/18/996207511/hospitals-serving-the-poor-struggled-during-covid-wealthy-hospitals-made-million

Tensley, B. (2020, April 6). *How coronavirus is deepening American inequality*. New York: CNN. https://www.cnn.com/2020/04/06/politics/coronavirus-equalizer-myth-race-income/index.html

Tribble, S. J. (2020, October 17). *Rural hospitals struggling financially because of COVID-19*. Washington, DC: National Public Radio. https://www.npr.org/2020/10/17/924868600/rural-hospitals-struggling-financially-because-of-covid-19

Trougakos, J. P., Chawla, N., & McCarthy, J. M. (2020). Working in a pandemic: Exploring the impact of COVID-19 health anxiety on work, family, and health outcomes. *Journal of Applied Psychology, 105*(11), 1234–1245. https://doi.org/10.1037/apl0000739

United Nations. (2020). *World social report 2020: Inequality in a rapidly changing* world. https://www.un.org/development/desa/dspd/world-social-report/2020-2.html

US Chamber of Commerce. (2020, August 30). *Coronavirus pandemic hits minority-owned small businesses disproportionally hard, new poll shows*. Washington, DC: Author. https://www.uschamber.com/press-release/coronavirus-pandemic-hits-minority-owned-small-businesses-disproportionately-hard-new

Vera, A., & Toropin, K. (2020, December 12). *Tensions over eviction of black-indigenous family in Portland reach boiling point as protesters clash with police*. New York: CNN. https://www.cnn.com/2020/12/12/us/red-house-portland-oregon-protests/index.html

Weill, J. A., Stigler, M., Deschenes, O., & Springborn, M. R. (2020). Social distancing responses to COVID-19 emergency declarations strongly differentiated by income. *PNAS, 117*(33), 19658–19660. https://doi.org/10.1073/pnas.2009412117

Witteveen, D., & Velthorst, E. (2020). Economic hardship and mental health complaints during COVID-19. *PNAS, 117*(44), 27277–27284. https://doi.org/10.1037/pnas.2009609117

Wolfe, D., & Dale, D. (2020, October 28). *'It's going to disappear': A timeline of Trump's claims that Covid-19 will vanish*. New York: CNN. https://www.cnn.com/interactive/2020/10/politics/covid-disappearing-trump-comment-tracker/index.html

Woodward, B. (2020). *Rage*. Simon & Schuster.

Woodward, C. (March 13, 2021). *Warp-speed spending and other surreal stats of COVID times*. : Associated Press. https://apnews.com/article/ca4d27105a7a897a737421eda8464c78

World Bank. (2020). *Reversal of fortune*. Washington, DC: Author. https://openknowledge.worldbank.org/bitstream/handle/10986/34496/9781464816024.pdf

Wu, C.-H., Wang, Y., Parker, S. K., & Griffin, M. A. (2020). Effects of chronic job insecurity on big five personality change. *Journal of Applied Psychology, 105*(11), 1308–1326. https://doi.org/10.1037/apl0000488

Yeyati, E. L., & Filippini, F. (2021, June 8). *Social and economic impact of COVID-19*. Washington, DC:Brookings.https://www.brookings.edu/research/social-and-economic-impact-of-covid-19/

Ziady, H. (2020, October 7). *Billionaires have never been richer despite the pandemic*. New York: CNN. https://www.cnn.com/2020/10/07/business/billionaires-ubs-report/index.html

Zidar, O. (2019). Tax cuts for whom? Heterogeneous effects of income tax changes on growth and employment. *Journal of Political Economy, 127*(3), 1437–1471.

Chapter 4
Colonial -Isms and COVID-19

Abstract Colonial societies have granted privileges and social benefits to a select few. Colonial hierarchical tenets elevated the importance of assigned, artificially constructed group membership in order to determine who was entitled to those entitlements. Outgroup membership has been defined by biased and stereotyped classifications referred to as "-isms" in this book (e.g., ableism, ageism, heterosexism, racism, sexism). People assigned to inferior -ism groups have been treated as second class citizens or worse during the history of these colonial nations. Furthermore, colonial ingroups have effectively used strategies to generate animosity between outgroups in those societies, such as colonial splitting, to further disempower those groups and protect personal privilege. As a result of the -ism classifications, minoritized groups entered the COVID-19 pandemic highly vulnerable and with significant disadvantage. Bias and discrimination targeting minoritized people hampered pandemic response and treatment in those communities. Colonial leaders found value and political gain in blaming minoritized groups and using colonial splitting across the spectra of -isms to their strategic advantage. Colonial hierarchies have resulted in significant damage to the psychological well-being of those nations, leaving all citizens vulnerable to the pandemics of the future.

A hallmark feature of colonialism is pitting disempowered groups against one another in order to weaken them financially, politically, physically, and emotionally. In a previous book, I refer to the intentional process of colonial forces pitting minoritized groups against one another as *colonial splitting* (Blume, 2020). Splitting is a psychological term describing behaviors that drive wedges between people, fostering an adversarial relationship amongst those to whom the splitting behavior has been directed. Splitting is inevitably manipulative and meant to empower the perpetrator at the expense of the victims of the splitting activities.

Colonial splitting flows from hierarchical beliefs that insist on defining people as superior-inferior. Power imbalances are such that ingroups have significant power to control and oppress outgroups financially and politically. However, privileged groups have surprisingly vulnerable positions in society due to the instability that colonial injustices have created, contributing to a perceived need to use

A. W. Blume, *Colonialism and the COVID-19 Pandemic*, International and Cultural Psychology, https://doi.org/10.1007/978-3-030-92825-4_4

manipulation to control outgroups. One inherent fear is that if outgroups wielded their collective group strengths together in society, they would represent a threat to the privilege of ingroups (Sidanius et al., 2017). Colonial splitting is used to keep minoritized groups disunited and disempowered. As a result, colonial societies are prone to civil unrest due to divisiveness. Collective distrust partly due to colonial splitting resulted in record sales of firearms in 2020 (Gibson, 2020).

-Isms and Colonial Splitting

Superior-inferior classifications have contributed to defining people by the perceived group membership. Those stereotyped categorizations are generated through the perceptual filters of explicit or implicit ethnic and racial biases (Greenwald & Banaji, 1995). One result of the stereotyping has been hierarchical classification of people by perceived group membership--referred to as *-isms* in this book. -Ism is a reference of a process of dehumanizing people who are members of groups not valued by the colonial worldview. -Isms refer to the common suffix used to define dehumanizing treatment of certain groups, such as the words of ageism, classism, racism, sexism, and other forms of biased and prejudicial treatment such as homophobia and bias toward religious minoritized groups. The consequences of -isms have been a variety of social inequities visited upon groups treated unjustly, such as economic inequities (Chap. 3), educational inequities (Chap. 5), and health inequities (Chap. 6). These dehumanizing -isms in colonial societies have created group pandemic vulnerabilities.

Deception is one aspect of colonial splitting (see also Chap. 1) used to manipulate the interpretations and behavioral responses of outgroups, leaving them significantly more vulnerable to the pandemic than they would have been otherwise. Deception capitalized on the pre-existing distrust between groups from centuries of colonial splitting. In 2020, the deceit was so widespread that former US president Barack Obama referred to it as "truth decay" (BBC, 2020a). In fact, "truth decay" has long been brazenly wielded by privileged colonial leaders with little concern about consequences to others, including during COVID-19.

Colonial splitting contributed to pre-pandemic relational psychopathology that hindered the mitigation and treatment of COVID-19. Although it may seem as if colonial splitting impacted only outgroups, SARS-CoV-2 thrived on colonial distrust and inequities. In the following sections, specific -isms will be discussed in the context of COVID-19, focusing on how mistreatment of outgroups has made all psychologically unwell and vulnerable.

Racism and COVID-19

On December 20, 2020, Dr. Susan Moore, a Black American physician, passed away from COVID-19, two weeks after she had shared publicly how a White physician had not taken her physical health complaints seriously (Watts & Hanna, 2021).

Dr. Moore's case represents a highly visible example of how implicit bias toward minoritized patients may hinder the quality of care of people from socially disempowered groups (FitzGerald & Hurst, 2017), even if they are fellow physicians, illustrating the depth of how systemic racism has created an inequitable health care. The story is a micro-example of a macro-problem: Treating certain groups in society as inferior, second-class citizens over the centuries has contributed to widespread racism infused into all the systems of society including health care (Blume, 2020). Later in the pandemic, the Editor of the Journal of the American Medical Association suggested that systemic racism did not exist in the medical profession (Tanner, 2021), demonstrating how ignorant many White health care professionals and researchers are of the inherent biases in health care and medicine. When making some medical decisions, physicians were reported to use a binary correction for race (Black vs. all other races), an algorithm widely reported during the pandemic (Smith & Spodak, 2021), not understanding the inherent problems with racialized approaches to medicine. Another examination found that hospitalized Blacks experienced significantly more adverse events than White patients in the same hospitals (Gangopadhyaya, 2021). Another study found that articles on racism were sparse in high impact medical journals and empirical studies related to racism and health extremely rare (Krieger et al., 2021), highlighting medical biases.

Spread of COVID-19 through Minoritized Communities Minoritized groups in the US were hospitalized and dying from COVID-19 at rates much higher than White Americans (American Public Media Research Lab Staff, 2021). The source of those differences are clearly the consequences of systemic racism that contributed to historically unequal treatment and social inequities infused into colonial cultures (Egede & Walker, 2020; Khazanchi et al., 2020; Salter et al., 2018). The impact of racism on the pandemic was obvious to Dr. Anthony Fauci who referred to those effects as "undeniable" (Associated Press, 2021b). The intersectional COVID-19 risks of age and race compounded negative consequences to older adult minoritized patients (Garcia et al., 2020). Colonial racism presented numerous barriers to addressing COVID-19 globally (Devakumar et al., 2020).

Racism in society also has placed minoritized group members at greater risk for COVID-19 due to unemployment and housing inequality. Systemic racism has made it more likely that minoritized workers are placed in harm's way on the job, perhaps even targeted with acts of bias (Miu & Moore, 2021). Racism has contributed to many minoritized people living in crowded communities or on isolated reservations with limited health care resources locally (Yearby & Mohapatra, 2020). As discussed in Chap. 1, colonial laws have perpetuated these racial inequalities over time (Echo-Hawk, 2013; Yearby & Mohapatra, 2020), contributing to significantly increased vulnerabilities to pandemics.

Colonial societies have created self-inflicted risks for social harm by decreasing social cohesiveness through acts of oppression and inequity. Strangely and shortsightedly, those with colonial privilege were so focused on the self-interests of the few they missed the essential life lesson that protecting the whole is necessary to protect the few. Systemic racism has created opportunity for pandemics like COVID-19, which capitalized on pre-existing inequities and colonial splitting and divisiveness that enhanced anger, distrust, fear, and hate. When populist-nationalistic political forces embraced colonial splitting tactics to deflect from responsibility and weaponize racism, widespread community spread and death were the results (Addo, 2020).

Racism and Civil Unrest During COVID-19 Systemic racism has contributed police killings of an unconscionable number of unarmed people of color in the US (Banks et al., 2006; Edwards et al., 2019), and that trend continued and perhaps worsened during the pandemic. In the US, the Black Lives Matter movement led to protests against police injustices, and the government responded harshly, including the highly visible use of force used to clear a pathway to a church for a presidential photo opportunity (Gjelten, 2020). In the nation of Colombia, a Black male was murdered allegedly for violating COVID-related protections, resulting in protests met by more violence from police (Grattan & Faiola, 2020). Although many of the global protests against racism and racist acts were attended by masked individuals, the sheer numbers of protestors in close proximity created greater health risks, especially to communities of color at higher risks of infection and severe consequences.

Xenophobia and COVID-19

One persistent act of racism during the pandemic was the xenophobic blaming of Asians and Asian Americans for causing and spreading COVID-19. The first expression of Asian xenophobia during the COVID-19 pandemic was assigning blame to China for the virus, which contributed to massive psychological stigma that was, ironically, warned about just prior to the COVID-19 pandemic (Taylor, 2019). Violence and discrimination against Chinese immigrants were common throughout US history, including lynchings and massacres and even exclusion from entering the country (Kao, 2021), so it was not a surprise that many acted hostilely toward Chinese Americans during COVID-19. Acts of discrimination and hate toward people who appeared to be Chinese followed the blaming, which meant in reality that anyone who was perceived to be Asian was targeted (Chen et al., 2020; Nguyen, 2021). Escalating violence was wielded toward Asian American individuals as a result of xenophobic hate (Kaur, 2021). The worst of the events occurred on March 16, 2021, when a White male murdered six Asian American women in the Atlanta, Georgia, metropolitan area, blaming sex addiction for the event but not accounting for probable racialized biases (Ramirez, 2021). By the summer of 2021, over 9000 incidents of anti-Asian intimidation or hate had occurred during the pandemic in the US (Tang, 2021). One study found that over 75% of a Chinese American sample had experienced anti-Chinese racism related to COVID-19 that was associated with psychological distress and mental health issues (Cheah et al., 2020). The Anti-Asian acts continued a historic pattern of blaming Asian Americans for epidemics and spreading diseases that has persisted since the first waves of immigration into the US (Chen et al., 2020; Noel, 2020).

Blaming immigrants for epidemics and pandemics has been a common practice in US history, and xenophobic polemics have been often weaponized as anti-immigration propaganda (Noel, 2020). Governor Greg Abbott of Texas blamed immigrants for spreading SARS-CoV-2 in his state, despite personally relaxing safety precautions in his state routinely against medical advice, and despite refusing federal aid to test those same immigrant applicants for COVID-19 to prevent spread (Alvarez, 2021). Xenophobic blaming of immigrants and refugees for COVID-19 and targeting them with discrimination and hate was not uniquely American and also occurred globally (UN Department of Global Communications, 2020).

Xenophobia is a fear-based response rooted in racist beliefs. Xenophobic beliefs are often leveraged in colonial splitting to dehumanize and disempower immigrant and refugees (Blume, 2020). As might be imagined, acts of xenophobia have contributed to significant distrust in perpetrators and victims. From the perspective of victims, being targeted by xenophobic bias contributes to and reinforces beliefs concerning distrust of social institutions such as health care. Being blamed falsely for a pandemic tends to push potential health care seekers underground, hindering the society's ability to adequately address the pandemic. Concerns about xenophobia in the US have contributed to a formal policy directive by the American Hospital Association (2020) on how to address the consequences of xenophobia on the pandemic response in hospital settings. Xenophobia was also observed in disseminated research of the COVID-19 pandemic, appropriately called out by fellow scientists who could see past the colonial lenses of scientific interpretation (Zeng et al., 2020)--a reminder of the insidious nature of racial bias in colonial societies and how scientists reared, educated, and trained in those societies cannot be truly objective (Blume, 2020).

Xenophobia and other forms of racial inequities have left immigrants and refugees vulnerable to COVID-19. Pre-pandemic economic and health inequities and being targeted for discrimination and hate have contributed to the increased risk to immigrants and refugees (World Health Organization[WHO], 2020). Refugee children may also be at risk due to crowded relocation settlements that promote spread of COVID-19 and other medical concerns and increased risk of suffering mental health consequences (Brickhill-Atkinson & Hauck, 2021). Close to 80 million people are known to be refugees globally. Significant virus spread has been found within many refugee camps, places with few mitigation resources available (US Global Leadership Coalition, 2020). Refugees have been treated as second class persons during the pandemic, often designated a lower priority population in hierarchical social systems that opt to address the needs of citizens first. Therefore, the primary responsibility for refugees has been left to the United Nations and various non-governmental organizations (NGOs).

The US populist government with white nationalistic sentiments engaged in zero tolerance policies toward immigrants during the early stages of the pandemic. Their policies included the separation of children from families and contributed to large numbers of detained and deported persons (Congressional Research Service, 2018).

The result was an immigration policy with little consideration for children or the spread of COVID-19 among those being detained. People were held in crowded conditions in US Immigration and Customs Enforcement (ICE) facilities where social distancing was impossible and mitigation measures minimal. Deportation to origin nations via flights, or transfer of individuals to different facilities, aided virus spread. Sometimes measurable fever would halt such transports (Loweree et al., 2020), but transmission remained a risk since the virus capably spread in asymptomatic individuals. The Trump administration resurrected a nineteenth century colonial law developed from xenophobic stereotypes to prevent immigration due to concerns about diseases. The law was used to justify expulsion of asylum seekers. However, a US federal court eventually blocked the expulsion of unaccompanied minors (BBC, 2020c).

Despite efforts to rid the US of "undesirable" immigration by white nationalistic standards, immigrants are very important contributors to the US economy. Almost 400,000 workers supplying food to the US population during COVID-19 were undocumented, and when those essential workers became ill from exposure to unsafe conditions, the food supply chain was interrupted (Foley, 2020; Jawetz, 2020; see also Chap. 3). Furthermore, undocumented immigrant workers were estimated to account for over 400,000 health care workers such as administrators, aides, custodial staff, doctors, and nurses necessary to adequately address the health needs of the US, including the COVID-19 pandemic. The irony of the US relying heavily upon hundreds of thousands of undocumented workers to perform necessary services to survive the pandemic while simultaneously hunting and deporting them represents a stunning example of hierarchical colonial hypocrisy. As expected, the pursuit of undocumented residents by ICE had the effect of pushing people under the radar--more likely to delay seeking and less likely to pursue health care when ill, enhancing spread and increasing mortality risks (Page & Flores-Miller, 2021). Xenophobia threatened the health and well-being of many essential US workers during COVID-19, self-inflicting harm on the whole of society.

Xenophobia derailed the response to the pandemic by setting up false narratives based on fear and blame, and by misleading the public as to the appropriate methods for addressing the pandemic. People of Asian descent as well as immigrants and refugees have been particularly targeted globally during the COVID-19 pandemic. Xenophobia opened the door to dysfunctional colonial deception and splitting to defend the self-interests of the privileged and to allow colonial leaders to deflect responsibility for coronavirus spread and public policy failures. In Indigenous psychology, a more functional response would be to address both externalized fear and artificial hierarchies in colonial societies to prevent xenophobic responses that hinder efficient and equitable pandemic response, including with COVID-19 (Blume, 2020). Xenophobia remains an inherent risk to responding effectively to future pandemics.

Populism, Nationalism, Racism, and Xenophobia

Populism is a political view that feigns to embrace common citizens in a social order, whereas nationalism is a political perspective that focuses on the self-interests and supremacy of a particular culture and nation. In connecting the dots, one can visualize how nationalism has broad appeal among colonial societies given common beliefs in national self-interests and cultural supremacy. Often populism and nationalism go hand in hand. Although populism certainly can take on any political perspective to suggest its support for "common" people, it typically embraces nationalism as a method for connecting with the needs of ingroups (Elias et al., 2020). In colonial nations, populism often embraces colonial values and tenets as the vehicle for advancing nationalism (Blume, 2020). Typically, in colonial nations, the "common" person is conceptualized as the descendants of European colonists.

Supremacy as valued by nationalism also make it easy for nationalists in colonial nations to hold racist and xenophobic views of outgroups. Populism and nationalism are often appealing perspectives during national times of crisis, such as a pandemic. As an example, a recent staff report from the Federal Reserve Bank of New York linked the rise of Nazi Germany in part due to the economic and social consequences of the Spanish Flu (Blickle, 2020; Derby, 2020). President Recep Tayyip Erdoğan of Turkey allegedly used COVID-19 as an excuse to move his nation toward authoritarianism (Kirisci, 2020). Pandemic populism and nationalism thrive on the tactics of divisiveness by asserting an us versus them mentality and by the practice of blaming others for social problems. Colonial splitting is a commonly used strategy to enhance that divisiveness. In the US, the Spanish flu pandemic happened in the context of nationalism and populism, and that pattern has repeated during the COVID-19 pandemic. Divisiveness and blame were common in both pandemics. One result of populist-nationalism has been a focus on national self-interests in the face of a global pandemic, diminishing cooperation within and between societies (Lasco, 2020). Another result has been an increase in distrust of others in those societies, resulting in a significant uptick in overtly racist and xenophobic activities (Elias et al., 2020).

Populist-nationalism during COVID-19 has been defiant against the practices of social distancing and wearing of masks—a way to express personal liberties of the common person (Lasco, 2020; Perry et al., 2020; Vieten, 2020). One can sense the underlying anger and frustration within the populism, where common citizens sense the injustices of their social orders--hence the experience of anger, fear, and frustration--but incorrectly blame outgroups for those injustices due to centuries of colonial splitting. The "common" American may correctly sense that they have not shared in the American dream, yet incorrectly blame other victims (outgroups) for circumstances perpetrated by the privileged of society--they do not understand that the culprit is the colonial social order in which they reside (Blume, 2020).

White Nationalism and Supremacy White nationalism and white supremacy, as foundational tenets of colonization (see Chap. 1), remain firmly ensconced into colonial social orders. The original constitution of the US was a document of white nationalism and white supremacy. The American civil war was fought because of disputes over slavery, which existed because of white supremacy values--the confederacy aimed to become a white nationalist nation. White supremacy is common in other nations as well and its expression has been thinly veiled in the activities of populist governments around the globe during the pandemic.

The Trump administration manipulated white nationalism to its political advantage, utilizing racism as a weapon for colonial splitting in a way that distracted from appropriately addressing the pandemic. In addition, the Trump administration encouraged white supremacist activism, which ultimately resulted in an insurrection and a second impeachment of the former president (Naylor, 2021; see also Chap. 9). As a result, the US experienced profound increases in white supremacy messaging (Anti-defamation League, 2021). Even as one arm of the US government was embracing the tenets of white nationalism and white supremacy, the Department of Homeland Security identified white supremacists as the most pressing terrorism threat to the country (Swan, 2020), which proved to be both accurate and prophetic. White supremacists also use bullying to their political advantage and social media has been an excellent and potentially anonymous way to bully minoritized groups. The anonymity of the internet provides cover for racist attacks on others that I refer to as *colonial sniping*—zoom-bombing during the pandemic was an excellent example of the tactic.

Guns as Symbolic of Colonial Fear and Fragility During the COVID-19 pandemic, record gun sales to first time owners occurred, suggesting the heightened level of fear and insecurity in the American social order (Arnold, 2020). The day after I wrote the previous sentence, new records for gun sales were reported in January, 2021, and records continued to be set for succeeding months well into 2021 Alcorn, 2021; Associated Press, 2021a). The open-carry of weapons at protests events were much more prominent, including at state capitol buildings and other government structures, and some were violent. Many protests occurred under the guise of expression of civil liberties by populist-nationalists, accompanied by further expressions of liberties through defiance of social distancing and masking.

From an IAPP perspective, the prominence of guns in the US during the pandemic was a symbol of colonial fear and fragility. Hierarchical social injustices contributed to a level of distrust so acute that many people felt the need to arm themselves, some for the first time. In addition, due to those same hierarchies, there was a racialized theme to the open-carry of weapons that was hard to miss. Colonial splitting has contributed to a splintered social order where individual rights have been taken more seriously than social responsibility. Splintered social orders were on display in the significant unrest during the pandemic and contributed to the lack of a cohesive vision and plan for addressing the COVID-19 pandemic. Additionally, the splintering of society has been mirrored in the health care system (see also Chap. 6). The lack of social cohesiveness in the midst of an interdependent threat like a pandemic left the US and other colonial nations in vulnerable positions. A collectivistic approach would have been much more psychologically functional under the circumstances of the pandemic than individualistic responses. Racism and xenophobia naturally contribute to the fragility of colonial societies through their us versus me mentalities. Guns cannot address the vulnerabilities of the colonialism, and historically, guns have made colonial nations much more unstable.

Whitewashing Enhances Distrust Whitewashing history, the process of rewriting history to favor a White American bias, is also another tactic favored by white supremacists. Whitewashing history is a form of cultural erasure. Nationalistic influences attempted to whitewash history in the US during the pandemic. As an example, in the fall of 2020, then President Trump ordered that a group called The President's Advisory 1776 Commission (2021) be constituted to create a report to reverse trends toward equity, diversity, and inclusion by appealing to the constitutional intent of the founding fathers. Of course, the constitution was never an inclusive document with some people being defined as 3/5 human and others not being considered human at all; women and people with certain religious beliefs were also excluded. The founding fathers embraced slavery and inequality as a compromise for unity. They were not concerned with providing life, liberty, and the pursuit of happiness to outgroups.

The *1776 commission* finished their work in great haste before President Trump's term expired and produced a report that reflected the biased perspectives of 1776, an era of "enlightenment" when bloodletting would have been a preferred method to address health problems. One can ascertain the problem with tackling a pandemic with a 1776 mindset. White nationalist activities often want to turn back the clock to the glory days of colonialism, so it is no surprise that the activity was encouraged by a nationalistic government led by a president who in 2016 indicated he was very skilled at promoting divisiveness and provoking rage in others (Woodward & Costa, 2016). One of the first actions of the Biden administration was to rescind the commission and the report (Kelly, 2021). Despite its rescission, the harm was done, because it sent yet another signal that certain groups are not welcomed or safe in the boundaries of a colonial nation—further eroding trust in the government at a time when collective trust was needed. Pandemic whitewashing of history by populist-nationalistic governments was not unique to the US. A similar UK report suggested it had no systemic racism, an assertion widely panned by multicultural researchers and others, yet compounding distrust, divisiveness, and inequities in that colonial nation nevertheless (John, 2021).

The Insidious Nature of White Supremacy White supremacy insidiously permeates the social structures and institutions of colonial societies. An example is the US criminal justice system that psychological research has demonstrated over and over again is negatively influenced by implicit bias against people of color (Banks et al., 2006; Staats et al., 2017). Historically, law enforcement was known to stand aside during racialized lynching events and to unleash their own violence during peaceful protests for justice and civil and human rights (Embrick, 2015; National Archives, n.d.; Waldrep, 2008). White supremacists leveraging law enforcement positions to carry forward their racist goals has continued to be a problem (Federal Bureau of

Investigation, 2006). Periodically, the reality of white supremacy in policing reveals itself. One such example was documented on a police camera that captured two law enforcement officers using racial epithets and other means to denigrate Black Americans, including the suggestion that slavery had been helpful to slaves (Fieldstadt, 2021). How reasonable is it for mainstream America to assume that people of color can trust in a criminal justice system enforced by officers with attitudes such as these?

White supremacy is at the heart of xenophobic fear and disgust toward immigrants and refugees. Disease threat has been historically weaponized against immigration and immigrant, complete with campaigns to generate public disgust of foreign immigrants and refugees as carrier of foreign germs (Markel & Stern, 2002). Since white supremacy perspectives assumes minoritized people are inferior, it is easy to view minoritized people as disposable. The white supremacy movement supporting eugenics is an excellent example of this perspective.

COVID-19 as an Instrument of Eugenics

Eugenics has been a historic consequence of colonial hierarchies. Eugenics takes racial superiority to a new level by suggesting that racial purity is desirable for a superior White race. Eugenics has been behind some of the worst atrocities of modern times, such as genocides, forced sterilizations, and segregation (e.g., Miller, 2019; Torpy, 2000). Nazi Germany is often held up as an example of a eugenic society, but much of what they learned was from US eugenicists. In fact, Hitler and Nazi Germany used the US treatment of Indigenous people as a blueprint for how to deal with people they considered to be inferior and expendable (Miller, 2019). Some methods used to address COVID-19 mimicked eugenic methodology to the great concern of minoritized groups. It is likely no surprise at this point that eugenic-like methods were often proposed and carried out by populist-nationalistic governments (e.g., Malinverni & Brigagão, 2020), reflecting foundational colonial values discussed in Chap. 1.

Infection-Acquired Herd Immunity as Covert Eugenics Herd immunity occurs when enough members of a population have attained sufficient antibodies to hinder viral spread. In the pandemics of the past, such as the Spanish Flu and the plagues of Europe, the only way to achieve that level of immunity was for a large population to develop antibodies through their sickness—to achieve infection-acquired herd immunity--contributing to huge numbers of fatalities and years of sickness. Today, we have the ability to achieve vaccine-acquired herd immunity more rapidly with significantly fewer fatalities if people are willing to get vaccinated.

Populist-nationalistic governments in colonial nations could not reconcile themselves to the idea that controlling the pandemic might require economic sacrifices. As an example, UK Prime Minister Boris Johnson reportedly resisted lockdowns in the fall of 2020 due to the economic consequences of the spring lockdowns, suggesting he would rather risk significant deaths to keep the economy open (BBC, 2021). To impose economic sacrifices to maintain the health and well-being of people was a cognitively-dissonant strategy for people committed to a colonial materialism as the measure of success, well-being, and happiness. Colonial societies had a pre-pandemic history of sacrificing others for material benefit to colonists, so it would be natural to consider a similar approach to protect the economic well-being of the privileged few during a pandemic.

Sweden early in the pandemic opted to pursue infection-acquired herd immunity in the absence of a vaccine, committing to keeping their economy open. However, even with efforts to control the pandemic through social distancing, masks, and handwashing, Sweden suffered significantly higher health consequences than other comparable European nations early in the pandemic (Jung et al., 2020). It took a while for the consequences to have an impact on policy, but eventually the experiment with pursuing infection-acquired herd immunity was abandoned, deemed a failure by Sweden's King Carl XVI Gustav (BBC, 2020d). From an Indigenous perspective, Sweden did not respect the power of nature as expressed through the power of the virus. Disrespect of nature has not gone well for human beings, as discussed in Chap. 2. However, the Swedish experiment was envied by populist-nationalists as a method for keeping the economy open at all costs and therefore remained a compelling model for some governments to pursue (e.g., Aschwanden, 2020).

One of several colonial nations interested in keeping the economy open without any further lockdowns was the US. The administration of the former US President Trump made a policy decision early in the pandemic to actively pursue infection-acquired herd immunity that minimized the possibility of economic sacrifice for the privileged—a policy that was confirmed through the release of certain documents and emails. In one such email, a former Trump health consultant suggested that the administration wanted people to become ill in order to advance the country toward infection-acquired herd immunity (Diamond, 2020). Ex-president Trump hinted the same in his interviews with Bob Woodward (2020), when he openly discussed publicly minimizing pandemic risks despite his own awareness of risks to the public.

Pursuing infection-acquired herd immunity alone would have resulted in extreme mortality rates, and projections suggested it likely would not work anyway (Brett & Rohani, 2020; Brumfel, 2020) As an example, the Spanish Flu was estimated to have killed 50–100 million people at a time when no influenza vaccines existed (Barry, 2018). It was no surprise that the US led the world with fatalities for a significant portion of the pandemic. Other populist-nationalistic societies had high fatality rates as well, given their priorities and strategies (WHO, 2021; Yeung et al., 2020). Other populist-nationalist nations chose to use colonial deception tactics to hide the extent of COVID-19 deaths, such as Russia (Troianovski, 2021). Most of the deaths would have been among minoritized groups viewed as expendable in colonial cultures. The pursuit of infection-acquired herd immunity exploits the -isms of society. Implicit in those policies is the eugenic belief that inferior people may be sacrificed for the good of the superior.

The Great Barrington Declaration Several months after the beginning of the pandemic, a document called *The Great Barrington Declaration* was released (Kulldorff et al., 2020), which delineated a blueprint for fully reopening economies and suggested that healthy adults could lead the way in achieving infection-acquired herd immunity through exposure. The declaration suggested that older adults would be protected but specifics on those protections were seriously lacking, plus it was not clear if older adults would be compliant with mitigation methods, especially with regard to wearing masks (Daoust, 2020). One problem with the declaration's position was that approximately 40–45% of carriers of the virus were asymptomatic and would have no idea when they placed high risk individuals in harm's way (Oren & Topol, 2020). Immunological experts widely panned the suggestion for infection-acquired herd immunity as a dangerous and unethical (Alwan et al., 2020; Howard, 2020; Yeung et al., 2020).

Experts estimated that as many as two million Americans might die in such an effort before achieving infection-acquired herd immunity (Howard, 2020). Dr. Anthony Fauci suggested the idea was fraught with risk, especially in terms of the ability to protect the most vulnerable to COVID-19 in the population (Yahoo News, 2020). Many vulnerable groups were not even discussed in the declaration. Researchers are unclear how long it would take to establish infection-acquired herd immunity, with some estimates being 2–3 years under ideal conditions, and no one was clear how long the immunity would last. A modern interpretation of immunity would be one achieved through exposure to vaccinations rather than infections, offering a much safer strategy to immunize the population (Aschwanden, 2020; Fontanet & Cauchmez, 2020; Rasmussen, 2020).

Another glaring flaw was that the declaration did not address minoritized groups at all, suggesting a lack of concern by the signers. Perhaps the oversight was inadvertent, but even if so, it would reflect a lack of consideration for what are commonly known population risk factors related to COVID-19. It is difficult to fathom how such an oversight would occur among medical experts without fully considering the role of implicit biases of colonial societies.

Many health disparity researchers quickly picked up on the inequities inherent in the Barrington declaration. Professionals familiar with the history of eugenics in medicine and psychology were able to see the push for infection-acquired herd immunity as yet another expression of that history of discounting minoritized groups (Ertuğrul, 2020; Gump, 2020; Mosley, 2020; Pilgrim, 2008). The authors of the declaration considered hierarchical self-interests but overlooked social responsibility, as would be expected in approaching the pandemic from a colonial mindset. The town of Great Barrington, Massachusetts, was so incensed by the naming of the document that their Selectboard (governmental council) wrote the authors a letter disavowing the declaration, indicating in the letter that the low rate of infection in their community was a function of a "collective value system" that valued and protected all citizens (Business Wire, 2020).

An excellent example of the selfishness of policies aligned with infection-acquired herd immunity occurred in the state of South Dakota, which did not enforce the recommendations of health experts to social distance and use face coverings. On the other hand, the sovereign nation of Cheyenne River was taking every precaution, understanding from an Indigenous point of view the inherent risks from pandemics and retraumatization by the experiences of COVID-19. The reservation went as far as closing highway traffic from South Dakota through the reservation in an attempt to protect the people. In the end, the community spread that surrounded the reservation was too much to keep out, and many were infected and died despite their best efforts to prevent South Dakota's problem from becoming their own (Levin & Lebeau, 2021). In an interconnected and interdependent existence, all people were vulnerable to the social irresponsibility of some.

Vaccinations (discussed in Chap. 7) hold the brightest promise for reducing the risk of community spread and potentially tracking economies to fully recover. Of course, the best way to provide herd immunity against future pandemics would be to promote health equity to substantially reduce risks before the next novel virus arrives (Williams & Cooper, 2020).

COVID-19 and Incarceration

Those incarcerated in prisons and jails represented another vulnerable population to the pandemic. The global incarcerated population has been estimated to be around 12 million, with over two million inmates located in the US (Burki, 2020a; Macmadu et al., 2020). Most of the incarcerated in the US are from minoritized groups (Macmadu et al., 2020), revealing yet another source of risk facing people of color during the pandemic. As discussed earlier, biases inherent in the criminal justice systems of colonial nations contribute to minoritized disparities in jails and prisons (Banks et al., 2006; Staats et al., 2017). An inequitable criminal justice system has resulted in inequitable health risks from SARS-CoV-2. Inmates have been historically exploited in different ways, including forced labor. In El Paso, Texas, during a severe wave of COVID-19, inmates moved bodies due to a shortage of staff (BBC, 2020b).

Jails and prisons are hotbeds of COVID-19 spread due to overcrowding that prevents social distancing, the lack of PPE resources, medical comorbidity, limited medical care and the risk of staffing shortages, and difficulties with sanitizing the environment (Akiyama et al., 2020; Alsan & Yang, 2020; Burki, 2020a; Hawks et al., 2020; Macmadu et al., 2020; Williams et al., 2020). The typical strategies of testing, contact tracing, use of PPE, and social distancing have been strongly recommended as ways to address the pandemic challenges in jails and prisons (Williams et al., 2020). Unfortunately, many of these recommendations were not implemented because of the limits of facility space and available resources. Another idea was to release low risk inmates to reduce crowding and spread (Akiyama et al., 2020; Williams et al., 2020), but the policy risked that implicit biases would guide decision making about who received an early release.

Many citizens see the care of prisoners as a low priority in hierarchical societies. Therefore, resources to support a health response were not forthcoming. That could have been the end of the story in a colonial society except that jail and prison staff were also at risk to COVID-19 spread (Alsan & Yang, 2020; Jiménez et al., 2020). In addition, one examination of national pre-pandemic data found that that a 0.1% increase in incarceration rates in an individual county was associated with a 6.5% increase in that same county of deaths due to infectious diseases (Kajeepeta et al., 2021), a reminder of the broad and interdependent impact of viruses. In reality, risk to our most vulnerable, including those who are incarcerated, is risk to us all. Certainly spread from staff to family members and communities occurred. From an Indigenous perspective, it is irrational and potentially pathological to deprioritize the needs of the most vulnerable under the assumption they are less worthy.

Sexism and COVID-19

Sexism is another -ism commonly experienced in colonial nations. Sexism arises from an artificially constructed colonial hierarchy that has favored males. Sexist beliefs and values in colonialism have justified the persistence of gender inequities in those societies for centuries. Sexism has interfered with women's participation of science, preventing unique perspectives from being heard, including during the pandemic (Buckee et al., 2020). Women have been disproportionately placed in harm's way as health care workers and caregivers to the ill (Spagnola et al., 2020; Wenham et al., 2020). Women experienced increased mental health challenges during the pandemic due to vicarious workplace trauma, increased family violence, and pregnancy and post-partum stressors (Almeida et al., 2020; Burki, 2020b; Evans et al., 2020). Stress due to pandemic caretaking roles also impacted women (Fisher et al., 2020).

Gender based inequities worsened as a result of the pandemic. Women entered the COVID-19 pandemic with known income and wealth disparities that hindered economic safety nets (Burki, 2020b). Women workers suffered significantly greater job losses than men during the COVID-19 pandemic, with many withdrawing from the work force due to caretaking responsibilities (Gould et al., 2020; Gould & Wilson, 2020; Silva & Miranda, 2021). White women had an unemployment rate of 15.8% in April, 2020, compared to 3% in February, 2020; Black women had a higher unemployment rate than White women, with 16.9% in April, 2020, compared to 5.3% in February (Gould & Wilson, 2020). Although the economy recovered some during the summer, Latina/x women were found to have an unemployment rate of 15.3% whereas White women had an unemployment rate at 10.3% in June, 2020 (Gould et al., 2020). A disproportionate number of Black and Latina/x women are single-heads of households (Gould et al., 2020; Gould & Wilson, 2020), leaving them with increased income vulnerability and less of a family financial safety net. In addition, many were negotiating parenting during a time of school shutdowns and online instruction. A US study found evidence that pandemic stressors impacting

Latina/x were of serious concern, and that increased perceived levels of social and emotional support for parents provided protection from mental health challenges (Brown et al., 2020).

On the other hand, sexism has also contributed to health disparities and very poor health outcomes among males over time (APA Working Group on Health Disparities in Boys and Men, 2018). The stereotyped roles of masculinity and hypermasculinity are partly to blame, contributing to unhealthy habits and risk taking with harmful consequences, including during the pandemic (Gupta, 2020; Reny, 2020). Appealing to masculinity was an important and unhealthy aspect of the US government's response during the early days of the pandemic (Kurtzleben, 2020; see also Chap. 9). As a result, masculinity and hypermasculinity during the COVID-19 pandemic contributed to significantly more men dying than women (Burki, 2020b; Spagnola et al., 2020; Wenham et al., 2020).

Sexism has proved to be a significant barrier to addressing COVID-19. Sexism has contributed to persistent economic inequities that left women economically vulnerable to the consequences of the pandemic. Sexism also has contributed to masculine and hypermasculine attitudes linked to pre-pandemic health comorbidities associated with COVID-19 hospitalizations and deaths and reckless behaviors that have placed everyone at risk. Sexism must be retired as a colonial value to be well-prepared to address the pandemics of the future.

Ageism and Colonialism

Early in the pandemic, evidence suggested that older adults were at significantly increased risk for severe consequences and death from the COVID-19 disease. Although the cut point for increased risk due to age was difficult to specifically define, it was generally recognized that people at around age 60 were at elevated risk for significant consequences (Banerjee, 2020). The increased risks to older adults from COVID-19 exposed significant age-related biases in colonial societies that have impacted the pandemic response and contributed to additional risks for health and mental health consequences as a result.

Colonial societies have always placed a high value on the ability of people to "pull their own weights," reflecting the importance of individualism and autonomy to those cultures (Blume, 2020). A substantial part of this focus on productivity is due to the importance of materialism to colonial societies. From a colonial perspective, older adults may be perceived as burdens on society, and certainly the warehousing of older adults in nursing homes and long-term care facilities serves as evidence that this may be the case. The needs of older adults tend to be overlooked in favor of the needs of younger adults, contributing to neglectful policies and a significant underuse of elder capital in terms of wisdom and experience.

Many proponents of infection-acquired herd immunity were willing to pursue that course despite obvious risks to older adults. Those who signed on to the Great Barrington Declaration superficially discussed the protection of older adults in society (Kulldorff et al., 2020), but clearly the intent of the declaration was meant to benefit the younger adults of American society who likely would have no or few symptoms. Infection-acquired herd immunity is the consequence of an archaic colonial value that defines value by age. Social media was a virtually anonymous venue for sharing ageist remarks during the pandemic, when younger citizens would refer to older adults as burdensome, expendable, and in derogatory terms (Jimenez-Sotomayor et al., 2020; Meisner, 2020; Monahan et al., 2020). In fact, a significant number of American citizens responded callously when confronted by the extreme death tolls of older adults, resisting social distancing and masking. As an Indigenous psychologist, I am relatively certain that the defiance occurred because colonial cultures are infused with ageist beliefs. Society would be much healthier if generational humility were exercised, with older generations valuing the fresh perspectives and novel ideas of younger generations, and younger generations valuing wisdom from experience of older generations.

Researchers identified how generational divisions were harmful to a healthy pandemic response. Ageist divisiveness was not only fostered through social media, but also through patronizing governmental policies favoring younger adults, triage health care practices that favored younger adults--including a decision by Tennessee to limit use of monoclonal antibody therapy (see also Chap. 9) to only the unvaccinated in the state (who tended to be younger) when treatment were strained by the delta variant surge (Siemaszko, 2021), and the utter neglect of residents in long-term care facilities (Fraser et al., 2020)—all examples of intergenerational colonial splitting sanctioned by colonial social orders. The ageism demonstrated during the pandemic showed that devaluing a life is not only dependent on ethnicity and race, but also dependent on one's age (Fraser et al., 2020).

Early in the pandemic, it became clear that residents of long-term care facilities were at risk for deadly spread of the coronavirus, with most residents being older adults. Not only was widespread anxiety and fear common as a mental health consequence, but also consequences of feeling isolated due to facility shutdowns to counteract spread (Chee, 2020). There was general concern for the mental health of older adults finding it necessary to distance themselves from others. Increased symptoms of anxiety, depression, and sleep disruption were identified in studies of older adults during the pandemic, as well as significant reduction in physical activity (Sepúlveda-Loyola et al., 2020). However, with those age-specific risks being noted, there was also evidence from research that older adults may have shown more resilience to those mental health concerns than younger populations (Vahia et al., 2020). From an IAPP perspective, the findings of potential resilience may reflect the experience and wisdom of elders that is traditionally revered in Indigenous cultures.

Family caregivers of older adults also experienced these same mental health symptoms for the same reasons. In addition, family caretakers experienced the symptoms of isolation and stress in the context of fatigue and strained finances, as well as a shortage of professional caretaker availability due to pandemic demands (Kent et al., 2020; Park, 2020). Professional caretakers also were reporting anxiety and depression as a result of work-related and personal challenges associated with the COVID-19 pandemic (Sun et al., 2020). The mental health consequences of

COVID-19 on caregivers generated concern for neglect and abuse of older adults under their care (Makaroun et al., 2020), which compounded the impact of the pandemic on the health and mental health of this demographic group. Targeted psychological support for older adults and caregivers may be an effective intervention for future pandemics.

The losses during the COVID-19 pandemic cannot be overstated. From an IAPP perspective, the loss of the tremendous wealth of experiences and wisdom of elders who passed during this pandemic was devasting. In addition, the survivors will be challenged by the long-term consequences of COVID-19. Researchers project that the health and mental health consequences of COVID-19 will impact older adults globally for years to come (Dhama et al., 2020). The long-term consequences of COVID-19 will continue for all age groups as people age, contributing to complexities in addressing older adult health for the foreseeable future.

True to Indigenous cultural beliefs, the COVID-19 pandemic has been met by extra protective measures in Indigenous Americans to preserve the cultural treasures that community elders embody. One measure was the policy of special protections for Indigenous language speakers in those communities, as well as for the carriers of traditions. Family members felt a higher responsibility to the community to protect their parents and grandparents for that reasons (Chinn, 2021). Contrary to the infection-exposed herd immunity policies pursued by certain privileged members of colonial society, Indigenous people understood their elders would not be protected unless the community stepped up to place their safety first. Elders are not expendable in Indigenous cultures. It is too great a risk to the community and its culture to consider such an individualized and libertarian approach.

Children and Ageism During COVID-19 At the other end of the age spectrum, children were also treated unfairly during the pandemic with their needs being considered secondary to the needs of adults. Children were treated somewhat carelessly because their mortality rates were lower than other age groups. However, several thousand confirmed deaths directly related to COVID-19 had occurred prior to the delta surge in 2021, and children were indirectly at risk from the increased violence toward children and because of poverty and hunger associated with the pandemic (UNICEF, 2021). Children were tremendously impacted by COVID-19 in important developmental ways and emergent needs during the pandemic were often neglected. Globally, over one million children were projected to have been orphaned by the spring of 2021 (Hillis, Unwin, et al., 2021), and over 120,000 US children had lost at least one primary caregiver to COVID-19, with estimates of a 15% increase of children being orphaned during the pandemic (Hillis, Blankinsop, et al., 2021). Clearly, the global psychological needs of children due to loss have been extraordinarily compounded by the consequences of the COVID-19 pandemic.

Decisions impacting children often were made with economic considerations being prioritized above the well-being of children. Other decisions were made that that benefitted adults but overlooked children, such as the CDC decision to reverse its policy on masking in May, 2021, rewarding vaccinated adults with no masking requirements yet increasing risks to children as a result who were unvaccinated

(CDC, 2021). Children have also long been ignored in major policy decisions in the colonial nations just like older adults. In the US, many school systems could not access the resources needed to adjust instruction during a pandemic, a sign that the society needs to re-evaluate its values concerning children. Education and the pandemic are discussed in detail in Chap. 5.

Colonial Ableism and COVID-19

As discussed in the ageism section, colonial perspectives have long devalued those who are considered not to be able to "pull their own weight" in society, and certainly those biases help to explain the focus on ableism in those societies. It is no surprise, then, that people with disabilities were highly neglected during the pandemic, with evidence that at home medical resources diminished due to pandemic demands as well as a paucity of research on the impact of the pandemic on people with disabilities (Lebrasseur et al., 2020). The interruption of health care services risked significant impact on health and mental health during the pandemic, although evidence on specifics was sparse (Lebrasseur et al., 2020; Turk & McDermott, 2020). People with disabilities were at great risk during the COVID-19 pandemic due to medical comorbidities that increase risk of severe symptoms and death, and historically have faced the stressful challenges of bias and discrimination (Sabatello, Landes, et al., 2020). Protections for people with disabilities were also not discussed in the Great Barrington Declaration, as another example of the callous disregard for the vulnerable in colonial societies.

Special concerns were expressed about how children with disabilities would be impacted by responses to the pandemic. For example, children with special educational needs did not necessarily get their needs met when schools migrated to web-based teaching (Constantino & Sahin, 2020). School systems with resources did better in addressing special needs than schools systems lacking resources, likely worsening existing educational and mental health inequities as a result (see also Chap. 5).

The lack of adequate resources to address the overwhelming medical challenges of the pandemic discussed in Chap. 3 highlighted many biases related to ableism in colonial cultures. One example was how the process for obtaining a vaccine often involved use of web sites that were not accessible for people with vision impairments or those without access to technology, leaving such citizens at a distinct disadvantage for accessing life-saving vaccines (Weber & Recht, 2021). Decisions were made with regard to triage of services (e.g., who was placed on ventilators) that did not respect disability or age (Andrews et al., 2020)--decisions that not only placed people with disabilities at risk for neglected or withdrawn care, but also placed health care providers in the positions of violating their own senses of morality to their own psychological peril (see Chap. 6). If colonial institutions had thoughtfully considered vaccine and medical resource planning and rollout and citizens had thoughtfully followed health guidelines, those with special needs would not have been triaged.

Ableism was yet another example of how hierarchical colonial beliefs proved to be barriers to a fair and just response to COVID-19. Those hierarchies have biased against people with disabilities in ways that have hindered appropriate protections for this vulnerable population, biases that need to be retired to improve health care in the next pandemic (Sabatello, Landes, et al., 2020). From an IAPP perspective, improving future pandemic responses will rely on a significant transformation of how people are valued in colonial societies—a movement from what they do and what they have to who they are—sacred creatures of a sacred creation. Re-evaluating what constitutes a valuable contribution to social orders is warranted.

COVID-19 and the Experiences of the Sexually Minoritized

Many sexual minoritized individuals have comorbid health conditions that placed them at high risk for serious COVID-19 illness (Heslin & Hall, 2021). In addition, societal stigma tended to hinder help seeking during the pandemic in ways that compounded symptom severity (Banerjee & Nair, 2020; Ruprecht et al., 2020). Members of sexual minoritized groups have long been marginalized in colonial societies, contributing to inequitable health care access and treatment (Phillips et al., 2020). During the COVID-19 pandemic, homophobia was obvious in the acts of certain leaders of populist-nationalistic governments, such as the use of a homophobic slur to describe social distancing in Brazil by President Jair Bolsonaro (Farzan & Berger, 2020). Further marginalization of sexual minoritized individuals hindered public health responses to address COVID-19 and enhanced distrust in colonial social systems.

Sexual minoritized cultures were seriously impacted by policies toward social distancing, leaving many sexually minoritized people feeling isolated. In addition, systemic homophobia exacerbated existing economic and health care inequities, and disrupted protective social safety nets, contributed to increase psychosocial stress and health risks that likely will persist for many years (Banerjee & Nair, 2020). Intersectionality of sexual minoritized status with other -isms discussed in this chapter have multiplied both risks and consequences, leaving many people to feel alone with their struggles, unsupported by others in society (Bowleg, 2020).

-Isms and Distrust

The feeling of isolation and aloneness was a profound experience for minoritized people during the pandemic and reflected the harsh impacts of colonial -isms on trust and well-being in many societies. A long history of colonial splitting had left many nations with high levels of divisiveness that detracted from any sense of social cohesiveness in addressing the collective and interdependent circumstances of a global pandemic. Addressing structural -isms in colonial social orders will require assuming responsibility for injustice of the social responsibilities and social transformation. Truth and reconciliation processes may be helpful to address both social responsibility and social transformation (Sabatello, Scroggins, et al., 2020).

An Indigenous Interpretation: Pandemics and -Isms

The colonial worldview assumes that hierarchies are natural and desirable, resulting in classifying the world according to superior-inferior categorizations. These categorizations have resulted in the -ism thinking discussed in depth in this chapter, and -isms have been used to oppress and exploit people historically. The historical circumstances of colonial -isms have been nothing short of hostile and disrespectful to others (see Table 4.1). The consequences to outgroup members of colonial societies have been widespread intergenerational income and wealth inequities that have left entire minoritized communities vulnerable to the pandemic. Colonial splitting and deception are used to maintain social hierarchies, resulting in widespread divisiveness and distrust. Divisiveness and distrust prevented coordinated and collective responses that would have benefitted the whole. The result was risk of sickness and death due to inconsiderate behavior that one might appropriately refer to as antisocial.

An IAPP perspective holds egalitarian assumptions about relationships with others, human and non-human. Respectful treatment of others is a logical outcome from assuming that the natural order that sustains humans and non-humans alike is sacred. Psychologically speaking, healthy relationships with others are essential to psychological well-being. As discussed in Chap. 1, colonial hierarchy, supremacy, and xenophobia contribute to belligerence rather than peace. Divisiveness and deception are toxic to relationships and will inevitably result in sickness. The consequences of the COVID-19 were essentially a failure of right relationships with others—nature, other humans, and even with the SARS-CoV-2 virus.

Colonialism also assumes that entities are independent of one another, but scientific evidence does not support this view. The preponderance of evidence from the

Table 4.1 Colonial tools for fostering divisions

Tactics	Risks to Pandemic Responses
Artificial -ism hierarchies	Social inequities
Blaming	Misinformation
Colonial splitting	Distrust
Deception, whitewashing history	Conspiracies, disinformation, manipulation
Populism/nationalism	Superiority, white supremacy
Unaddressed inequities	Collective vulnerabilities
Xenophobia	Externalized anxiety, anger, and fear
Collective impact	Loss of social cohesion

life sciences supports the Indigenous views that the natural world is interdependent, so each entity is dependent on one another rather than independent. Interdependence is the source of great strength and resilience when relationships are healthily in balance and harmonious, or of great weakness and risk when imbalanced, disharmonious, and driven by individual needs and wants. The consequences of colonialism were the result of people errantly assuming independence from others. The COVID-19 pandemic was a global lesson of what happens when humans assume they are independent from an interdependent existence. One can assume independence and act upon on that assumption, but the act may not necessarily be socially responsible in the context of an interdependent reality.

Many Indigenous communities feel a special responsibility to the most vulnerable in those communities. It was often the responsibility of Indigenous warriors to not only protect the peace but also to protect and provide for the vulnerable (Aiello et al., 2021). The health of the community would be measured by the health and well-being of its most vulnerable member. Shame would be over the community if some were needlessly neglected. If colonial societies operated under such assumptions, the historical abuses of -isms would not have been perpetrated, and the social orders would be stronger and safer for all as a result. If colonial societies had consistently addressed the pandemic with care and respect for the most vulnerable in their communities, there likely would have been significantly less trauma and grief into the foreseeable future. Psychological wellness of societies from an IAPP perspective depends upon protecting and providing for the most vulnerable. We have a lot of work to do to protect the most vulnerable from the wielding of -isms before the next pandemic threat arises.

References

Addo, I. Y. (2020). Double pandemic: Racial discrimination amid coronavirus disease 2019. *Social Sciences & Humanities Open, 2*, 100074. https://doi.org/10.1016/j.ssaho.2020.100074

Aiello, M., Bismar, D., Casanova, S., Casas, J. M., Chang, D., Chin, J. L., Comas-Diaz, L., Salvo Crane, L., Demir, Z., Garcia, M. A., Hita, L., Leverett, P., Mendez, K., Morse, G. S., Shodiya-Zumault, S., O'Leary, S. M., Weil, M. C., & Blume, A. W. (2021). Protecting and defending our people: Nakni tushka anowa (a warrior's path). *Journal of Indigenous Research, 9*, 8. https://digitalcommons.usu.edu/kicjir/vol9/iss2021/8

Akiyama, M. J., Spaulding, A. C., & Rich, J. D. (2020). Flattening the curve for incarcerated populations—Covid-19 in jails and prisons. *The New England Journal of Medicines, 382*, 2075–2077. https://www.nejm.org/doi/full/10.1056/NEJMp2005687

Alcorn, C. (2021, May 4). *Gun background checks soared in April*. New York: CNN. https://www.cnn.com/2021/05/04/business/gun-sales-april-illinois/index.html

Almeida, M., Shrestha, A. D., Stojanac, D., & Miller, L. J. (2020). The impact of the COVID-19 pandemic on women's mental health. *Archives of Women's Mental Health, 23*, 741–748. https://doi.org/10.1007/s00737-020-01092-2

Alsan, M., & Yang, C. (2020, June 8). *Study of COVID-19 in correctional facilities*. Chicago: National Commission on Correctional Health Care. https://www.ncchc.org/study-of-covid-19-in-correctional-facilities

Alvarez, P. (2021, March 5). *Texas Gov. Abbott stalled federal offer to test migrants then blamed them for spreading Covid.* New York: CNN. https://www.cnn.com/2021/03/04/politicis/abbott-migrants-covid-testing/index.html

American Hospital Association. (2020). *Acknowledging and addressing racism and xenophobia.* Author. https://www.aha.org/covid19

American Public Media Research Lab Staff. (2021, January 7). *The color of coronavirus: COVID-19 deaths by race and ethnicity in the U.S.* St. Paul. MN: Author. https://www.apmresearchlab.org/covid/deaths-by-race

Andrews, E. E., Ayers, K. B., Brown, K. S., Dunn, D. S., & Pilarski, C. R. (2020). Nobody is expendable: Medical rationing and disability justice during the COVID-19 pandemic. *American Psychologist, 76*(3), 451–461. https://doi.org/10.1037/amp0000709

Anti-defamation League. (2021). *White supremacist propaganda spikes in 2020.* Author. https://www.adl.org/white-supremacists-propaganda-spikes-2020

APA Working Group on Health Disparities in Boys and Men. (2018). *Health disparities in racial/ethnic and sexual minority boys and men.* Washington, DC: APA. Retrieved from http://www.apa.org/pi/health-disparities/resources/race-sexuality-men.aspx

Arnold, C. (2020, July 16). *Sales of guns to first time owners rise amid COVID-19 pandemic.* Washington, DC: National Public Radio. https://www.npr.org/2020/07/16/891758050/sales-of-guns-to-first-time-owners-rise-amid-covid-19-pandemic

Aschwanden, C. (2020, October 21). *The false promise of herd immunity for COVID-19.* London: Nature. https://www.nature.com/articles/d41586-020-02948-4

Associated Press. (2021a, February 4). *Gun sales hit high in January, continuing 2020 surge.* New York: Author. https://apnews.com/article/sports-coronavirus-pandemic-philanthropy-gun-politics-economy-8450c7b642c9fccdd1031842898cfcd9

Associated Press. (2021b, May 16). *Fauci says pandemic exposed 'undeniable effects of racism'.* New York: Author. https://apnews.com/article/ga-state-wire-race-and-ethnicity-coronavirus-pandemic-lifestyle-health-105c4a5a0eea3550804093b137532e67

Banerjee, D. (2020). 'Age and ageism in COVID-19': Elderly mental health-care vulnerabilities and needs. *Asian Journal of Psychiatry, 51*, 102154. https://doi.org/j.ajp.2020.102154

Banerjee, D., & Nair, V. S. (2020). "The untold side of COVID-19": Struggle and perspectives of the sexual minorities. *Journal of Psychosexual Health, 2*(2), 113–120. https://doi.org/10.1177/2631831820939017

Banks, R. R., Eberhardt, J. L., & Ross, L. (2006). Discrimination and implicit bias in a racially unequal society. *California Law Review, 94*(4), 1169–1190.

Barry, J. M. (2018). *The great influenza: The story of the deadliest pandemic in history.* Penguin Books.

BBC. (2020a, November 15). *Obama on division, 'crazy conspiracies' and 'truth decay'.* : Author. https://www.bbc.com/news/av/world-us-canada-54946926

BBC. (2020b, November 17). *Coronavirus: Five signs that show how bad El Paso's outbreak is.* London: BBC. https://www.bbc.com/news/world-us-canada-54966876

BBC. (2020c, November 18). *Judge rules US can't use Covid-19 to expel migrant children.* London: Author. https://www.bbc.com/news/world-us-canada-54995415

BBC. (2020d, December 17). *Coronovirus: Swedish King Carl XVI Gustaf says coronavirus approach 'has failed'.* : Author. https://www.bbc.com/news/world-europe-55347021

BBC. (2021, April 27). *Covid: Boris Johnson's 'bodies pile high' comments prompt criticism.* https://www.bbc.com/news/uk-politics-56890714

Blickle, K. (2020). *Pandemics change cities: Municipal spending and voter extremism in Germany, 1918–1933.* https://www.newyorkfed.org/medialibrary/media/research/staff_reports/sr921.pdf

Blume, A. W. (2020). *A new psychology based on community, equality, and care of the earth: An indigenous American perspective.* ABC-CLIO/Praeger.

Bowleg, L. (2020). We're not all in this together: On COVID-19, intersectionality, and structural inequality. *American Journal of Public Health, 110*(7), 917. https://doi.org/10.2105/AJPH.2020.305766

Brett, T. S., & Rohani, P. (2020). Transmission dynamics reveal the impracticality of COVID-19 herd immunity strategies. *PNAS, 117*(41), 25897–25903. https://doi.org/10.1073/pnas.2008087117

Brickhill-Atkinson, M., & Hauck, F. R. (2021). Impact of COVID-19 n resettled refugees. *Primary Care: Clinics in Office Practice, 48*, 57–66. https://doi.org/10.1016/j.pop.2020.10.0001

Brown, S. M., Doom, J. R., Lechuga-Peña, S., Watamura, S. E., & Koppels, T. (2020). Stress and parenting during the global COVID-19 pandemic. *Child Abuse & Neglect, 110*, 104699. https://doi.org/10.1016/j.chiabu.2020.104699

Brumfel, G. (2020, July 24). *Without a vaccine, researchers say, herd immunity may never be achieved.* Washington, DC: National Public Radio. https://www.npr.org/sections/health-shots/2020/07/24/891448860/without-a-vaccine-researchers-say-herd-immunity-may-never-be-achieved

Buckee, C., Hedt-Gauthier, B., Mahmud, A., Martinez, P., Tedijanto, C., Murray, M., Khan, R., Menkir, T., Li, R., Suliman, S., Fosdick, B. K., Cobey, S., Rasmussen, A., Popescu, S., Cevik, M., Dada, S., Jenkins, H., Clapham, H., Mordecai, E., & Dhatt, R. (2020, May 15). *Women in science are battling both Covid-19 and the patriarchy*. London: Time Higher Education. https://www.timeshighereducation.com/blog/women-science-are-battling-both-covid-19-and-patriarchy#%20

Burki, T. (2020a). Prisons are "in no way equipped" to deal with COVID-19. *Lancet, 395*, 1411–1412. https://www.thelancet.com/journals/lancet/article/PIIS0140-6736(20)30984-3/fulltext

Burki, T. (2020b). The indirect impact of COVID-19 on women. *Lancet Infection, 20*, 904–905. https://doi.org/10.1016/S1473-3099(20)30568-5

Business Wire. (2020, November 6). *Herd immunity 'declaration' and use of town name draw official condemnation by Great Barrington leadership*. New York: Author. https://www.businesswire.com/news/home/20201106005053/en/

CDC. (2021, May 13). *Interim public health recommendations for fully vaccinated people*. Atlanta: Author. https://www.cdc.gov/coronavirus/2019-ncov/vaccines/fully-vaccinated-guidance.html

Cheah, C. S. L., Wang, C., Ren, H., Zong, X., Cho, H. S., & Xue, X. (2020). *Pediatrics, 146*(5), e2020021816. https://doi.org/10.1542/peds.2020-021816

Chee, S. Y. (2020). COVID-19 pandemic: The lived experiences of older adults in aged care homes. *Millennial Asia, 11*(3), 299–317. https://doi.org/10.1177/0976399620958326

Chen, H. A., Trinh, J., & Yang, G. P. (2020). Anti-Asian sentiment in the United States—COVID-19 and history. *The American Journal of Surgery, 220*, 556–557. https://doi.org/10.1016/j.amjsurg.2020.05.020

Chinn, N. (2021, January 2). *The Navajo nation faces a battle to protect its elders and traditions as Covid-19 deaths spike*. New York: CNN. https://www.cnn.com/2021/01/02/us/navajo-nation-coronavirum-toll/index.html

Congressional Research Service. (2018, July 20). *The trump administration's "zero tolerance" immigration enforcement* policy. Washington, DC: Author. https://crsreports.congress.gov.r45266

Constantino, J. N., & Sahin, M. (2020). The impact of COVID-19 on individuals with intellectual and developmental disabilities: Clinical and scientific priorities. *American Journal of Psychiatry, 177*(11), 1091–1093. https://doi.org/10.1176/appi.ajp.2020.20060780

Daoust, J.-F. (2020). Elderly people and responses to COVID-19 in 27 countries. *PLoS One, 15*(7), e0235590. https://doi.org/10.1371/journal.pone.0235590

Derby, M. S. (2020, May 4). *New York fed paper finds pandemic a century ago fueled Nazi rise*. New York: Wall Street Journal. https://www.wsj.com/articles/new-york-fed-paper-finds-pandemic-a-century-ago-fueled-nazi-rise-11588629945

Devakumar, D., Shannon, G., Bhopal, S. S., & Abubakar, I. (2020). Racism and discrimination in COVID-19 responses. *Lancet, 395*, 1194. https://doi.org/10.1016/S0140-6736(20)30792-3

Dhama, K., Patel, S. K., Kumar, R., Rana, J., Yatoo, M. I., Kumar, A., Tiwari, R., Dhama, J., Natesan, S., Singh, R., & Harapan, H. (2020). Geriatric population during the COVID-19 pandemic: Problems, considerations, exigencies, and beyond. *Frontiers in Public Health, 574198*. https://doi.org/10.3389/fpubh.2020.574198

Diamond, D. (2020, December 16). *'We want them infected': Trump appointee demanded 'herd immunity' strategy, emails reveal*. Arlington, VA: Politico. https://www.politico.com/news/2020/12/16/trump-appointee-demanded-herd-immunity-strategy-446408

Echo-Hawk, W. R. (2013). *In the light of justice: The rise of human rights in native America*. Fulcrum.

Edwards, F., Lee, H., & Esposito, M. (2019). Risk of being killed by police use of force in the United States by age, race-ethnicity, and sex. *PNAS, 116*(34), 16793–16798. https://doi.org/10.1073/pnas.1821204116

Egede, L. E., & Walker, R. J. (2020). Structural racism, social risk factors, and Covid-19—A dangerous convergence for black Americans. *New England Journal of Medicine, 383*, e77. https://doi.org/10.1056/NEJMp2023616

Elias, A., Ben, J., Mansouri, F., & Paradies, Y. (2020). Racism and nationalism during and beyond the COVID-19 pandemic. *Ethnic and Racial Studies*. https://doi.org/10.1080/01419870.2020.1851382

Embrick, D. G. (2015). Two nations, revisited: The lynching of black and Brown bodies, police brutality, and racial control in 'post-racial' Amerikkka. *Critical Sociology, 41*(6), 835–843. https://doi.org/10.1177/0896920515591950

Ertuğrul, T. (2020). *Sweden's coronavirus fight strategy and bitter memories of past eugenic practices*. Ankara: Center for Eurasian Studies. https://avim.org.tr/en/Analiz/SWEDEN-S-CORONAVIRUS-FIGHT-STRATEGY-AND-BITTER-MEMORIES-OF-PAST-EUGENIC-PRACTICES-1

Evans, M. L., Lindauer, M., & Farrell, M. E. (2020). A pandemic within a pandemic—Intimate partner violence during Covid-19. *New England Journal of Medicine, 383*(24), 2302–2304. https://doi.org/10.1056/NEJMp2024046

Farzan, A. N., & Berger, M. (2020, November 11). *Bolsonaro says Brazilians must not be 'sissies' about coronavirus, as 'all of us are going to die one day'*. Washington, DC: Washington Post. https://www.washingtonpost.com/world/2020/11/11/bolsonaro-coronavirus-brazil-quotes/

Federal Bureau of Investigation. (2006, October 17). *White supremacist infiltration of law enforcement*. Washington, DC: Author. https://www.documentcloud.org/documents/60-FBI-White-Supremacist-Infiltration-of-Law.html

Fieldstadt, E. (2021, February 1). *Georgia police chief, officer ousted after video of racist remarks on slavery, Stacey Abrams*. New York: NBC News. https://www.nbcnews.com/news/us-news/georgia-police-chief-officer-ousted-afer-video-racist-remarks-slavery-n1256350

Fisher, J., Languilaire, J.-C., Lawthom, R., Nieuwenhuis, R., Petts, R. J., Runswick-Cole, K., & Yerkes, M. A. (2020). Community, work, and family in times of COVID-19. *Community, Work, & Family, 23*(3), 247–252. https://doi.org/10.1080/13668803.2020.1756568

FitzGerald, C., & Hurst, S. (2017). Implicit bias in healthcare professionals: A systematic review. *BMC Medical Ethics, 18*, 19. https://doi.org/10.1186/s12910-017-0179-8

Foley, R. J. (2020, May 5). *Nearly 1,400 Tyson workers at 3 Iowa plants get coronavirus*. New York: Associated Press. https://apnews.com/article/c8286cc4dd670e88850ad33e977866a4

Fontanet, A., & Cauchmez, S. (2020). COVID-19 herd immunity: Where are we? *Nature Reviews: Immunology, 20*, 583–584. https://doi.org/10.1038/s41577-020-00451-5

Fraser, S., Lagacé, M., Bongué, B., Ndeye, N., Guyot, J., Bechard, L., Garcia, L., Taler, V., Adam, S., Beaulieu, M., Bergeron, C. D., Boudjemadi, V., Desmette, D., Donizetti, A. R., Éthier, S., Garon, S., Gillis, M., Levasseur, M., Tougas, F., & CCNA Social Inclusion and Stigma Working Group. (2020). Ageism and COVID-19: What does our society's response say about us? *Age and Ageing, 49*, 692–695. https://doi.org/10.1093/ageing/afaa097

Gangopadhyaya, A. (2021). *Do black and white patients experience similar rates of adverse safety events at the same hospital?* Washington, DC: Urban Institute. https://www.urban.org/research/

publication/do-black-and-white-patients-experience-similar-rates-adverse-safety-events-same-hospital

Garcia, M. A., Homan, P. A., García, C., & Brown, T. H. (2020). The color of COVID-19: Structural racism and the disproportionate impact of the pandemic on older black and Latinx adults. *Journals of Gerontology: Social Sciences, 76*(3), e75–e80. https://doi.org/10.1093/geronb/gbaa114

Gibson, K. (2020, November 3). *U.S. gun sales surge to record high in 2020*. New York: CBS News. https://www.cbsnews.com/news/gun-sales-record-high-2020/

Gjelten, T. (2020, June 1). *Peaceful protesters tear-gassed to clear way for trump church photo-op*. Washington, DC: National Public Radio. https://www.npr.org/2020/06/01/867532070/trumps-unannounced-church-visit-angers-church-officials

Gould, E., Perez, D., & Wilson, V. (2020, August 20). *Latinx workers—Particularly women—Face devasting job losses in the COVID-19 recession*. Washington, DC: Economic Policy Institute. https://www.epi.org/197015

Gould, E., & Wilson, V. (2020, June 1). *Black workers face two of the most lethal preexisting conditions for coronavirus—Racism and economic inequality*. Washington, DC: Economic Policy Institute. https://www.epi.org/publications/black-workers-covid/

Grattan, S., & Faiola, A. (2020, October 6). *In Colombia, a death in police custody follow a history of brutality*. Washington, DC: Washington Post. https://www.washingtonpost.com/world/the_americas/colombia-police-protest-javier-ordonez/2020/10/05/c8f2df86-0438-11eb-897d-3a6201d6643f_story.html

Greenwald, A. G., & Banaji, M. R. (1995). Implicit social cognition: Attitudes, self-esteem, and stereotypes. *Psychological Review, 102*, 4–27. https://doi.org/10.1037/0033-295X.102.1.4

Gump, B. B. (2020, November 6). *The Great Barrington declaration: When arrogance leads to recklessness*. U.S. News and World Report. https://www.usnews.com/news/healthiest-communities/articles/2020-11-06/when-scientists-arrogance-leads-to-recklessness-the-great-barrington-declaration

Gupta, A. H. (2020, October 22). *How an aversion to masks stems from 'toxic masculinity'*. New York: New York Times. https://www.newyorktimes.com/2020/10/22/us/masks-toxic-masculinity-covid-men-gender.html

Hawks, L., Woolhandler, S., & McCormick, D. (2020). COVID-19 in prisons and jails in the United States. *JAMA Internal Medicine, 180*(8), 1041–1042. https://www.jamanetwork.com/

Heslin, K. C., & Hall, J. E. (2021, February 5). *MMWR, 70*(5), 149–154. https://doi.org/10.15585/mmwr.mm7005a1

Hillis, S. D., Blankinsop, A., Villaveces, A., Annor Libard, L., Masseti, G. M., Demissie, Z., Mercy, J. A., Nelson, C. A., Cluver, L., Flaxman, F., Sherr, L., Donnelly, C. A., Ratmann, O., & Unwin, H. J. T. (2021). COVID-19-associated orphanhood and caregiver death in the United States. *Pediatrics*. https://doi.org/10.1542/peds.2021-053760

Hillis, S. D., Unwin, H. J. T., Chen, Y., Cluver, L., Sherr, L., Goldman, P. S., Ratmann, O., Donnelly, C. A., Bhatt, S., Villaveces, A., Butchart, A., Bachman, G., Rawlings, L., Nelson, C. A., & Flaxman, S. (2021). Global minimum estimates of children affected by COVID-19 associated orphanhood and deaths of caregivers: A modelling study. *Lancet, 398*, 391–402. https://doi.org/10.1016/S0140-6736(21)01253-8

Howard, J. (2020, October 14). *A herd immunity strategy to fight the pandemic can be 'dangerous,' experts say. Here's why.* : CNN. https://www.cnn.com/2020/09/01/health/herd-immunity-coronavius-pandemic-explainer-wellness/index.html

Jawetz, T. (2020, September 28). *Immigrants as essential workers during COVID 19: Testimony before the U.S. house judiciary subcommittee on immigration and citizenship*. Washington, DC: Center for American Progress. https://www.americanprogress.org/issues/immigration/reports/2020/09/28/490919/immigrants-essential-workers-covid-19/

Jiménez, M. C., Cowger, T. L., Simon, L. E., Behn, M., Cassarino, N., & Bassett, M. T. (2020). Epidemiology of COVID-19 among incarcerated individuals and staff in Massachusetts jails and prisons. *JAMA Network Open, 3*(8), e2018851. https://doi.org/10.1001/jamanetworkopen.2020.18851

Jimenez-Sotomayor, M. R., Gomez-Moreno, C., & Soto-Perez-de-Celis, E. (2020). Coronavirus, ageism, and twitter: An evaluation of tweets about older adults and COVID-19. *Journal of the American Geriatric Society, 68*, 1661–1665. https://doi.org/10.1111/jgs.16508

John, T. (2021, March 31). *Campaigners slam UK government report into racial disparities as a 'whitewash'*. New York: CNN. https://www.cnn.com/2021/03/31/uk.uk-racial-disparity-report-intl-gbr/index.html

Jung, F., Krieger, V., Hufert, F. T., & Küpper, J.-H. (2020). Herd immunity or suppression strategy to combat COVID19. *Clinical Hemorheology and Microcirculation, 75*, 13–17. https://doi.org/10.3233/CH-209006

Kajeepeta, S., Mauro, P. M., Keyes, K. M., El-Sayed, A. M., Rutherford, C. G., & Prins, S. J. (2021). Association between county jail incarceration and cause-specific county mortality in the USA, 1987-2017: A retrospective, longitudinal study. *The Lancet Public Health*. https://doi.org/10.1016/S2468-2667(20)30283-8

Kao, A. C. (2021). Invisibility of anti-Asian racism. *AMA Journal of Ethics, 23*(7), E507–E511. https://doi.org/10.1001/amajethics.2021.507

Kaur, H. (2021, March 4). *The history of attacks against Asian Americans is complicated. Addressing it will be, too*. New York: CNN. https://www.cnn.com/2021/03/04/us/asian-american-racism-violence-response-tmd/index.html

Kelly, C. (2021, January 20). *Biden rescinds 1776 commission via executive order*. New York: CNN. https://www.cnn.com/2021/01/20/politics/biden-rescind-1776-commission-executive-order/index.html

Kent, E. E., Ornstein, K. A., & Dionne-Odom, J. N. (2020). The family caregiving crisis meets an actual pandemic. *Journal of Pain and Symptom Management, 60*(1), e66–e69. https://doi.org/10.1016/j.jpainsymman.2020.04.006

Khazanchi, R., Evans, C. T., & Marcelin, J. R. (2020). Racism, not race, drives inequity across the COVID-19 continuum. *JAMA Network Open, 3*(9), e2019933. https://doi.org/10.1001/jamanetworkopen.2020.19933

Kirisci, K. (2020, May 8). *The coronavirus has led to more authoritarianism for Turkey*. Washington, DC: Brookings Institute. https://www.brookings.edu/blog/order-from-chaos/2020/05/08/the-coronavirus-has-led-to-more-authoritarianism-for-turkey/

Krieger, N., Boyd, R. W., De Maio, F., & Maybank, A. (2021, April 20). Medicine's privileged gatekeepers: Producing harmful ignorance about racism and health. *Health Affairs*. https://doi.org/10.1377/hblog20210415.305480

Kulldorff, M., Gupta, S., & Bhattacharya, J. (2020, October 4). *Great Barrington Declaration*. https://gbdeclaration.org

Kurtzleben, D. (2020, October 28). *Trump has weaponized masculinity as president. Here's why it matters*. Washington, DC: National Public Radio. https://www.npr.org/2020/10/28/928336749/trump-has-weaponized-masculinity-as-president-heres-why-it-maters

Lasco, G. (2020). Medical populism and the COVID-19 pandemic. *Global Public Health, 15*(10), 1417–1429. https://doi.org/10.1080/17441692.2020.1807581

Lebrasseur, A., Fortin-Bédard, N., Lettre, J., Bussières, E.-L., Best, K., Boucher, N., Hotton, M., Beulieu-Bonneau, S., Mercier, C., Lamontagne, M.-E., & Routhier, F. (2020). Impact of COVID-19 on people with physical disabilities: A rapid review. *Disability and Health Journal, 14*, 101014. https://doi.org/10.1016/j.dhjo.2020.101014

Levin, J., & Lebeau, D. (2021, February 3). *Covid's South Dakota rampage created a failed experiment on herd immunity*. New York: Bloomberg News. https://www.bloomberg.com/news/features/2021-02-03/covid-19-retreats-in-kristi-noem-s-south-dakota-because-so-many-got-infected

Loweree, J., Reichlin-Melnick, A., & Ewing, W. A. (2020). *The impact of COVID-19 on non-citizens and across the U.S. immigration system: March-September, 2020*. Washington, DC:

American Immigration Council. https://www.americanimmigrationcouncil.org/research/impact-covid-19-us-immigration-system

Macmadu, A., Berk, J., Kaplowitz, E., Mercedes, M., Rich, J. D., & Brinkley-Rubinstein, L. (2020). COVID-19 and mass incarceration: A call for urgent action. *The Lancet Public Health, 5*, e571–e572. https://doi.org/10.1016/S2468-2667(20)30231-0

Makaroun, L. K., Bachrach, R. L., & Rosland, A.-M. (2020). Elder abuse in the time of COVID-19—Increased risks for older adults and their caregivers. *American Journal of Geriatric Psychiatry, 28*(8), 876–880. https://doi.org/10.1016/j.jagp.2020.05.017

Malinverni, C., & Brigagão, J. I. M. (2020). COVID-19: Scientific arguments, denialism, eugenics, and the construction of the antisocial distancing discourse in Brazil. *Frontiers in Communication, 5*, 582963. https://doi.org/10.3389/fcomm.2020.582963

Markel, H., & Stern, A. M. (2002). The foreignness of germs: The persistent association of immigrants and disease in American society. *The Milbank Quarterly, 80*(4), 757–788.

Meisner, B. A. (2020). Are you OK, boomer? Intensification of ageism and intergenerational tensions on social media amid COVID-19. *Leisure Sciences.* https://doi.org/10.1080/01490400.2020.1773983

Miller, R. J. (2019, August 14). *Nazi Germany and American Indians. Indian country today*. Phoenix: Indian Country Today. https://indiancountrytoday.com/opinion/nazi-germany-and-american-indians-Uha07e3luUCaeLq1nJP5-Q

Miu, A. S., & Moore, J. R. (2021). Behind the masks: Experiences of mental health practitioners of color during the COVID-19 pandemic. *Academic Psychiatry.* https://doi.org/10.1007/s40596-021-01427-w

Monahan, C., Macdonald, J., Lytle, A., Apriceno, M. B., & Levy, S. R. (2020). COVID-19 and ageism: How positive and negative responses impact older adults in society. *American Psychologist, 75*(7), 887–896. https://doi.org/10.1037/amp0000699

Mosley, M. (2020, November 18). COVID-19 and eugenics in 2020. *Emergency Medicine News, 42*(11B). https://doi.org/10.1097/01.EEM.0000723320.81180.97

National Archives. (n.d.). *Confrontations for justice: John Lewis, march from Selma to Montgomery, 1965*. Author. https://www.archives.gov/exhibits/eyewitness/html.php?section=2

Naylor, B. (2021, January 11). *Impeachment resolution cites Trump's 'incitement' of capitol insurrection*. Washington, DC: National Public Radio. https://www.npr.org/sections/trump-impeachment-effort-live-updates/2021/01/11/955631105/impeachment-resolution-cites-trumps-incitement-of-capitol-insurrection

Nguyen, D. (2021, February 11). *Attacks on older Asians stoke fear as lunar new year begins*. New York: Associated Press. https://apnews.com/article/us-news-okaland-san-francisco-coronavirus-pandemic-cfd77ca7d4b0c63890f2a087c160d03a

Noel, T. K. (2020). Conflating culture with COVID-19: Xenophobic repercussions of a global pandemic. *Social Sciences & Humanities Open, 2*, 100044. https://doi.org/10.1016/j.ssaho.2020.100044

Oren, D. P., & Topol, E. J. (2020). Prevalence of asymptomatic SARS-CoV-2 infection. *Annals of Internal Medicine, 173*, 362–367. https://doi.org/10.7326/M20-3012

Page, K. R., & Flores-Miller, A. (2021). Lessons we've learned—Covid-19 and the undocumented Latinx community. *New England Journal of Medicine, 384*, 5–7. https://doi.org/10.1056/NEJMp2024897

Park, S. S. (2020). *Caregivers' mental health and somatic symptoms during COVID-19 the journals of gerontology, series B, gbaa121*. https://doi.org/10.1093/geronb/gbaa121

Perry, S. L., Whitehead, A. L., & Grubbs, J. B. (2020). Culture wars and COVID-19 conduct: Christian nationalism, religiosity, and Americans' behavior during the coronavirus pandemic. *Journal for the Scientific Study of Religion, 59*(3), 405–416.

Phillips, G., Felt, D., Ruprecht, M. M., Wang, X., Xu, J., Pérez-Bill, E., Bagnarol, R. M., Roth, J., Curry, C. W., & Beach, L. B. (2020). Addressing the disproportionate impacts of the COVID-19

pandemic on sexual and gender minority populations in the United States: Actions toward equity. *LGBT Health, 7*(6), 279–282. https://doi.org/10.1089/gbt.2020.0187
Pilgrim, D. (2008). The eugenic legacy in psychology and psychiatry. *International Journal of Social Psychiatry, 54*(3), 272–284. https://doi.org/10.1177/0020764008090282.
Ramirez, M. (2021, March 18). *Who gets to decide what is racism, hate? Atlanta shootings renew debate over white violence, privilege*. Washington, DC: USA Today. https://www.usatoday.com/story/news/2021/03/18/atlanta-victims-were-killed-white-violence-racism-many-insist/4751240001/
Rasmussen, A. L. (2020). Vaccination is the only acceptable path to herd immunity. *Med, 1*, 21–23. https://doi.org/10.1016/j.medj.2020.12.004
Reny, T. T. (2020). Masculine norms and infectious disease: The case of COVID-19. *Politics and Gender, 16*(4), 1028–1035. https://doi.org/10.1017/S1743923X20000380
Ruprecht, M. M., Wang, X., Johnson, A. K., Xu, J., Felt, D., Ihenacho, S., Stonehouse, P., Curry, C. W., DeBroux, C., Costa, D., & Phillips, G. (2020). Evidence of social and structural COVID-19 disparities by sexual orientation, gender identity, and race/ethnicity in an urban environment. *Journal of Urban Health*. https://doi.org/10.1007/s11524-020-00497-9
Sabatello, M., Landes, S. D., & McDonald, K. E. (2020). People with disabilities in COVID-19: Fixing our priorities. *The American Journal of Bioethics, 20*(7). https://doi.org/10.1080/15265161.2020.1779396
Sabatello, M., Scroggins, M. J., Goto, G., Santiago, A., McCormick, A., Morris, K. J., Daulton, C. R., Easter, C. L., & Darien, G. (2020). Structural racism in the COVID-19 pandemic: Moving forward. *The American Journal of Bioethics*. https://doi.org/10.1080/15265161.2020.1851808
Salter, P. S., Adams, G., & Perez, M. J. (2018). Racism in the structure of everyday worlds: A cultural-psychological perspective. *Current Directions in Psychological Science, 27*(3), 150.155. https://doi.org/10.1177/0963721417724239
Sepúlveda-Loyola, W., Rodríguez-Sánchez, I., Pérez-Rodríguez, P., Ganz, F., Torralba, R., Oliveira, D. V., & Rodríguez-Mañas, L. (2020). The journal of nutrition. *Health, & Aging, 24*, 938–947. https://doi.org/10.1007/s12603-020-1500-7
Sidanius, J., Cotterill, S., Sheehy-Skeffington, J., Kteily, N., & Carvacho, H. (2017). Social dominance theory: Explorations in the psychology of oppression. In C. G. Sibley & F. K. Barlow (Eds.), *The Cambridge handbook of the psychology of prejudice (pp. 149–187)*. Cambridge University Press. https://doi.org/10.1017/9781316161579.008
Siemaszko, C. (2021, September 21). *Tenessee limiting monoclonal antibody treatment to unvaccinated residents*. New York: NBC News. https://www.nbcnews.com/news/us-news/tennessee-limiting-monoclonal-antibody-treatment-unvaccinated-residents-n1279740
Silva, D., & Miranda, L. (2021, February 6). *About 275,000 women left workforce in January in 'critical' pandemic trend, experts say*. New York: NBC News. https://www.nbcnews.com/us-news/about-275-000-women-left-workforce-january-critical-pandemic-trend-n1256942
Smith, J., & Spodak, C. (2021, April 27). *Black or 'other'? Doctors may be relying on race to make decisions about your health*. New York: CNN. https://www.cnn.com/2021/04/25/health/race-correction-in-medicine-history-refocused/index.html
Spagnola, P. A., Manson, J E., & Joffe, H. (2020). Sex and gender differences in health: What the COVID-19 pandemic can teach us. *Annal of Internal Medicine, 173*(50, 385–386. https://doi.org/10.7326/M20-1941.
Staats, C., Capatosto, K., Tenny, L., & Mamo, S. (2017). *State of the science: Implicit bias review*. Columbus, OH: Kirwan Institute. http://kirwaninstitute.osu.edu/wp-content/uploads/2017/11/2017-SOTS-final-draft-02.pdf
Sun, N., Wei, L., Shi, S., Jiao, D., Song, R., Ma, L., Wang, H., Wang, C., Wang, Z., You, Y., Liu, S., & Wang, H. (2020). *American Journal of Infection Control, 48*, 592–598. https://doi.org/10.1016/j.ajc.2020.03.018
Swan, B. W. (2020, September 4). *DHS draft document: White supremacists are greatest terror threat*. Arlington, VA: Politico. https://www.politico.com/news/2020/09/04/white.supremacists-terror-threat-dhs-409236

Tang, T. (2021, August 12). *More than 9,000 anti-Asian incidents since pandemic began*. New York: Associated Press. https://apnews.com/article/lifestyle-joe-biden-health-coronavirus-pandemic-race-and-ethnicity-d3a63408021a247ba764d40355ecbe2a

Tanner, L. (2021, March 26). *Editor sidelined after medical journal racism podcast outcry*. New York: Associated Press. https://apnews.com/article/race-and-ethnicity-5b2c36f977f5d665513e4ea04a5fad77

Taylor, S. (2019). *The psychology of pandemics: Preparing for the next global outbreak of infectious disease*. Cambridge Scholars Publishing.

The President's Advisory 1776 Commission. (2021). *The 1776 report*. https://f.hubspotusercontent10.net/hubfs/397762/The%20President%E2%80%99s%20Advisory%201776%20Commission%20-%20Final%20Report.pdf

Torpy, S. J. (2000). Native American women and coerced sterilization: On the trail of tears in the 1970s. *American Indian Culture and Research Journal, 24*(2), 1–22.

Troianovski, A. (2021, April 10). *'You can't trust anyone': Russia's hidden Covid toll is an open secret*. New York: New York Times. https://www.nytimes.com/2021/04/10/world/europe/covid-russia-death.html

Turk, M. A., & McDermott, S. (2020). The COVID-19 pandemic and people with disability. *Disability and Health Journal, 13*, 100944. https://doi.org/10.1016/j.dhjo.2020.100944

UN Department of Global Communications. (2020, May 11). *COVID-19: UN counters pandemic-related hate and xenophobia*. New York: United Nations. https://www.un.org/en/coronavirus/covid-19-un-counters-pandemic-related-hate-and-xenophobia

UNICEF. (2021). *COVID-19 and children*. New York: Author. https://data.unicef.org/covid-19-and-children/

US Global Leadership Coalition. (2020, December 8). *COVID-19 brief: Impact on refugees*. Washington, DC: Author. https://www.usglc.org/coronavirus

Vahia, I. V., Jeste, D. V., & Reynolds, C. F. (2020). Older adults and the mental health effects of COVID-19. *JAMA, 324*(22), 2253–2254. https://doi.org/10.1001/jama.2020.21753

Vieten, U. M. (2020). The "new normal" and "pandemic populism": The COVID-19 crisis and anti-hygienic mobilization of the far-right. *Social Sciences, 9*, 165. https://doi.org/10.3990/soc.sci9090165

Waldrep, C. (2008). National policing, lynching, a constitutional change. *The Journal of Southern History, 74*(3), 589–626. https://www.jstor.org/stabl/27650230

Watts, A., & Hanna, J. (January 8, 2021). *Indiana health system says experts will examine Covid-19 death of black doctor who accused staff of racist treatment*. New York: CNN. https://www.cnn.com/2021/01/08/us/black-doctor-susan-moore-covid/index.html

Weber, L., & Recht, H. (2021, February 25). *Covid vaccine websites violate disability laws, create inequity for the blind*. San Francisco: Kaiser Health News. https://khn.org/news/article/covid-vaccine-websites-violate-disability-laws-create-inequity-for-the-blind/

Wenham, C., Smith, J., & Morgan, R. (2020). COVID-19: The gendered impacts of the outbreak. *Lancet, 395*, 846–847. https://doi.org/10.1016/S0140-6736(20)30526-2

WHO. (2020). A*partTogether survey: Preliminary overview of refugees and migrants self-reported impact of COVID-19*. Geneva: Author. https://apps.who.int/iris/handle/10665/337931

WHO. (2021, February 20). *Situation by country, territory, and area*. Geneva: Author. https://covid19.who.int/table

Williams, B., Ahalt, C., Cloud, D., Augustine, D., Rorvig, L. & Sears, D. (2020, March 26). *Correctional facilities in the shadow of COVID-19: Unique challenges and proposed solutions*. Health Affairs Blog. https://www.healthaffairs.org/do/10.1377/hblog20200324.784502/full/

Williams, D. R., & Cooper, L. A. (2020). *JAMA, 323*(24). https://jamanetwork.com/

Woodward, B. (2020). *Rage*. Simon & Schuster.

Woodward, B., & Costa, R. (2016, April 2). *Transcript: Donald trump interview with bob Woodward and Robert Costa*. Washington, DC: Washington Post. https://www.washingtonpost.com/news/post-politics/wp/2016/04/02/transcript-donald-trump-interview-with-bob-woodward-and-robert-costa/

Yahoo News. (2020, October 15). *Fauci on herd immunity: 'Quite frankly, that is nonsense'*. : Author. https://news.yahoo.com/fauci-herd-immunity-quite-frankly-131828997.html
Yearby, R., & Mohapatra, S. (2020). Law, structural racism, and the COVID-19 pandemic. *Journal of Law and the Biosciences, 7*(1), 1–20. https://doi.org/10.1093/jlb/lsaa036
Yeung, J., Renton, A., & Dewan, A. (2020, October 14). *The latest on the coronavirus pandemic*. New York: CNN. https://www.cnn.com/wolrd/live-news/coronavirus-pandemic-10-14-20-intl/h_571c71aa21a9a2a0d0aadd95af67a022
Zeng, G., Wang, L., & Zhang, Z. (2020). Prejudice and xenophobia in COVID-19 research manuscripts. *Nature Human Behaviour, 4*, 879. https://doi.org/10.1038/s41562-020-00948-y

Chapter 5
Colonialism, COVID-19, and Education

Abstract Educational disparities are commonly experienced in colonial nations by the outgroups of those societies. Although educational attainment holds the promise of social advancement for some in those societies, education also has been historically used as a tool of colonial assimilation and a method to erase Indigenous cultures. Educational systems in the US have never been equal, with students of color often studying in schools that were excluded from the mainstream, under-resourced, and understaffed. Schools and families of minoritized students were ill-prepared for closures and online instruction, often lacking in computing skills and equipment and wifi capabilities. Children globally were at increased risk for dropping out of school, poverty, hunger, and poor health during COVID-19. Colonial nations have not typically prioritized the needs of children and students when compared to other age demographics, and the persistent lack of investment in resources for children has been a significant barrier to pandemic education and protecting children's health and well-being. Psychological wellness for future generations, especially with consideration for the next pandemic, requires that the needs of education and children be prioritized. Indigenous psychology suggests that protection of the most vulnerable is foundational to establishing equitable, educated, and healthy societies.

Education has been cited as one of the great tools for correcting inequities and injustices in colonial societies, providing significant hope to those aspiring to advance themselves in those societies. However, the hopes associated with education have been often incongruent with the realities of education for many people living in colonial nations. Social hierarchies have contributed to privileged and non-privileged educational tracks with widely variable resources. Education has also been used to advance colonial interests rather than the interests of minoritized groups, contributing to widespread distrust of colonial educational systems. Consequentially, educational institutions and systems were generally ill prepared for responding to an enduring crisis such as COVID-19, as will be discussed subsequently.

A. W. Blume, *Colonialism and the COVID-19 Pandemic*, International and Cultural Psychology, https://doi.org/10.1007/978-3-030-92825-4_5

The Difficult History of Colonial Education

Indigenous people have first-hand knowledge of how colonial educational systems have been instrumental to subverting people and cultures. In many colonial nations, including the US, education was used as a tool of oppression—of indoctrination. Residential or boarding schools were created to facilitate the assimilation of Indigenous people into the colonial cultures. The stated goals of boarding schools were to erase Indigenous culture and language use in children, and to mold those children into benign residents within the social order. Children were forced, many times under armed guards, to leave their families and their communities for the schools, sometimes not seeing family for years. Residential schools in the US treated children harshly, often severely punishing use of traditional language and cultural practices. Indigenous children were physically and sexually abused, and many died at the schools (Dunbar-Ortiz, 2014; Nies, 1996). The mental health consequences of residential schools have been profound and widespread (Bombay, Matheson, & Anisman, 2014, 2017). Residential schools contributed to distrust of educational institutions by Indigenous people, dissuading many from pursuing advanced education. Additionally, US mainstream education is poorly matched to Indigenous culture, and racism contributes to unsafe school climates (Blume, 2020).

Hierarchical interpretations of colonialism were superimposed on educational systems resulting in inequities from the beginning. Black and Latinx students were tracked into a separate and unequal educational system due to segregation (US Department of Education, 1994). Institutions serving minoritized populations have been historically under-funded and under-resourced. Significant educational disparities have resulted, impacting outgroup children for many years, and contributing to significant economic disadvantages (APA Presidential Task Force on Educational Disparities, 2012; Schmaling, Blume, Engstrom, Paulos, & De Fina, 2017).

Segregation and boarding schools created a culture of distrust in education among minoritized groups in the US, but there were also other concerns, such as eugenics and its impact on education (Winfield, 2012). Eugenics proponents, including many educators, errantly believed in racial differences in intelligence favoring the White race (Helms, 2012; Lowe, 1980), a belief used to support different standards and expectations for the education of White and minoritized students. Differential treatment of minoritized students has been persistent. Black, Indigenous, and Latinx students in the US have been assigned to special education class at significantly higher rates that White students (Chinn & Hughes, 1987), suggesting implicit biases against students of color, as well as inherent biases in mainstream psychological assessment.

Educational disparities faced by minoritized children typically result in economic and health disparities over the course of a lifetime, evidence that the so-called playing field in in the US is not and has never been level. Finances, health, and mental health have been impacted negatively by an inability to receive a quality education and all the benefits that might bring. Colonial educational hierarchies have been maintained to benefit the privileged few. The promise of education offers hope to disadvantaged outgroups, but many have not been able to leverage education to their financial advantage. Education as the ticket to social equity has been promoted as a false panacea to address inherent inequities of colonial social orders. Educational dreams clash with contemporary realities in which many minoritized workers must rely on the gig economy or frontline service jobs (Chap. 3), risking exposure to COVID-19.

What to Do with the Children?

One of the most striking public policy debates during the COVID-19 involved addressing the education of children. The debate was divided along the competing interests of economy and education--the difficulty was that many colonial societies seemed unable or unwilling to offer the protections needed to students and their instructors to safely offer quality education. One irony was the assumption that widespread quality education could be offered during the pandemic. To sell the belief that quality education was an attainable goal under crisis conditions, one would have to overlook longstanding pre-pandemic disparities in education.

Children have been undervalued members of colonial societies for most of their histories. Colonial societies value people who "contribute" to society, a euphemism for *gainful* work to advance society. Settler families often had many children to contribute to the workings of the family. Historically, children have been viewed as assets in the labor force until recently in some nations. True to the colonial values, what a person contributes in the here and now is what seems to account for a person's value to the economic order of materially driven cultures. For many years, children were expected to work gainfully and often exploited for their labor. Child labors laws became necessary to protect children from the exploitation of adults who desired their cost-effective productivity, and those lawful protections of the human rights of children are not universal even today. When humane treatment of children became more common colonial societies, their value as cheap labor was diminished. From a material point of view, children transitioned from a source of cheap labor to a potential economic liability.

Of course, loving families saw more in their children than labor, but others who make policy decisions regarding children have continued to prioritize the needs of other age demographics before the needs of children. For example, US children represent one-third of people living in poverty and the number without health insurance rose significantly pre-pandemic (Alker, 2019; Haider, 2020). The US federal budget designated only 9% of its expenditures to benefit children pre-pandemic (Hahn, Lou, & Isaacs, 2020), not much of an investment in America's future. If children were a national priority, public school systems would want for nothing, children would not go hungry, and children's health flush with funding. Which brings us back to the circumstances of COVID-19 and schools.

Colonial policymakers during the pandemic showed little evidence of prioritizing the needs of children. Populist-nationalist leaders consistently prioritized economic needs over the needs of children (Krieg, 2020). With the Trump administration flaunting masks and social distancing openly, it was problematic to reopen US schools safely. Non-masking by the Trump family resulted in complaints toward Jared Kushner and Ivanka Trump by parents from their children's private school. Kushner and Trump withdrew their children from the school rather than change their stances on masks and social distancing (Bennett, 2020).

The US strategy was to try to reopen schools despite the lack of resources to protect children or teachers (Valant, 2020). The CDC provided guidelines for safely reopening schools (as well as camps and childcare centers) that were widely rejected, ignored, and even buried from the public by political leaders. Another example of the disregard policymakers had for the health needs of children occurred much later in the pandemic, when the highly contagious delta variant asserted itself and schools were on the verge of opening for 2021 fall sessions. During the delta variant surge, children were much more likely to require emergency care or hospitalization in low vaccination-rate states (Siegel et al., 2021), of which Florida was one. Florida Governor Ron DeSantis forbid masking mandates by school districts at that time, threatening to end state funding if his executive order was violated. He justified the order by prioritizing the liberties of parents rather than the collective good of students, many that were unvaccinated (Reuters, 2021). Brazil, also governed by a populist-nationalist leader, closed schools indefinitely and the economy open with few restrictions (Barbara, 2021). In both nations, economic expediency won out over the needs of children. Meanwhile, due to circumstances of the pandemic, 24 million children globally were projected to drop out of school (National Geographic Society, 2021).

The lack of money and resources that prevented many colonial nations from delivering quality public education during the pandemic will seriously impact educational progress for years. Public schools already had suffered tremendous pre-pandemic losses in money and resources during the Great Recession. Fewer teachers and diminishing resources in US K-12 public education have forced larger class sizes and smaller levels of support in districts, with 37 states showing evidence of spending less supporting school districts between 2009–2017, likely due to reduced tax revenue (Baker & Di Carlo, 2020). Private schools, which tend to serve families of privilege, had plenty of resources when compared to public schools and were not subject to the whims of politics for their funding (Kuriloff, 2020).

Pandemic learning was negatively impacted by a lack of preparation and resources, but learning for minoritized students was particularly difficult given pre-existing resource inequities (Challenge Success & NBC News, 2021; Dorn, Hancock, Sarakatsannis, & Viruleg, 2020). Advances in mathematics were notably lower the fall, 2020, then in previous years (Kuhfeld, Tarasawa, Johnson, Ruzek, & Lewis, 2020). The resources needed to conduct face-to-face teaching safely, or to provide quality remote learning capabilities, challenged all but the most privileged of schools. The quality of online teaching was also at the mercy of the Wi-Fi, internet, and computer capabilities of families, with low SES families at particular risk for being inadequately equipped for online instruction (McKenzie, 2020). Over 30% of all children globally were unable to access online learning during the height the pandemic (UNICEF, 2020). Digital resource inequities constitute another global divide of those who benefit from digital privileges and harm to those who do not.

Pressures to reopen schools were understandable given concerns that pre-existing inequities placed huge numbers of students at risk for worsening education achievement gaps, with many being minoritized students (Mulvihill, Sainz, & Kunzelman, 2021). The question remained whether school reopening could be done quickly or safely given resource challenges. New guidelines were released by the CDC concerning school reopening in early 2021 (CDC, 2021), which included guidelines about what level of community spread was safe for reopening, guidelines for mitigation methods that were difficult for minoritized cash-strapped schools to meet, and guidelines that did not adequately address vaccinating all teachers (Ali & Siemaszko, 2021; Inside Higher Ed, 2021). At the time the new guidelines were released, almost 90% of K-12 children lived in "red" zones where reopening was not recommended due to level of community spread (McPhillips, 2021). Schools that reopened were predominantly White, while instruction of minoritized students were much more likely online (Associated Press, 2021). Resource-challenged schools were damned if they reopened and damned if they did not. To prepare for future pandemics, economic and digital resource inequities must be addressed (Canvas., 2020).

Pre-existing teacher and education support staff shortages were profoundly exacerbated by all the challenges discussed above. Waves of retirements and resignations resulted due to the stressors of the COVID-19 pandemic. Psychological stress and burnout were commonly acknowledged. In an unusual twist on the realities of education, resources to hire personnel were widely available but skilled labor was not interested (Gecker, 2021). The implications of the shortages of skilled and experienced teachers and staff will have broad negative impact on K-12 education for many years to come, and those consequences will also ultimately health and psychological well-being of future generations.

Higher Education and COVID-19

Colleges and universities enrollments fall during the pandemic and revenues drop as a result of shutdowns that closed or restricted dormitory capacity, food services, and athletics (Richmond & Hollingsworth, 2020). Public universities suffered significant financial stress due to the financial pressures on states and municipalities that were losing tax revenue. Economic pressures on public higher education have accumulated for years due to reduced state and municipality budgets and anti-tax initiatives, and the movement to online instruction compounded those economic challenges for some (Whitford, 2021). Like K-12 institutions, higher education entered the pandemic on already shaky financial foundations.

When the pandemic emerged, colleges and universities tried many strategies to address instruction, from remaining open to various hybrid formulations of online instruction. Perhaps with some desperation, many institutions attempted to reopen with social distancing in the fall of 2020 resulting in community viral spread. Social distancing and masking recommendations largely ignored by students, much to the dismay of many local communities (Richmond & Hollingsworth, 2020). Like many other colonial citizens, some college students demonstrated complete disregard for protecting others at risk in those communities.

When vaccinations arrived, the strategy for reopening higher education were much different than for K-12. Faculty members in higher education were not prioritized for vaccinations like K-12 instructors were (Inside Higher Ed, 2021), ensuring online higher education instruction for a longer period of time. Universities and colleges were not universal in their approach to mandating vaccines or other mitigation measures, resulting in confusion and inconsistent compliance, complicated by the spread of the delta variant (Redden, 2021). Falling enrollment, failed reopening policies, and non-compliance with mitigation measures including vaccinations enhanced the financial stressors that colleges and universities faced, including upon their often-expensive athletic programs.

Athletics and Pandemic Health

Athletics are important parts of the culture of schools and provide a sense of school identity and cohesiveness that is appealing to students, their families, and alumni. High school athletics in many small towns function as sources of collective entertainment for citizens. There is certainly great value for athletics under these conditions. However, athletics may be prioritized to the detriment of the education mission of higher education. Athletics at any level may contribute tremendous interpersonal benefits *and* tremendous financial shortcomings to the institution, especially where imbalances favor athletics over academics. During the COVID-19 pandemic, there was evidence that student athletic events were proceeding somewhat recklessly in certain areas of the US despite the numerous signs of risks to some participants.

There are great reasons to have athletic programs, especially in support of student athletes. However, financial pressures on both students and institutions have encouraged looking at athletics as a potential source of income and revenue respectively (Kearns, Bachynski, & Caplan, 2020). Some students view athletics as a ticket out of poverty, and it may be true for a very talented few. Sadly, many will not achieve that goal and one hopes that they have also invested time in their education just in case. The promises of riches through athletics is part of the cluster of economic myths in colonial societies that stand akin to the myth of the American dream (Blume, 2020). Colleges and universities have been forced by the circumstances of colonial social orders to seek financial security through business interests in elite athletic programs and to license sports gear that may benefit them financially.

The high transmissibility of SARS-CoV-2 created significant challenges for student athletic programs. The pandemic significantly impacted athletic seasons and reduced revenue as a result (Anderson, 2020). Team contact sports do not facilitate social distancing on the field or in the locker room. Fitness centers were found to be high risk places for spread (Chang et al., 2020), and so there was no reason to doubt that other athletic training facilities would represent virus spreading risks, too. However, the financial pressures on athletic programs and student athletes forced consideration of competing despite the risks.

The National Collegiate Athletics Association conducted a study intended to assess the consequences of COVID-19 closures in April and May, 2020, on collegiate athletes. The study found that, not surprisingly, that the closures had been associated with loss of fitness and with mental health symptoms (NCAA Research, 2020). These findings were very similar to what was being seen in the larger public in the US. The overall take away was that student athletes were negatively impacted from the COVID-19 shutdowns, implying that shutting down athletics were not helpful to student athletes. One can imagine these findings being used to advocate for reopening athletic events as in the best interests of the colleges and universities, and perhaps also to the student athletes. Not surprisingly, collegiate athletics did reopen with the rest of society in the summer and fall of 2020, with mixed results. Many teams had issues with viral spread. Games and matches were cancelled, with some schools playing only a small portion of their schedules (e.g., Kearns et al., 2020). Some schools and individual athletes that opted out during that time for safety reasons. One athlete, allegedly dismissed from his team after opting out, is suing his former coach (Schrotenboer, 2021).

Unfortunately, the NCAA data on student athlete well-being were only a small part of the research findings on student athletes and the coronavirus. A college football player in Pennsylvania tragically died from COVID-19 that may have been contracted on campus, believed to be the first collegiate athlete to have passed (Witz, 2020). Many college students are young adults, a time when risk-taking and novelty-seeking is common. Just like other university students, college athletes take risks and see themselves as invulnerable, and therefore often will not abide by recommended health precautions. During that time, there was an ageist perception that younger adults were not vulnerable to COVID-19 like older adults that was probabilistically true generally for the age group but not necessarily true for high risk individuals of that age group.

Health researchers eventually found evidence of health concerns not reflected in the NCAA study for student athletes (NCAA Research, 2020), research that suggested certain student athletes were vulnerable. Emerging research confirmed cardiovascular risks to student athletes, research so compelling that the Director of the National Institute of Health, Francis Collins, posted a blog warning of the cardiological risks associated with COVID-19 among student athletes (Collins, 2020). Researchers who were investigating student athletes recovering from asymptomatic, mild, or moderate symptoms of COVID-19 found that over half were showing signs of abnormal echocardiograms and a significant minority were showing symptoms of myocarditis that threatened further cardiovascular complications under the stress of physical exertion (Brito et al., 2020). Researchers identified several predictors for post-COVID-19 complications to young athletes, such as asthma, diabetes, and hypertension (Harmon et al., 2020). Despite the potential risks, many athletes wanted to return to sports after COVID-19, so physicians developed a plan to determine when an athlete might return safely to sport activities after experiencing myocarditis (Kim et al., 2020). What remains unknown is whether these COVID-19 related cardiovascular events are precursors to longer-term cardiovascular problems. Myocarditis from COVID-19 was found not only to be a health risk for collegiate athletes but also for high school athletes (Kearns et al., 2020).

College student athletes also experienced long-term consequences of COVID-19, such as respiratory symptoms. There were isolated incidences of high school students being placed on ventilators with the associated potential consequences (Kearns et al., 2020). As a result of these health consequences, guidelines were also developed for high school student athletes returning from COVID-19 to control the cardio-health risks of subsequent exertion (Drezner et al., 2020). High school coaches with COVID-19 also experienced cardiovascular and respiratory distress with a few passing away as a result (Kearns et al., 2020).

Health and Mental Health Consequences of COVID on Children and Youth

The COVID-19 pandemic and its disruptions to the normal routines of children and parents seriously impacted family health and mental health. A survey conducted in 2020 found that 10% of parents and their children reported worsening mental health symptoms. In addition, work loss during the pandemic threatened insurance coverage for over two million children and increased food insecurity was a concern for 11% of US families with children (Patrick et al., 2020). The pandemic also significantly stressed relationships between children and parents (Challenge Success & NBC News, 2021). For example, mental health problems and suicide in children have occurred at alarming rates, attributed solely to the changes in lifestyle and education (Kyodo News, 2021; Leicester, 2021). In addition, there was both evidence and concern that the level of exposure to computer and phone screens during the pandemic would contribute to significant and dysfunctional changes in children's vision (Goshua, 2021; Wang et al., 2021).

Early data from the pandemic suggested that children might be impervious to the effects of the coronavirus, but that was also a time when children were not in school. Although younger children were less likely to have serious symptoms, some children suffered from robust immune responses with substantial inflammation that risked death from multisystem inflammatory syndrome, and in a rare instance resulted in a child being paralyzed (Bhojwani, 2021; LeRovere et al., 2021). The risks of long-term COVID-19 health related consequences to children from robust immune responses are still not well-understood but worrisome enough to be investigated by NIH (2021). Lower SES children globally also risked suffering indirect health consequences due to economic inequities. Poverty interacting with the circumstances of COVID-19 compounded malnutrition and hunger and stressed the already limited health care resources for children in many nations (Richards, Abdi, Stephenson, Northcote, & Mathieson, 2020; Roberton et al., 2020). Intergenerational poverty is a significant concern as impoverished children become adults (Wagmiller & Adelman, 2009).

Mental health was impacted by the challenging circumstances of education, with girls and minoritized students experiencing high levels of psychological stress as a result (Challenge Success & NBC News, 2021). Access to mental health services via hospital emergency departments during the US shutdown in the spring, 2020, remained comparable to visits in 2019, despite the significant reduction of overall pediatric visits to emergency departments (Leeb et al., 2020). Emergency department mental health visits rose significantly after the 2020 shutdowns in the US for both children aged 5–11 and youth over age 11 (Einhorn, 2020). Anxiety and depression in children and youth during the pandemic increased (Kumar & Naya, 2020), with enhanced concerns for child suicide globally (Kyodo News, 2021; Loades et al., 2020). In a survey study of the mental health of youth aged 11–17 assessed in May–November, 2020, the most cited reasons for self-reported anxiety and depression included coronavirus, current events, financial concerns, grief and loss, loneliness and isolation, and racism—stressors associated with the COVID-19 pandemic (Mental Health America, 2020). Prolonged loneliness is also a risk factor for many mental health problems including depression (National Science Foundation, 2016).

Immediate and long-term health and mental health consequences will impact education for years to come. Already financially stressed schools will be further challenged by post-pandemic health and mental health demands going forward. One can imagine that the financial resources of nations will be significantly challenged post-pandemic. It remains an open question if the financial concerns of education will become a higher priority in colonial cultures in the context of post-pandemic financial stress. Given the depth of COVID-19 consequences to minoritized communities and schools, economic inequities will likely persist well into the future without radical change to priorities (Dorn et al., 2020; Fox, 2020).

A Question of Values and Priorities: An Indigenous Interpretation

Colonial education was not intended to be of equitable quality and accessibility across all students. If education were considered to be an absolute right in the US from its inception, it would have been mentioned in the constitution or the bill of rights, but it was not. Schools have been used as a colonial method to control, assimilate, and isolate outgroup students from the mainstream, often resulting in abuses and consequential distrust of educational institutions. Separate and unequal educational systems created neglected schools that serve minoritized students. Simultaneously under-funded and under-resourced, educational systems have

Table 5.1 Colonial myths and education—a report card on US progress

Colonial myth	Colonial reality
American dream is attainable	Very few have shared in the dream over time because of systemic barriers
Education is highly valued in the US	The amount of resources dedicated to education, especially to public education, do not support this myth
Education is the ticket out of poverty	Class mobility has become significantly rarer over time in the US—poverty will likely worsen post-pandemic
Education levels the playing field	Inequities ensure that educational experiences are not equivalent—COVID-19 highlighted inherent inequities
School athletics are the ticket to success	Mixed outcomes—true for the very elite--the educational opportunity is helpful for some who are not among the very elite but not for all
US education is the best in the world	Outcomes do not support this myth—access to world class education in the US is reserved for the privileged
US values its children	Certainly not a top priority for care, funding, and resources—policies during COVID-19 often did not reflect valuing children

contributed to inequitable student outcomes that perpetuated other social inequities. Despite mythic beliefs in the power of education to lift up outgroup students, the reality of educational disparities has been mostly dream-dashing rather than dream-fulfilling (see Table 5.1).

Weaknesses in educational systems were apparent during the COVID-19 pandemic. Schools were ill equipped for prolonged closures and students fell through the cracks. Quality education was extremely difficult and unlikely during the pandemic simply because quality education was difficult and unlikely for many students pre-pandemic. The pandemic exacerbated pre-existing educational disparities, with minoritized students at greater risk for falling through the educational cracks of online instruction. Colonial educational inequities will be exacerbated for years to come, challenging already financially-strapped schools and families.

Indigenous Americans find psychological value in viewing children as sacred--in protecting the sacred treasure of our collective future. In order to promote psychological wellness over time, an investment in children is not only necessary, it is also wise. The best way to positively impact the future is to treat our children with sacred respect—to make children a social priority in order to advance psychological well-being intergenerationally. Healthy children in turn help to create healthy generations. Safe children will help to create a safe world.

Indigenous education emphasizes connectivity with nature as an important for learning and storytelling as a method for instruction. Emphasizing education through connectivity with nature would present more opportunities to get out into the ventilated real world for a more authentic learning experience under healthier conditions. Fresh air educational experiences likely would promote the ability to meet in-person safely when indoor experiences may not be safe. Storytelling to educate students would transmit cultural history intergenerationally in order to prevent colonial amnesia about the past, including pandemics (see also Chap. 11).

To prepare for future pandemics, education systems must be decolonized of their hierarchies that favor some and harm others. Resources should be free-flowing to benefit all students. Cutting edge technology and educational methods should be equally available. Investing in schools should be considered a top priority rather than an afterthought. Educators need to also decolonize hierarchical teaching methods that favor some groups over others, and coursework and textbooks transformed into multicultural perspectives that match to the educational needs of all students. An equitable education should be a right rather than privilege. If we are interested in advancing psychological wellness in the world, providing equitable education for all would be healthy step in the right direction.

References

Ali, S. S., Siemaszko, C. (2021, February 12). Teachers give thumbs up to new CDC roadmap for reopening schools during pandemic. NBC News. https://www.nbcnews.com/news/us-news/teachers-give-thumbs-new-cdc-roadmap-reopening-schools-during-pandemic-n1257749

Alker, J. (2019, October 29). The number of uninsured children is on the rise. Georgetown University Center for Children and Families. https://ccf.georgetown.edu/2019/10/29/the-number-of-uninsured-children-in-on-the-rise-acs/

Anderson, G. (2020, April 24). Pandemic hits college sports. Inside Higher Ed. https://www.insidehighered.com/news/2020/04/24/financial-crisis-related-coronavirus-hits-athletic-departments

APA Presidential Task Force on Educational disparities. (2012). *Ethnic and racial disparities in education: Psychology's contribution to understanding and reducing disparities*. American Psychological Association. https://www.apa.org/ed/resources/racial-disparities.pdf

Associated Press. (2021, March 24). School survey shows 'critical gaps' for in-person learning. Author. https://apnews.com/article/joe-biden-us-news-race-and-ethnicity-coronavirus-pandemic-72aa9af9ca082769e4fb2e8ae478c3d3

Baker, B. D., & Di Carlo, M. (2020). *The coronavirus pandemic and K-12 education funding*. Albert Shanker Institute. https://www.shankerinstitute.org/resource/coronavirus-pandemic-and-k-12-education-funding

Barbara, V. (2021, January 25). I can't believe I need to say this, but we need schools more than bars: What we're facing in Brazil is an educational catastrophe. The New York Times. https://www.nytimes.com/2021/01/25/opinion/brazil-schools-coronavirus.html?auth=login-email&login=email

Bennett, K. (2020, November 13). Ivanka Trump and Jared Kushner's children withdrawn from school after administrators raised concerns about adherence to Covid precautions. CNN. https://www.cnn.com/2020/11/13/politicis/jared-kushner-ivanka-trump-children-school-covid/index.html

Bhojwani, J. (2021, September 16). Covid likely led to a rare disorder that left 8-year old girl paralyzed. CNN. https://www.nbcnews.com/news/us-news/covid-likely-led-rare-disorder-left-8-year-old-girl-n1279336

Blume, A. W. (2020). *A new psychology based on community, equality, and care of the earth: An indigenous American perspective*. ABC-CLIO/Praeger.

Bombay, A., Matheson, K., & Anisman, H. (2014). The intergenerational effects of Indian residential schools: Implications for the concept of historical trauma. *Transcultural Psychiatry, 51*(3), 320–338. https://doi.org/10.1177/1363461513503380

Bombay, A., Matheson, K., & Anisman, H. (2017). Perspectives on intergenerational transmission of trauma: The case of Aboriginal peoples in Canada. In T. V. Cooper, M. C. Skewes, K. B. Schmaling, & A. W. Blume (Eds.), *Social issues in living color: Challenges and solu-*

tions from the perspective of ethnic minority psychology: Promoting health and well-being (pp. 171–196). Praeger/ABC-CLIO.

Brito, D., Meester, S., Yanamala, N., Patel, H. B., Balcik, B. J., Casaclang-Verzosa, G., Seetharam, K., Riveros, D., Beto, R. J., Balla, S., Monseau, A. J., & Sengupta, P. P. (2020). High prevalence of pericardial involvement in college student athletes recovering from COVID-19. Journal of the American College of Cardiology: Cardiovascular Imaging. https://doi.org/10.1016/j.jcmg.2020.10.023.

Canvas. (2020). *State of student success and engagement in higher education: 2020 global research study and trends*. Infrastructure. https://www.instructure.com/en-au/canvas/resources/all/state-of-student-success-engagement

CDC. (2021, February 12). K-12 operational strategy. Author. https://urldefense.com/v3/__https://www.cdc.gov/coronavirus/2019-ncov/community/schools-childcare/operation-strategy.html__;!!JmPEgBY0HMszNaDT!4ka-kPVLlcMhJGIjzV-yfgZFM3mL9UdGuMoiggojw3Fsulqk8owdqW6VDX8iMqan$.

Challenge Success and NBC News. (2021, May 14). *Kids under* pressure. Stanford University Graduate School of Education. https://challengesuccess.org/resources/kids-under-pressure-a-look-at-student-well-being-and-engagement-during-the-pandemic/

Chang, S., Pierson, E., Koh, P. W., Gerardin, J., Redbird, B., Gursky, D., & Leskovec, J. (2020). Mobility network models of COVID-19 explain inequities and inform reopening. *Nature*. https://doi.org/10.1038/s41586-020-2923-3

Chinn, P. C., & Hughes, S. (1987). Representation of minority students in special education classes. *Remedial and Special Education, 8*(4), 41–46. https://doi.org/10.1177/074193258700800406

Collins, F. (2020, October 1). COVID-19 can damage hearts of some college athletes. National Institutes of Health. https://directorsblog.nih.gov/2020/10/01/covid-19-can-damage-hearts-of-some-college-athletes/

Dorn, E., Hancock, B., Sarakatsannis, J., & Viruleg, E. (2020, December 8). COVID-19 and learning loss—Disparities grow and students need help. McKinsey and Company. https://www.mckinsey.com/industries/public-and-social-sector/our-insights/covid-19-and-learning-loss-disparities-grow-and-students-need-help

Drezner, J. A., Heinz, W. M., Asif, I. M., Batten, C. G., Fields, K. B., Raukar, N. P., Valentine, V. D., & Walter, K. D. (2020). Cardiopulmonary considerations for high school student-athletes during the COVID-19 pandemic: NFHS-AMSSM guidance statement. *Sports Health, 12*(5), 459–461. https://doi.org/10.1177/1941738120941490

Dunbar-Ortiz, R. (2014). *An indigenous peoples' history of the United States*. Beacon Press.

Einhorn, E. (2020, December 15). *Covid is having a devastating impact on children--and the vaccine won't fix everything*. https://www.nbcnews.com/news/education/covid-having-devastating-impact-children-vaccine-won-t-fix-everything-n1251172

Fox, M. (2020, December 9). How the pandemic will affect Black and Latino children's education and wealth for years to come. NBC News. https://www.nbcnews.com/news/nbcblk/how-pandemic-will-effect-black-latino-children-s-education-wealth-n1250598

Gecker, J. (2021, September 23). COVID-19 creates dire US shortage of teachers, school staff. : Associated Press. https://apnews.com/article/business-science-health-education-california-b6c495eab9a2a8f1a3ca068582c9d3c7

Goshua, A. (2021, February 22). 'A doozy of a year': Experts worry screen time during Covid-19 could increase vision problems in kids. STAT News. https://www.statnews.com/2021/02/22/a-doozy-of-a-year-experts-worry-screen-time-during-covid-19-could-increase-vision-problems-in-kids/

Hahn, H., Lou, C., & Isaacs, J. B. (2020). *How much does the federal government spend on programs for children?* Urban Institute. https://www.urban.org/sites/default/files/publication/102752/how-much-does-the-federal-government-spend-on-programs-benefiting-children.pdf

Haider, A. (2020, January 12). The basic facts about children in poverty. Center for American Progress. https://www.americanprogress.org/issues/poverty/reports/2021/01/12/494506/

basic-facts-children-poverty/#:~:text=In%202019%2C%2014.4%20percent%20of,below%20 the%20official%20poverty%20measure.

Harmon, K. G., Pottinger, P. S., Baggish, A. L., Drezner, J. A., Luks, A. M., Thompson, A. A., & Swaminathan, S. (2020). Comorbid medical conditions in young athletes: Considerations for preparticipation guidance during the COVID-19 pandemic. *Sports Health, September–October.* https://doi.org/10.1177/1941738120939079

Helms, J. E. (2012). A legacy of eugenics underlies racial-group comparisons in intelligence testing. *Industrial and Organizational Psychology, 5*(2), 176–179. https://doi.org/10.1111/j.1754-9434.2012.01426.x

Inside Higher Ed. (2021, February 15). *Vaccines for educators—but not all educators*. Author. https://www.insidehighered.com/news/2021/02/15/evolving-patchwork-approaches-how-states-prioritize-educators-covid-vaccines-raises?utm_source=Inside+Higher+Ed&utm_campaign=447e236cbd-DNU_2021_COPY_02&utm_medium=email&utm_term=0_1fcbc04421-447e236cbd-197467985&mc_cid=447e236cbd&mc_eid=ecf63688ce.

Kearns, L., Bachynski, K., & Caplan, A. L. (2020, November 26). Add Covid-related myocarditis, mechanical ventilation, and death to this year's football risks. STAT News. https://www.statnews.com/2020/11/26/myocarditis-mechanical-netilation-death-join-football-risks-covid-19/

Kim, J. H., Levine, B. D., Phelan, D., Emery, M. S., Martinez, M. W., Chung, E. H., Thompson, P. D., & Baggish, A. L. (2020). Coronavirus disease 2019 and the athletic heart. Emerging perspectives on pathology, risks, and return to play. *JAMA Cardiology,* e1–e9. https://doi.org/10.1001/jamacardio.2020.5890.

Krieg, G. (2020, July). 'Normally, people don't play with kids' lives': Trump's push to reopen schools becomes another partisan fight. CNN. https://www.cnn.com/2020/07/14/politics/trump-schools-reopening/index.html.

Kuhfeld, M., Tarasawa, B., Johnson, A., Ruzek, E., & Lewis, K. (2020). *Learning during COVID-19: Initial findings on students' reading and math achievement and growth.* NWEA Research. https://www.nwea.org/research/publication/learning-during-covid-19-initial-findings-on-students-reading-and-math-achievement-and-growth

Kumar, A., & Naya, K. R. (2020). COVID-19 and its mental health consequences. *Journal of Mental Health, 180*(6), 817–818. https://doi.org/10.1080/09638237.2020.1757052

Kuriloff, P., (2020, December 3). Covid disrupted American kids' schools. It might be a chance to change them for the better. : NBC News. https://www.nbcnews.com/think/opinion/covid-disrupted-american-kids-schools-it-might-be-chance-change-ncna1248824

Kyodo News. (2021, February 15). Juvenile suicides in Japan hit record-high 479 in 2020. Kyodo News. https://english.kyodonews.net/news/2021/02/2b5a05d20889-juvenile-suicides-in-japan-hit-record-high-479-in-2020.html

Leeb, R. T., Bitsko, R. H., Radhakrishnan, L., Martinez, P., Njai, R., Holland, K. M. (2020, November 13). Mental health-related emergency department visits among children aged <18 years during the COVID-19 pandemic—United States, January 1-October 17, 2020. MMWR, 69(45), 1675–1680. https://doi.org/10.15585/mmwr.mm6945a3.

Leicester, J. (2021, March 12). Global rise in childhood mental health issues amid pandemic. Associated Press. https://apnews.com/article/global-rise-childhood-mental-health-pandemic-8329ceff77ac8e1e0f90a32214e7def1

LeRovere, K. L., Riggs, B. J., Poussaint, T. Y., Young, C. C., Newhams, M. M., Maamari, M., Walker, T. C., Singh, A. R., Dapul, H., Hobbs, C. V., McLaughlin, G. E., Son, M. B. F., Maddux, A. B., Clouser, K. N., Rowan, C. M., McGuire, J. K., Fitzgerald, J. C., Gertz, S. J., Shein, S.L. …Randolph, A. G. (2021). Neurologic involvement in children and adolescents hospitalized in the United States for COVID-19 or multisystem inflammatory syndrome. *JAMA Neurology* https://doi.org/10.1001/jamaneurol.2021.0504.

Loades, M. E., Chatburn, E., Higson-Sweeney, N., Reynolds, S., Shafran, R., Brigden, A., Linney, C., McManus, M. N., Borwick, C., & Crawley, E. (2020). Rapid systematic review: The impact of social isolation and loneliness on the mental health of children and adolescents in the context of COVID-19. *Journal of the American Academy of Child & Adolescent Psychiatry, 59*(11), 1218–1239.e3. https://doi.org/10.1016/j.jaac.2020.05.009

Lowe, R. (1980). Eugenics and education: A note on the origins of the intelligence testing movement in England. *Educational Studies, 6*(1), 1–8. https://doi.org/10.1080/0305569800060101

McKenzie, L. (2020). *Bridging the digital divide: Lessons from COVID-19*. Inside Higher Ed. https://www.insidehighered.com/content/bridging-digital-divide-lessons-covid-19

McPhillips, D. (2021, February 15). Nearly all US kids live in red zones under new DCD schools guidance. CNN. https://www.cnn.com/2021/02/12/health/us-kids-red-zones-cdc-school-guideline/index.html

Mental Health America. (2020, December 9). Young people's mental health in 2020: Hope, advocacy, and action for the future. Author. https://www.mhanational.org/research-reports/young-peoples-mental-halth-2020-hope-advocacy-and-action-future

Mulvihill, G., Sainz, A., & Kunzelman, M. (2021, January 31). Push to reopen schools could leave out millions of students. Associated Press. https://apnews.com/article/joe-biden-anthony-fauci-coronavirus-pandemic-infectious-diseases-us-news-eaa4fefe24af8649990e0f0e50ef5dd1

National Geographic Society. (2021, June). The year that isolates us. *National Geographic, 238*(7), 78.

National Science Foundation. (2016, February 3). The profound power of loneliness. National Science Foundation. https://www.nsf.gov/discoveries/disc_summ.jsp?cntn_id=137534

NCAA. (2020). *NCAA student-athlete COVID-19 well-being study*. https://www.ncaa.org/about/resources/research/ncaa-student-athlete-covid-19-well-being-study

Nies, J. (1996). Native American history: A chronology of a culture's vast achievements and their links to world events. Ballantine Books.

NIH. (2021, February 16). Longitudinal study follows multisystem inflammatory syndrome in children (MIS-C). Author. https://www.nhlbi.nih.gov/news/2021/longitudinal-study-follows-multisystem-inflammatory-syndrome-children-mis-c

Patrick, S. W., Henkhaus, L. E., Zickafoose, J. S., Lovell, K., Halvorson, A., Loch, S., Letterie, M., & Davis, M. M. (2020). Well-being of parents and children during the COVID-19 pandemic: A national survey. *Pediatrics, 146*(4), e2020016824. https://doi.org/10.1542/peds.2020-016824

Redden, E. (2021, July 16). A waiting game. Inside Higher Ed. https://www.insidehighered.com/news/2021/07/16/all-eyes-vaccination-rates-colleges-mandating-covid-shots

Reuters (2021, July 30). Florida governor blocks school mask mandates, says parents can choose. Author. https://www.reuters.com/world/us/florida-gov-desantis-issue-order-giving-parents-choice-mask-children-school-2021-07-30/

Richards, K., Abdi, M., Stephenson, H., Northcote, C., & Mathieson, K. (2020). *Nutrition critical: Why we must all act now to tackle child malnutrition*. Save the Children. https://resourcecentre.savethechildren.net/library/nutrition-critical-why-we-must-act-now-tackle-child-malnutrition

Richmond, T., & Hollingsworth, H. (2020, September 26). US colleges struggle to salvage semester amid outbreaks. Associated Press. https://apnews.com/article/virus-outbreak-college-football-football-archive-2fec1a5f332f0ad1508e0a94f94ec048

Roberton, T., Carter, E. D., Chou, V. B., Stegmuller, A. R., Jackson, B. D., Tam, Y., Sawadogo-Lewis, T., & Walker, N. (2020). Early estimates of the indirect effects of the COVID-19 pandemic on maternal and child mortality in low-income and middle-income countries: A modelling study. *Lancet Global Health, 8*, e901–e908. https://doi.org/10.1016/S2214-109X(20)30229-1

Schmaling, K. B., Blume, A. W., Engstrom, M. R., Paulos, R., & De Fina, S. (2017). Leaky educational pipeline for racial/ethnic minorities. In A. Czopp (Ed.), *Social issues in living color: Challenges and solutions from the perspective of ethnic minority psychology, Vol. 2* (pp. 103–122). *Societal and global issues*. A. W. Blume, Series Ed.). Praeger.

Schrotenboer, B. (2021, September 1). Washington State coach Nick Rolovich sued by former player Kassidy Woods. USA Today. https://www.usatoday.com/story/sports/ncaaf/pac12/2021/09/01/washington-state-coach-nick-rolovich-sued-ex-player-kassidy-woods/5683198001/

Siegel, D. A., Reses, H. E., Cool, A. J., Shapiro, C. N., Hsu, J., Boehmer, T. K., Cornwell, C. R., Gray, E. B., Henley, S. J., Lochner, K., Suthar, A. B., Lyons, B. C., Mattockes, L., Hartnett, K., Adjemian, J., van Santen, K. L., Sheppard, M., Soetebier, K. A., … Taizes, E. (2021). Trends in COVID-19 cases, emergency department visits, and hospital admissions among children and adolescents aged 0–17 years-United States, August 2020–August 2021. *MMWR, 70*, 1249–1254. https://doi.org/10.15585/mmwr.mm7036e1

UNICEF. (2020). *COVID-19: Are children able to continue learning during school closures?* Author. https://data.unicef.org/resources/remote-learning-reachability-factsheet/

US Department of Education. (1994). *Education reforms and students at risk: A review of the current state of the art*. Author. https://www2.ed.gov/pubs/EdReformStudies/EdReforms/chap1b.html

Valant, J. (2020, July 29). School reopening plans linked to politics rather than public health. Brookings Institute. https://www.brookings.edu/blog/brown-center-chalkboard/2020/07/29/school-reopening-plans-linked-to-politics-rather-than-public-health/

Wagmiller, R. L., & Adelman, R. M. (2009). *Childhood and intergenerational poverty*. National Center for Children in Poverty. https://www.nccp.org/wp-content/uploads/2020/05/text_909.pdf

Wang, L., Musch, D. C., Wei, N., Qi, X., Ding, G., Li, X., Li, J., Song, L., Zhang, L., Ning, Y., Zeng, X., Hua, N., Li, S., & Qian, X. (2021). Progression of myopia in school-aged children after COVID-19 home confinement. *JAMA Ophthalmology*. https://doi.org/10.1001/jamaophthalmol.2020.6239

Whitford, E. (2021, May 5). Public higher ed funding still has not recovered from 2008 recession. Inside Higher Ed. https://www.insidehighered.com/news/2020/05/05/public-higher-education-worse-spot-ever-heading-recession

Winfield, A. G. (2012). Resuscitating bad science: Eugenics past and present. In W. H. Watkins (Ed.), *The assault on public education* (pp. 143–159). Teachers College Press.

Witz, B. (2020, September 23). College football's worst fear in the pandemic: The death of a player. New York Times. https://www.nytimes.com/2020/09/23/sports/ncaafootball/college-football-death-jamain-stephens-html

Chapter 6
Health Inequity and COVID-19

Abstract Intergenerationally persistent health disparities and inequities among minoritized citizens of colonial nations have worsened during the COVID-19 pandemic. The SARS-CoV-2 virus opportunistically and severely attacked those with premorbid health and mental health conditions, contributing to disparities of COVID-19 incidence, hospitalizations, and death among people of color. The COVID-19 disease has been found to produce a range of respiratory and cardiovascular symptoms, as well as loss of taste and smell, damage to organs, and immune-related inflammatory responses. The COVID-19 disease also has been linked to significant mental health consequences, such as anxiety and depression, and cognitive symptoms that may range from memory problems and brain fog to psychotic symptoms. Many people also have long-term presentation of symptoms that are poorly understood. Colonial health care systems were ill-prepared for a sustained global health crisis and responded without a unified approach or vision. Health and mental health care providers have experienced significant psychological consequences and burnout as a result of being overworked, under protected and supported, and even abused by the public. The global psychological consequences from COVID-19 present tremendous long-term challenges to psychologists and other health care professionals.

The first few chapters of this book have highlighted a sad and important truth concerning minoritized people: For many, COVID-19 was not the most imminent threat to their lives due to pre-existing inequities. Many outgroup families also faced tremendous economic challenges going into the pandemic that were also compounded by the pandemic, and others faced the challenges of bias, discrimination and stigma that threatened health and safety. Some have suffered the challenges of environmental degradation as well, which also have threatened health and well-being. Many of those pre-existing inequities conspire together to create risks for pre-existing health inequities as well, inequities with heightened risks for other health risks.

Very early in the pandemic it became apparent that the coronavirus was an opportunistic virus that preyed on those with other health problems. The SARS-CoV-2 virus is extremely efficient as a contagion and stealth in that its spread can occur

A. W. Blume, *Colonialism and the COVID-19 Pandemic*, International and Cultural Psychology, https://doi.org/10.1007/978-3-030-92825-4_6

without symptoms. As discussed previously, the virus was also able to capitalize on the existing inequities that left certain groups of people more vulnerable, such as minoritized outgroups and older adults. The inequities created by colonialism have contributed to intergenerational health disparities that are a primary risk factor for serious symptoms and risk of death from COVID-19. Before discussing the association of health disparities with the COVID-19 pandemic, the symptoms of COVID-19 and the nature of health and mental health disparities will be briefly reviewed to provide a foundation for understanding the potential health impact of the virus over time.

Review of COVID-19 History and Concerns

Well before the emergence of SARS-CoV-2, many Americans were rightfully concerned about the certain problems in society without necessarily linking those concerns to a pandemic per se. In December of 2019, the Pew Research Center released a poll on what Americans saw as the major problems facing the US. Notably, affordable health care was the number one concern, followed by drug addiction, affordable higher education, the federal budget deficit, climate change, economic inequities, racism, immigration, terrorism, sexism, and jobs (Pew Research Center, 2019), issues discussed at length in this book. Americans had some inkling that injustices and inequities left the nation vulnerable but were unable to see the larger picture of their commonalities. Amidst those vulnerabilities SARS-CoV-2 arrived.

The SARS-CoV-2 virus that causes COVID-19 is certainly not the most lethal virus seen in recent times. Hemorrhagic viruses such as those that cause Ebola or Marburg diseases have known fatality rates greater than 24% and perhaps closer to 53.8% for Marburg and 65% for Ebola, but as blood borne pathogens, they do not spread as easily as SARS-CoV-2 and often kill a host before spread is possible (Nyakarahuka et al., 2016). And SARS-Cov-2 is not the only significant viral pandemic in recent time—HIV has plagued humans for generations now although recent treatments such have allowed people to live with the virus for many years and have reduced spread and mortality rates significantly (Bosh et al., 2020). However, SARS-CoV-2 has the potential for droplet and airborne transmission at relatively short distances, making it much more efficient at spread than HIV, and up to half of all those infected may be asymptomatic (Centers for Disease Control [CDC], 2020a), making it a potentially lethal and stealth virus.

The symptoms of COVID-19 have been unusual and pervasive, sometimes common cold like and other times much more severe and unpredictable. At first it was believed that COVID-19 was primarily a respiratory disease, but it has also shown symptoms common to vascular diseases (NIH, 2020; Siddiqi et al., 2021). As a coronavirus, SARS-CoV-2 is in the same virus family as the common cold (National Institutes of Health [NIH], 2020). Common symptoms include nasal symptoms, potentially high fever, coughing and trouble breathing, sore throat, headaches, myalgia and other physical pain, sometimes gastrointestinal symptoms, and a pronounced loss of smell and taste (CDC, 2020b). However, as discussed earlier in the book, COVID-19 also may present with potentially severe cardiovascular symptoms. In addition, there is evidence that SARS-CoV-2 attack cells of the pancreas, and may be linked to new onset of diabetes (Wu et al., 2020). People with COVID-19 have succumbed from a wide range of causes including respiratory distress, pneumonia, organ failure, heart attacks, strokes, and inflammatory immune reactions often seen in children (NIH, 2020; Galeotti & Bayry, 2020; Siddiqi et al., 2021; Zimmermann & Curtis, 2020).

Asymptomatic infectious carriers contributed to widespread community spread, often without detection. In December, 2019, before its stealth nature was known by scientists, it was believed that COVID-19 cases were confined to China. The first known cases in the US occurred in Washington state in late February, 2020. However, when asymptomatic spread became apparent, researchers began to look back in time for evidence of SARS-CoV-2. What they found was startling to some, with evidence that COVID-19 was spreading in Europe in December, 2019 (Fox, 2020), and that two patients died in California from previously undetected COVID-19 in January, 2020 (Hanna et al., 2020). The first US wave in early 2020 brought significant challenges such as finding places to store and bury bodies (Anderson, 2021). In 2020, a study found evidence of excessive outpatient clinic and hospital visits for respiratory discomfort and cough that was significantly higher than the annual expected rate in the Los Angeles metropolitan area beginning in late December, 2019, and extending into February, 2020 (Elmore et al., 2020). Later in 2021, researchers reported finding blood samples with antibodies for SARS-CoV-2 among people living in the US Midwest in late 2019, suggesting inland spread much earlier than originally suspected (Althoff et al., 2021). That evidence would correspond with lab results from three deer in the US unexpectedly showed antibodies to SARS-CoV-2 in January, 2020 (Maron, 2021). Finding cases earlier than previously thought is not unusual when investigating a pandemic. For example, the first US patient with AIDS has been traced back to the late 1960s (Highleyman, 1999), and evidence suggests that people in Africa were infected as early as the late 1950s (Zhu et al., 1998). It would not be surprising to eventually find historic COVID-19 cases that occurred before December, 2019. In addition, a forensic medicine study found genetic evidence of a coronavirus epidemic in eastern Asia approximately 20,000 years ago (Souilmi et al., 2021).

Globally, there had been over 220 million confirmed infections by August, 2021, and nearly 4.5 million deaths (WHO, 2021). At the time I wrote this sentence, the US surpassed 500,000 known deaths from the COVID-19 on February 22, 2021 (ironically George Washington's birthday anniversary—see Fig. 6.1), with over 100,000 of those deaths occurring in a little over a month during early 2021 amidst a significant COVID-19 surge that coincided with colder weather and holiday gatherings (Hanna & Wolfe, November 13, 2020; Hollingsworth & Webber, 2021; Vera et al., 2021). The losses were so pronounced in the US that the country's life expectancy decreased more than one year in a matter of six months (Arias et al., 2021; Marchione, 2021). The reduction in American life expectancy is difficult to conceptualize, but even more so when considering that during the same six months, Black American life expectancy fell 2.7 years (Arias et al., 2021; Marchione, 2021). The

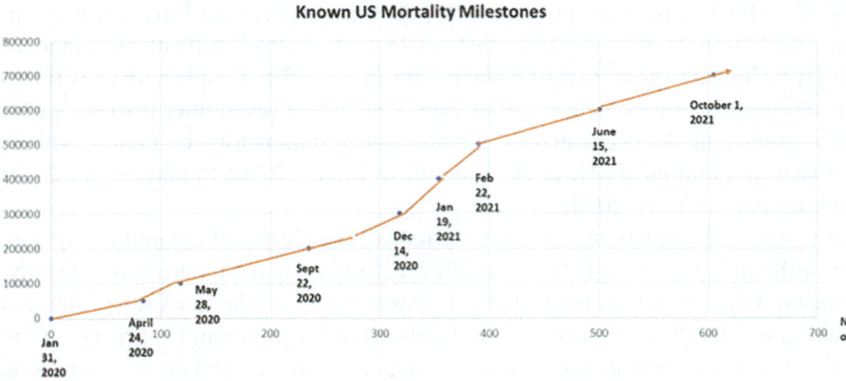

Fig. 6.1 US mortality milestones for COVID-19 as of August, 2021. Note: The death toll was likely much higher than the official tally since many deaths related to SARS-CoV-2 were recorded as deaths due to other causes and due to certain states underreporting their data

US suffered a greater loss of life expectancy than other high-income nations likely due to systemic racism and health disparities (Woolf et al., 2021).

By late summer 2021, 1 out of every 500 US citizens had died from COVID-19 and the US official death toll exceeded that of the Spanish Flu pandemic (Holcombe, 2021; Johnson, 2021)—tolls that were likely significantly undercounted for both pandemics. The delta variant surge capitalized on the large numbers of unvaccinated, with another surge of mortalities and hospitalizations so intense that Idaho was forced to ration health care (Boone, 2021). Those who were lost to COVID-19 were honored in the fall of 2021 with what grew to be over 700,000 white flags spread across 20 acres of the US Capitol Mall (Reuters, 2021). The loss of human capital and complicated grief will be major psychological concerns globally post-pandemic (Pearce et al., 2021).

Medical comorbidities also complicated the picture in terms of mortalities attributed to COVID-19. In many US states, causes of death have been assigned to the pre-existing medical condition rather than COVID-19, and there were likely many COVID-19 deaths never diagnosed. The CDC compared the US mortality rate during the pandemic with the expected mortality rate from non-pandemic data, resulting in an estimate of excess deaths that would not have been expected in a non-pandemic year. The total suggests how many deaths may have been misattributed to pre-existing medical conditions or to undiagnosed COVID-19. Between February, 2020, and February, 2021, there were at least 143,000 excess deaths over the expected mortality rate (CDC, 2021a), suggesting over 600,000 people had passed in the US due to COVID-19 by February, 2021.

The stresses of the pandemic also contributed to other causes of death. I remember noticing early in the pandemic that people were driving very recklessly on empty highways. Racing on the freeways seemed more common than before the pandemic, and drivers appeared to be taking more dramatic chances in passing and weaving between slower cars. More than once I uttered the sentiment that such and such driver acted as if they did not care about life. These observations were highly subjective, yet data have consistently supported the subjective observations. Although US drivers drove significantly fewer miles in 2020 and the first part of 2021, deaths from motor vehicle accidents were significantly higher due to risky behaviors, such as substance use, high speed, and neglecting seatbelts (Associated Press, 2021b). Perhaps some accidents were linked to depression during the pandemic, or perhaps even to cognitive consequences of SARS-CoV-2 that are discussed subsequently.

The development of treatments and vaccinations to address COVID-19 provided tools to contain the spread and potentially prevent high mortality (see Chap. 7). It had been hoped that with the help of vaccine-assisted herd immunity that eventually the threat will be reduced, perhaps becoming a seasonal annoyance rather than a pandemic threat (Lavine et al., 2021), but that level of vaccination was threatened by hesitancy and misinformation. However, the breadth of spread has also enhanced the likelihood of mutated variants of the virus, some that may hinder the work of vaccines (CDC, 2021c). New variants increased reinfection rates, potentially thwarting efforts toward collective immunity as was seen in South America (Andina Agencia Pruana de Noticias, 2021; Associated Press, 2021a; Kupferschmidt, 2021; Sabino et al., 2021). In the US, reinfections are of concern, but since those data were not tracked well, it was unclear how widespread the problem might be (Aleccia, 2021). An additional risk is that people could be infected by more than one variant at a time (Roberts, 2021).

Researchers found that asymptomatic carriers of the disease were not as likely to develop antibodies as those with palpable symptoms (He et al., 2021), suggesting they may be at risk for reinfection. New variants also caused reinfection concerns, with some researchers are projecting that COVID-19 may have seasonal waves lasting into 2022 and beyond requiring continued social distancing (Kissler et al., 2020). Allowing uncontrolled spread of the virus has contributed greatly to uncertainty and stress in the US.

Colonial Health Care Systems Deliver Colonial Responses

One of the most interesting outcomes during the pandemic was how poorly the US health care system responded to address COVID-19. The wholly inadequate response was diagnostic of underlying colonial tenets that created a flawed US health care system. In addition, the US populist-nationalist government early in the pandemic fully embraced colonial tenets as its way to govern, diminishing hope for a collectively-oriented public health approach.

The US health care system was exposed not as one unified system but as many splintered units, reflected the colonial individualism of the US. Cities, counties, states, and the federal government all have their own health care systems. The federal system advises what they should do, but in reality, the splintered health care entities make their own decisions concerning what to abide by and what to ignore.

There was no centralized coordination that encouraged national cooperation or collaboration in the process. Evidence of the weaknesses of splintered US health care systems was obvious in the national outcomes from COVID-19.

The splintered systems encouraged competition among the various health entities much more easily than collaboration. Examples of the lack of cooperation abound--competitive PPE and medical equipment purchases for which health care systems bid against one another to drive up medical costs, varied safety guidelines state by state working at cross-purposes to prevent spread, vaccine delivery systems that were both competitive and uneven, and public confusion because there were many different competing messages about what to do and what not to do. The result was one mixed-up mess and thousands of unnecessary casualties.

The populist-nationalist government of former-President Trump believed strongly in pandemic responses that elevated liberty and individualism, compounding the weaknesses of the health care systems. No consistent federal processes were in place to promote unity across the splintered health care systems. In addition, there was an effort to take away federal protections for pre-existing health conditions and other policies, potentially contributing to less insurance coverage among people already at risk (Abelson & Goodnough, 2021).

American health care seems to be good at inventions and innovation (a.k.a., the science) but poor at collective processes (a.k.a., policies and responses; see also Chap. 7). In the context of a pandemic--an interdependent health threat--the splintered individualized systems were not up to the collective task. The health care systems also were doomed to fail because of the sheer number of pre-existing colonial inequities and in the face of exercises of personal liberty to thwart the pandemic response (see also Chap. 9). With so many different systems in a hierarchical society, inequities across the many systems was inevitable. Health care systems often reflect the disparities inherent in the geographical areas they serve—disparities that are discussed later in this chapter. Without a compete transformation of the health care systems, it is likely that the deadly mistakes of COVID-19 will be repeated during future pandemics.

COVID-19 Symptoms and Their Relevance to Psychological Health

The psychological consequences of social isolation and social chaos in the US were predictable. The stress of the COVID-19 pandemic contributed to a wide variety of psychological symptoms. A majority of Americans surveyed reported feeling lonely, miserable, restless, unhappy, and unsupported (APA, 2020b). Those unpleasant circumstances alone warranted concerns of psychological consequences from the pandemic, but there was more.

Another unpleasant surprise from COVID-19 was its mental health symptoms. A large retrospective cohort study found that people with pre-existing mental disorders were at increased risk for SARS-CoV-2 infection independent of other health diagnoses. Investigators also found that COVID-19 was much more likely to precede an initial diagnosis for anxiety or depression than several other acute diagnoses such as gall bladder or kidney stones, broken bones, and infections including influenza (Taquet et al., 2020).

The COVID-19 disease seems to attack the brain, particularly the hippocampus, contributing to potential memory problems post-infection (Ritchie et al., 2020). In a study investigating the impact of COVID-19 on the brain, large cells from bone marrow (referred to as megakaryocytes) that create platelets for clotting were unexpectedly found in brain capillaries of COVID-19 victims (Nauen et al., 2021). People who were placed on ventilators were also susceptible to cognitive problems post-infection (Ritchie et al., 2020). Inflammatory responses of the immune system have been linked to potential post-infection cognitive difficulties (Zhou et al., 2020). The COVID-19 disease also has been linked to the onset of psychotic symptoms in a small minority of patients (Parra et al., 2020). Perhaps stress triggered a first break, but there were other risks for psychotic symptoms, such as inflammation, the virus overwhelming the central nervous system, or use of corticosteroids (Parra et al., 2020). Not only was COVID-19 linked to psychotic symptoms, but also a pre-pandemic diagnosis of a schizophrenia spectrum disorder may have increased mortality by two-fold (Nemani et al., 2021).

Regardless of cause, COVID-19 risks cognitive dysfunction that may require long-term psychological and medical care. Long-term COVID-19 symptoms may include cognitive decline, but the course of the decline is not well-understood. Long-term research is needed to determine if there are increased risks for Alzheimer's (Heneka et al., 2020; Ritchie et al., 2020).

The COVID-19 pandemic has complicated the work of mental health professionals in other ways. Very early in the pandemic the alarm was being sounded about the potential for a mental health pandemic that may continue for years post-pandemic (APA, 2020a; Pfeifferbaum & North, 2020). One systematic review of research found evidence that the pandemic had contributed to worsening symptoms in people with pre-pandemic mental health issues, in addition to the onset of new mental health concerns. The same review study found an uptick in anxiety, depressive, and post-traumatic stress symptoms during the pandemic, as well as a decreased public sense of psychological wellness (Vindegaard & Benros, 2020). Alcohol use with its potential long-term health and mental health consequences was up significantly in the US in 2020 (APA, 2021; Pollard et al., 2020; Ridout et al., 2021). Concerns have also been expressed about US weight gain (APA, 2021; Ridout et al., 2021). Emergency departments in the US were seeing significantly more opioid overdoses in 2020 when compared to 2019 (Holland et al., 2021). Mental health professionals speculated as to whether hoarding behaviors and sanitizing routines of the pandemic would become obsessive-compulsive behaviors post-pandemic for many (Fontenelle & Miguel, 2020; Nowak et al., 2020).

There was also great concern that economic and health related stress, substance misuse, and the sequestering of families during the pandemic would contribute to increased family violence. Unfortunately, the circumstances of the pandemic seemed to have contributed to less help seeking related to violence (Evans et al., 2020; Holland et al., 2021; Lawson et al., 2020). Increased child abuse might have gone unnoticed when comparing declining 2020 emergency department visits to 2019 data, but the 2020 overall ratio of visits related to child abuse increased compared to 2019 (Swedo et al., 2020).

Depression in particular was of increasing concern during the COVID-19 pandemic (APA, 2021; Fitzpatrick et al., 2020; Holland et al., 2021; Ridout et al., 2021). One small study early in the pandemic found a significant association between self-reports of depressive symptoms and indicators of immune response to the coronavirus (Yuan et al., 2020). Emergency departments saw a significant increase in visits associated with suicide attempts in 2020 when compared to 2019 (Holland et al., 2021). Mental health symptoms related to COVID-19 tended to lag behind the infection, hence there were concerns that post-pandemic depression and suicide may lag and persist for years (Fitzpatrick et al., 2020; Sher, 2020).

Global concerns regarding severe and persistent mental health consequences from COVID-19 also emerged (e.g., Kumar & Nayar, 2020). Early in the pandemic, researchers from Italy reported high rates of mental health symptoms, including psychological stress and post-traumatic symptoms (Rossi et al., 2020). Spanish researchers found similar findings with regard to post-traumatic symptoms, as well as a significant association of pandemic loneliness to anxiety, depression, and post-traumatic symptoms (González-Sanguino et al., 2020). Canadian researchers found their citizens were drinking and using cannabis more. They also found that the number of Canadians experiencing high levels of depression had doubled and the numbers of citizens experiencing high levels of anxiety had increased by a factor of four as the safety net for addressing these mental health issues had declined (Dozois & Mental Health Research Canada, 2020). Evidence from Canada also suggested greater obsessive-compulsive symptomology during the pandemic as contrasted with pre-pandemic (Abba-Aji et al., 2020). Given the breadth of the global mental health consequences of COVID-19, mental health resources will be stressed globally for the foreseeable future. In the US, the brunt of mental health consequences will fall on those experiencing physical health disparities: minoritized individuals (APA, 2020a).

Long-term physical health symptoms and their psychological impact Recovery for some with COVID-19 has been slow, with significant long-term symptoms that negatively impact quality of life and health, as well as long-term cognitive and mental health issues (Morley, 2020). Long-term physical health problems being observed over the "long-haul" in some patients often referred to as *long COVID* (del Rio et al., 2020). Little is known about the long-term consequences of COVID-19, but early research found that brain fog, profound fatigue, and the loss of taste and smell may occur, and *long-hauler symptoms* may seriously impact quality of life (Logue et al., 2021). Persistent long-hauler symptoms included breathing problems, fatigue, and sleep dysfunction (Nasserie et al., 2021). Gastrointestinal complaints and periodic fever, as well as anxiety and depression, may also persist for months after infection (Marshall, 2020; Peris et al., 2021). Mental health consequences were being found several months after COVID-19 infection, especially among those who initially had severe symptoms (Taquet et al., 2021).

The significance of long-hauler symptoms on the health, mental health, and well-being prompted the NIH has announced an initiative to study and address the long-term symptoms of COVID-19 (Collins, 2021). The coronavirus can negatively impact every major organ, including the heart as discussed in Chap. 5, and may feature a variety of other unpleasant symptoms such as pain, fatigue, fever, breathing problems, and periodic coughing (Carfi et al., 2020; Morley, 2020). Autoimmune and inflammatory reactions may continue post-infection, flaring symptoms periodically. Children have been at risk for inflammatory reactions post-infection that can be life threatening (Galeotti & Bayry, 2020). Additionally, although children tended to have less severe presentations of COVID-19, some children may have longer-term breathing problems (Zimmermann & Curtis, 2020). Some people report their long-term loss of smell and taste sometimes contributed to a significant loss in appetite (Abo Aljadavel et al., 2021; Carfi et al., 2020), although many patients with COVID-19 eventually recovered their senses of smell (Lechien et al., 2021). Long-term health consequences of COVID-19 threaten happiness, well-being, and quality of life. Mental health care professionals should expect new and significant challenges in caring for these victims over the courses of their lifetimes.

The mental health consequences to health care providers The coronavirus also has contributed to a wounded and dispirited health care workforce. Many of the consequences were avoidable with better protections earlier in the pandemic. The need for more attention to the mental health consequences to frontline health and mental health care providers was raised relatively early in the pandemic when it was clear that PPE resources were limited and demand for care was extreme. Readers might remember that many frontline physical and mental health care workers are minoritized individuals (see Chap. 3). Health care providers were psychological distressed by the circumstances of the pandemic and found to have increased symptoms of anxiety, depression, and sleep deficits (Vindegaard & Benros, 2020). By 2021, health care professionals in six nations reported significant problems with sleeplessness and burnout (Kim et al., 2021); over 75% of American health care workers also reported feeling burned out (Kirzinger et al., 2021). One large study of health and mental health care professionals conducted early in the pandemic found that over one-third of the sample reported significant mental health symptoms, anxiety and depression—over 5% reported suicidal ideations and 14% traumatization (Young et al., 2020). Many were also psychologically stressed by racist acts on and off the job (Miu & Moore, 2021).

Health and mental health care professionals were confronted with daily ethical dilemmas and multiple traumas that contributed to vicarious trauma (the trauma of others as re-experienced through the eyes of first responders and frontline care workers). One study found that experiencing vicarious trauma was significantly associated with psychological distress from violating personal ethics concerning professional behavior (Litam & Balkin, 2020). Unfortunately, many terrible ethical decisions re-emerged during the delta variant surge, when hospitals were overwhelmed once again to the point of preventing care of non-COVID-19 patients with life threatening conditions (Neumann, 2021; Stone, 2021). Many health and mental health care professionals were placed in lose-lose circumstances that violated their own moral sensibilities, a psychological wounding that likely compounded their experiences of vicarious trauma. Those who care for others may require care themselves as a result of COVID-19. The mental health wounding of frontline care providers, many who are minoritized individuals, complicates addressing post-pandemic disparities.

Social Inequities Contribute to COVID-19 Disparities

Social inequities have significantly contributed to health disparities. The Healthy People 2030 initiative to address health disparities discusses important social determinants of health and wellness (Healthy People 2030, 2021). Several determinants are discussed at some length in this book, including economic stability, quality and accessibility of education, and quality and accessibility of health care (see Chaps. 3, 4, 5, and 7). Minoritized individuals were significantly more likely to experience economic, education, and health inequities, and hence, pre-pandemic health disparities. Another social determinant of health disparities--neighborhood cohesion and stability--typically is a function of economic stability (Healthy People 2030, 2021). There is also evidence that high incarceration rates of people of color may be associated with greater community health disparities (Dumont et al., 2013). Superimposed on economic, education, and health inequities are also risks from discrimination and racism (CDC, 2021d).

Disparities in the incidence and prevalence of COVID-19 mirrored pre-existing health disparities in minoritized communities, as did hospitalization and mortality rates (Turner-Mesa et al., 2020). Neighborhood instability increased COVID-19 risks, which in turn further challenged neighborhood stability--as did stigma related to sickness, disease, and stereotypes (Turner-Mesa et al., 2020). Interestingly, stigma was also a very large barrier to addressing the Spanish Flu Pandemic of the last century (Barry, 2018), another lesson that was lost over time. Disparities in chronic diseases were associated with significant risk for suffering severe and potentially life-threatening consequences of COVID-19—diseases such as chronic respiratory disease, diabetes, hypertension, liver diseases, and autoimmune diseases—were widespread among minoritized groups pre-pandemic (Moore et al., 2020). Many of these individuals, despite health risks, were forced by economic inequities to continue to work despite risk of virus exposure as essential yet disposable workers (CDC, 2021d).

The effects of COVID-19 mirrored and worsened existing health disparities among minoritized groups (van Dorn et al., 2020). In addition, rural pre-pandemic inequities were exacerbated by the monetary costs of COVID-19 (Summers-Gabr, 2020), threatening adequate rural health care well into the future. Worsening disparities among minoritized and rural Americans greatly reduce pandemic readiness and enhance vulnerabilities to a next pandemic.

Social inequities were also predictive of population health disparities observed in past pandemics, such as the "Spanish" Flu Pandemic and the more recent 2009 H1N1 pandemic (Bambra et al., 2020). Sadly, despite the evidence of vulnerability from the past, inequities have actually worsened. The COVID-19 disparities serve as another reminder that in order to effectively address the next pandemic, social inequities and injustices of colonial societies need to be urgently addressed. Perhaps the horror of COVID-19 will be the impetus to address health inequities (Hooper et al., 2020). Will we act more wisely after the COVID-19 pandemic?

The Devastation of COVID-19 on Minoritized Communities

The impact of COVID-19 to the health and well-being of US minoritized communities has been disastrous. During the first wave in the spring of 2020, it became apparent that US minoritized groups were taking the brunt of the pandemic. The CDC reported in the summer of 2021 that the ratio of American Indian and Alaska Natives who had known cases were 1.7 times that of White Americans, of Black Americans it was 1.1 times that of White Americans, and of Latinx people it was 1.9 times that of White Americans. The ratio of American Indian and Alaska Natives who were hospitalized due to COVID-19 were 3.4 times that of White Americans, of Black Americans it was 2.8 times that of White Americans, and of Latinx people it was 2.8 times that of White Americans. Mortality ratios due to COVID-19 for American Indian and Alaska Natives were 2.4 times that of White Americans, of Black Americans it was 2.0 times that of White Americans, and of Latinx people it was 2.3 times that of White Americans (CDC, 2021b). For children, adolescents, and young adults, COVID-19 incident disparities for people were greatest for Indigenous, Latinx, and Pacific Islander Americans (Van Dyke et al., 2021). Each of these figures may be confounded by under reporting, which commonly occurs when investigating health disparities and health trends for minoritized groups.

One particularly hard-hit US metropolitan area was El Paso, TX, a Latinx majority city that experienced overflowing hospitals and resorted to make-shift morgues, including refrigerated trailers, for the storage of bodies (BBC, 2020). Louisiana was another hard-hit area early in the pandemic. A study examined mortality differences between Black and White Americans in Louisiana during that time and found that almost 77% of people who were hospitalized and over 70% who passed away were Black (Price-Haywood et al., 2020). Asian American communities on the US coasts have also been significantly impacted, their circumstances compounded by significant levels of xenophobia (della Cava, 2020). Native Hawaiians, who also face the same inequities as other Indigenous groups, experienced significant rates of COVID-19 in many western states, and during the 2021 delta surge, rates of infection spiked (Kaholokula et al., 2020; Kelleher, August 27, 2021). Indigenous Americans on different US reservations experienced devasting levels of infection

(Hatcher et al., 2020). The events of COVID-19 were a form of Indigenous déjà vu given the 500-year history of neglect and devastation by viruses. Even when national data were broken out by race and ethnicity, data for Indigenous groups were often not reported (Conger et al., 2020).

Ethnic and racial disparities were also seen in COVID-19 deaths among US long-term care facilities, a particularly vulnerable living situation. Data from 13,312 long-term care facilities were examined, revealing that facilities with higher proportions of non-White residents experienced the greatest mean number of cases and deaths (Gorges & Konetzka, 2021). Older minoritized adults were not the only ones at risk. Disparities in COVID-19 were found in every age group for American Indians, Alaska Native, Black Americans, and Asian Americans and Pacific Islanders when compared to White Americans, with the most pronounce disparities found for the age 25–54 age group. The same study also found that Black and Latinx study participants lost seven times more and American Indians and Alaska Natives nine times more of their expected years of life before age 65 than White Americans (Bassett et al., 2020).

Racial and ethnic disparities in mental health symptoms were also found. One would expect that the physical health disparities of COVID-19 would also contribute to mental health disparities, due to the cognitive impacts of SARS-CoV-2 and its long-hauler symptoms discussed earlier. With the large numbers of US COVID-19 cases and racialization of the pandemic, there was great concern that disparities in depression, suicide, and substance abuse were seriously impacting minoritized groups (Czeisler et al., 2020; Novacek et al., 2020). Concern for COVID-19 mental health disparities was not limited to the US. As an example, a study from Quebec found that minoritized participants were much more likely to experience significant mental health consequences during COVID-19 than White Canadians (Miconi et al., 2020), due to the same colonial inequities, discrimination, and stigma related to pre-pandemic disparities in the US. Indigenous American and Pacific Islander college students reported the highest rate of negative mental health consequences of any ethnicity or race at 71%, and LGBTQ students also reported greater mental health needs than sexual majority students (Anderson, 2021).

Disparities in Trust of American Health Care

Addressing health disparities related to COVID-19 will be an uphill battle due to the longstanding distrust in colonial social systems including health care. For much of its history, American health care systems have not provided quality or ethical health care for many minoritized individuals. The exploitive history by health researchers and practitioners has both contributed to and prevented treatment of health disparities over time (Institute of Medicine, 2003). Skepticism of minoritized communities to health care advice from the mainstream scientific community was predictable, especially in the context of populist-nationalist governments, flaunting divisions and fanning distrust by highlighting -isms (see also Chap. 7).

Defending the Well-being of the Most Vulnerable: An Indigenous Interpretation

Pandemics have a way of highlighting the health vulnerabilities of colonialism that has left most of the world vulnerable. Many people do not have the resources to appropriately protect themselves from viruses. The -isms of colonialism have marginalized a significant portion of the population from wellness and quality care resulting in numerous health disparities that increase pandemic risks. The consequences of COVID-19 will negatively impact health and mental health for years, especially minoritized communities, providing constant reminders of how hurtful, unjust, and wasteful the consequences of colonial values can be.

The COVID-19 pandemic has cost the nations of the world dearly, illustrating the global risks of not addressing known vulnerabilities to health. The risks that health inequities present to economies and national security have been known for some time (Robert Wood Johnson Foundation, 2017). Many colonial nations have not addressed national health and wellness in such a way to diminish national security risks to those nations (Katz & Singer, 2007). Researchers have suggested that the US, as an example, has been underinvesting in the health of its citizens for years, and this underfunding in combination with other inequities in society created national vulnerabilities during the COVID-19 pandemic (Maana & Galea, 2020).

Pandemics are a significant risk to national and international peace and well-being, as illustrated by the events during the COVID-19 pandemic and by the events of other pandemics (Barry, 2018; White House, 2021). The extent of damage from the COVID-19 pandemic has called into question whether countries have the ability to rebound quickly from such a crisis (Daszak et al., 2021). Health inequities naturally increase the risks for pandemics of the future and complicate their mitigations, creating global security risks as a result (Quinn & Kumar, 2014). If colonial nations are truly concerned about national security, they should focus inwardly to tackle the significant inequities within their own borders, including health disparities. Colonial nations have misplaced their priorities of national self-interests toward perceived threats outside the borders rather than self-inflicted problems within their borders.

The WHO reported well-before the COVID-19 pandemic that a complete transformation of how social orders operate will be needed to achieve health equity (WHO, 2008). Colonial assumptions will need to be retired that overtly or tacitly support hierarchical societies. Dr. Anthony Fauci stated that it will take an intergenerational commitment to adequately address health disparities in the US (BET, 2020). Furthermore, minoritized health and mental health care professionals experienced significant wounding during the COVID-19 pandemic due to be targeted with acts of bias and discrimination at the exact time they are so needed to help with the long-term care of other wounded people (Miu & Moore, 2021).

An IAPP view is that societies are only as strong as our most vulnerable. We were not very strong in our pandemic responses because the most vulnerable were left behind years before and societies never bothered to restore them to wellness. A wise course of action would be to create a happy and healthy society that never leaves behind people again. Decolonizing how health and wellness are approached requires decolonizing the processes and institutions of colonial societies—replacing hierarchies with equitable health care as a priority of society. A unified, collective approach to wellness is a necessary protection from future pandemic risks.

References

Abba-Aji, A., Li, D., Hrabok, M., Shalaby, R., Gusnowski, A., Vuong, W., Surood, S., Nkire, N., Li, X.-M., Greenshaw, A. J., & Agyapong, V. I. O. (2020). COVID-19 pandemic and mental health: Prevalence and correlates of new-onset obsessive-compulsive symptoms in a Canadian province. *International Journal of Environmental Research and Public Health, 17*, 6986. https://doi.org/10.3390/ijerph17196986

Abelson, R., & Goodnough, A. (2021, March 22). *If the supreme court ends Obamacare, here's what it would mean*. New York Times. https://www.nytimes.com/article/supreme-court-obamacare-case.html?0p19G=2103

Abo Aljadavel, D., Jalilvand, H., Abdi, M., & Jahandideh, H. (2021). The course of parosmia improvement in patients with COVID-19 in Iran. *Depiction of Health, 11*(4), 402–412. http://doh.tbzmed.ac.ir

Aleccia, J. N. (2021, February 7). *Covid reinfections may be more common than realized. Why isn't the US tracking them?* NBC News. https://www.nbcnews.com/health/health-news/covid-reinfections-may-be-more-common-realized-why-isn-t-n1256898

Althoff, K. N., Schlueter, D. J., Anton-Culver, H., Cherry, J., Denny, J. C., Thomsen, I., Karlson, E. W., Havers, F. P., Cicek, M. S., Thibodeau, S. N., Pinto, L. A., Lowy, D., Malin, B. A. Ohno-Machado, L., Williams, C., Goldstein, D., Kouame, A., Ramirez, A., Roman, A., …Schully, S. D. (2021). Antibodies to SARS-CoV-2 in all of us research program participants, January 2–March 18, 2020. *Clinical infectious Diseases*. https://doi.org/10.1093/cid/ciab519

Anderson, G. (2021, February 17). *Indigenous and LGBTQ students' mental health most hurt by pandemic*. Inside Higher Ed. https://www.insidehighered.com/quicktakes/2021/02/17/indigenous-and-lgbtq-students-mental-health-most-hurt-pandemic#:~:text=Indigenous%20students%20reported%20the%20highest,Center%20for%20Collegiate%20Mental%20Health

Andina Agencia Peruana de Noticias. (2021, February 12). *What is known about COVID-19 reinfection cases in Peru?* Author. https://andina.pe/ingles/noticia-what-is-known-so-far-about-covid19-reinfection-cases-in-peru-833533.aspx

APA. (2020a, May 27). *Written testimony of the American Psychological Association submitted to the House Ways and Means Committee. Hearing: The disproportionate impact of Covid-19 on communities of color*. Author. https://www.apaservices.org

APA. (2020b, October 20). *Stress in America 2020 survey signals growing national mental health crisis*. Author. https://www.apa.org/news/press/releases/2020/10/stress-mental-health-crisis

APA. (2021, March 11). *One year on: Unhealthy weight gains, increased drinking reported by Americans coping with pandemic stress*. Author. https://www.apa.org/news/press/releases/stress/2021/one-year-pandemic-stress

Arias, E., Tejada-Vera, B., & Ahmad, F. (2021). *Provisional life expectancy estimates for January through June, 2020*. CDC NVSS Vital Statistics Rapid Release Report No. 010. https://www.cdc.gov/nchs/products/index.htm

Associated Press. (2021a, January 31). *The latest: Many Peruvians ignore new virus lockdown orders*. Author. http://apnews.com/article/europe-pakistan-coronavirus-pandemic-china-938eb46da9dbb6151758799a61a307c0

Associated Press. (2021b, September 2). *NHTSA: Traffic deaths rise again as drivers take risks*. Associated Press. https://apnews.com/article/business-health-coronavirus-pandemic-traffic-ccd5fc85f8f2c0a6c8772595858099a3

Bambra, C., Riordan, R., Ford, J., & Matthews, F. (2020). The COVID-19 pandemic and health inequalities. *Journal of Epidemiology and Community Health, 74*, 964–968. https://doi.org/10.1136/jech-2020-214401

Barry, J. M. (2018). *The great influenza: The story of the deadliest pandemic in history*. Penguin Books.

Bassett, M. T., Chen, J. T., & Krieger, N. (2020). Variation in racial/ethnic disparities in COVID-19 mortality by age in the United States: A cross-sectional study. *PLoS Medicine, 17*(10), e1003402. https://doi.org/10.1371/journal.pmed.1003402

BBC. (2020, November 17). *Coronavirus: Five signs that show how bad El Paso's outbreak is*. BBC. https://www.bbc.com/news/world-us-canada-54966876

BET. (2020, July 29). *Dr. Fauci on why the coronavirus is wreaking havoc on Black communities*. Author. https://www.bet.com/video/news/national/2020/covid-19-vaccine-dr-fauci-why-black-people-are-wary-after-tuskegee-experiment.html

Boone, R. (2021, September 7). *Idaho hospitals begin rationing health care amid COVID surge*. Associated Press. https://apnews.com/article/business-health-public-health-coronavirus-pandemic-idaho-db21f9a14254996144e78aafb1518259

Bosh, K. A., Johnson, A. S., Hernandez, A. L., Prejean, J., Taylor, J., Wingard, R., Valleroy, L. A., & Hall, H. I. (2020). Vital signs: Deaths among persons with diagnosed HIV infection, United States, 2010-2018. *Morbidity and Mortality Weekly Report, 69*(46), 1717–1724. https://www.cdc.gov/mmwr/volumes/69/wr/mm6946a1.htm

Carfi, A., Bernabei, R., & Landi, F. (2020). Persistent symptoms in patients after acute COVID-19. *JAMA, 324*(6), 603–605. https://doi.org/10.1001/jama.2020.12603

CDC. (2020a, October 5). *Scientific brief: SARS-CoV-2 and potential airborne transmission*. https://www.cdc.gov/coronavirus/2019-ncov/more/scientific-brief-sars-cov-2.html

CDC. (2020b, December 22). *Symptoms of coronavirus*. Author. https://www.cdc.gov/coronavirus/2019-ncov/symptoms-testing/symptoms.html

CDC. (2021a, February 17). *Excess deaths associated with COVID-19*. Author. https://cdc.gov/nchs/nvss/vsrr/covid19/excess_deaths.htm

CDC. (2021b, July 16). *Risk for COVID-19 infection, hospitalization and death by race/ethnicity*. Author. https://www.cdc.gov/coronavirus/2019-ncov/covid-data/investigations-discovery/hospitalization-death-by-race-ethnicity.html

CDC. (2021c, February 12). *About variants of the virus that causes COVID-19. About variants of the virus that causes COVID-19*. Author. https://cdc.gov/coronavirus/2019-ncov/transmission/variant.html

CDC. (2021d, February 12). *Health equity considerations and racial and ethnic minority groups*. Author. https://www.cdc.gov/coronavirus/2019-ncov/community/health-equity/race-ethnicity.html

Collins, F. S. (2021, February 23). *NIH launces new initiative to study "Long COVID"*. National Institutes of Health. https://www.nih.gov/about-nih/who-we-are/nih-director/statements/nih-launches-new-initiative-study-long-covid

Conger, K., Gebeloff, R., & Oppel, R. A. (2020, July 30). *Native Americans feel devastated by the virus yet overlooked in the data*. New York Time. https://www.nytimes.com/2020/07/30/us/native-americans-coronavirus-data.html

Czeisler, M. E., Lane, R. I., Petrosky, E., Wiley, J. F., Christensen, A., Njai, R., Weaver, M. D., Robbins, R., Facer-Childs, E. R., Barger, L. K., Czeisler, C. A., Howard, M. E., & Rajaratnam, S. M. W. (2020). Mental health, substance use, and suicidal ideation during the COVID-19 pandemic--United States, June 24–30, 2020. *MMWR, 69*(32), 1049–1057. https://doi.org/10.15585/mmwr.mm6932a1

Daszak, P., Keusch, G. T., Phelan, A. L., Johnson, C. K., & Osterholm, M. T. (2021). Infectious disease threats: A rebound to resilience. *Health Affairs, 40*(2), 204–211. https://doi.org/10.1377/hlthaff.2020.01544

del Rio, C., Collins, L. F., & Malani, P. (2020). Long-term consequences of COVID-19. *JAMA, 324*(17), 1723–1724. https://doi.org/10.1001/jama.2020.19719

della Cava, M. (2020, October 19). *Asian Americans in San Francisco are dying at alarming rates from COVID-19: Racism is to blame*. USA Today. https://www.usatoday.com/story/news/2020/10/19/coronavirus-asian-americans-racism-death-rates-san-francisco/3710108001/

Dozois, D. J. A., & Mental Health Research Canada. (2020). Anxiety and depression in Canada during the COVID-19 pandemic: A national survey. *Canadian Psychology/Psychologie Canadienne*. https://doi.org/10.1037/cap0000251

Dumont, D. M., Allen, S. A., Brockmann, B. W., Alexander, N. E., & Rich, J. D. (2013). Incarceration, community health, and racial disparities. *Journal of Health Care for the Poor and Underserved, 24*(1), 78–88. https://muse.jhu.edu/article/496934

Elmore, J. G., Wang, P.-C., Kerr, K. F., Schriger, D. L., Morrison, D. E., Brookmeyer, R., Pfeiffer, M. A., Payne, T. H., & Currier, J. S. (2020). Excess patient visits for cough and pulmonary disease at a large US health system in the months prior to the COVID-19 pandemic: Time-series analysis. *Journal of Medical Internet Research, 22*(9), e21562. https://doi.org/10.2196/21562

Evans, M. L., Lindauer, M., & Farrell, M. E. (2020). A pandemic within a pandemic—Intimate partner violence during Covid-19. *New England Journal of Medicine, 383*, 2302–2304. https://doi.org/10.1056/NEJMp2024046

Fitzpatrick, K. M., Harris, C., & Drawve, G. (2020). How bad is it? Suicidality in the middle of the COVID-19 pandemic. *Suicide & Life-Threatening Behavior, 50*, 1241–1249. https://doi.org/10.1111/sltb.12655

Fontenelle, L. F., & Miguel, E. C. (2020). The impact of coronavirus (COVID-19) in the diagnosis and treatment of obsessive-compulsive disorder. *Depression and Anxiety*, 510–511. https://doi.org/10.1002/da.23037

Fox, M. (2020, May 5). *French doctors say they found a Covid-19 patient from December*. CNN. https://www.cnn.com/2020/05/04/health/france-coronavirus-december-death-intl/index.html

Galeotti, C., & Bayry, J. (2020). Autoimmune and inflammatory diseases following COVID-19. *Nature Reviews Rheumatology, 16*, 413–414. https://doi.org/10.1038/s41584-020-0448-7

González-Sanguino, C., Ausín, B., Castellanos, M. A., Saiz, J., López-Gómez, A., Ugidos, C., & Muñoz, M. (2020). Mental health consequences during the initial stage of the 2020 Coronavirus pandemic (COVID-19) in Spain. *Brain, Behavior, and Immunity, 87*, 172–176. https://doi.org/10.1016/j.bbi.2020.05.040

Gorges, R. J., & Konetzka, T. (2021). Factors associated with racial differences in deaths among nursing home residents with COVID-19 infection in the US. *JAMA Network Open, 4*(2), e2037431. https://doi.org/10.1001/jamanetworkopen.2020.37431

Hanna, J., & Wolfe, D. (2020, November 13). *These charts show how serious this fall's Covid-19 surge is in the US*. CNN. https://www.cnn.com/2020/11/12/health/coronavirus-fall-surge-statistics/index.html

Hanna, J., Moon, S., & Chan, S. (2020, April 22). *2 Californians died of coronavirus weeks before previously known 1st US death*. CNN. https://www.cnn.com/2020/04/22/us/california-deaths-earliest-in-us/index.html

Hatcher, S. M., Agnew-Brune, C., Anderson, M., Zambrano, L. D., Rose, C. E., Jim, M. A., Baugher, A., Liu, G. S., Patel, S. V., Evans, M. E., Pindyck, T., Dubray, C. L., Rainey, J. J., Chen, J., Sadowski, C., Winglee, K., Penman-Aguilar, A., Dixit, A., … McCollum, J. (2020). COVID-19 among American Indian and Alaska native persons--23 states, January 31–July 3, 2020. *MMWR, 69*(34), 1166–1169. https://doi.org/10.15585/mmwr.mm6934e

He, Z., Ren, L., Yang, J., Guo, L., Feng, L., Ma, C., Wang, X., Leng, Z., Tong, X., Zhou, W., Wang, G., Zhang, T., Guo, Y., Wu, C., Wang, Q., Liu, M., Wang, C., Jia, M., & Hu, X.… Wang, C. (2021). Seroprevalence and humoral immune durability of anti-SARS-CoV-2 antibodies in Wuhan, China: A longitudinal, population-level, cross-sectional study. *Lancet, 397*, 1075–1084. https://doi.org/10.1016/S0140-6736(21)00238-5

Healthy People 2030. (2021). *Social determinants of health*. Author. https://health.gov/healthypeople/objectives-and-data/social-determinants-health

Heneka, M. T., Golenbock, D., Latz, E., Morgan, D., & Brown, R. (2020). Immediate and long-term consequences of COVID-19 infections for the development of neurological disease. *Alzheimer's Research & Therapy, 12*, 69. https://doi.org/10.1186/s13195-020-00640-3

Highleyman, L. (1999). First AIDS case in 1969. *BETA, 12*(4), 5.

Holcombe, M. (2021, September 15), *1 in every 500 US resident have died of Covid-19*. CNN. https://www.cnn.com/2021/09/15/health/us-coronavirus-wednesday/index.html

Holland, K. M., Jones, C., Vivolo-Kantor, A. M., Idaikkdar, N., Zwald, M., Hoots, B., Yard, E., D'Inverno, A., Swedo, E., Chen, M. S., Petrovsky, E., Board, A., Martinez, P., Stone, D. M., Law, R., Coletta, M. A., Adjemian, J., Thomas, C., Puddy, R. W., … Houry, D. (2021). Trends in US emergency department visits for mental health, overdose, and violence outcomes before and during the COVID-19 pandemic. *JAMA Psychiatry*. https://doi.org/10.1001/jamapsychiatry.2020.4402

Hollingsworth, H., & Webber, T. (2021, February 22). *US tops 500,000 virus deaths, matching the toll of 3 wars*. Associated Press. https://apnews.com/article/us-over-500k-coronavirus-deaths-4ffa86c709f6a843de9cf0711e7215cf

Hooper, M. W., Nápoles, A. M., & Pérez-Stable, E. J. (2020). *JAMA, 323*(24), 2466–2467. https://doi.org/10.1001/jama.2020.8598

Institute of Medicine. (2003). *Unequal treatment: Confronting racial and ethnic health disparities in healthcare*. The National Academies Press.

Johnson, C. K. (2021, September 20). *COVID has killed as many Americans as the 1918–19 flu*. Associated Press. https://apnews.com/article/science-health-pandemics-united-states-coronavirus-pandemic-c15d5c6dd7ece88d0832993f11279fbb

Kaholokula, J. K., Samoa, R. A., Miyamoto, R. E. S., Palafox, N., & Daniels, S.-A. (2020). COVID-19 special column: COVID-19 hits Native Hawaiian and Pacific Islander communities the hardest. *Hawai'i Journal of Health & Social Welfare, 79*(5), 143–146.

Katz, R., & Singer, D. A. (2007). Health and security in foreign policy. *Bulletin of the World Health Organization, 85*(3), 166–244. https://www.who.int/bulletin/volumes/85/3/06

Kelleher, J. S. (2021, August 27). *COVID-19 surge pummels Hawaii and its native population*. Associated Press. https://apnews.com/article/lifestyle-health-coronavirus-pandemic-hawaii-097137d852609f37e4aada899da5938f

Kim, H., Hegde, S., LaFiura, C., Raghavan, M., Luong, E., Cheng, S., Rebholz, C. M., & Seidelmann, S. B. (2021). COVID-19 illness in relation to sleep and burnout. *BMJ Nutrition, Prevention & Health*, 000228. https://doi.org/10.1136/bmjnph-2021-000228036889/en/.

Kirzinger, A., Kearney, A., Hamel, L., & Brodie, M. (2021). *KFF/the Washington post frontline health care workers survey*. Kaiser Family Foundation. https://www.kff.org/report-section/kff-the-washington-post-frontline-health-care-workers-survey-toll-of-the-pandemic/

Kissler, S. M., Tedijanto, C., Goldstein, E., Grad, Y. H., & Lipsitch, M. (2020). Projecting the transmission dynamics of SARS-CoV-2 through the postpandemic period. *Science, 368*, 860–868. https://doi.org/10.1126/science.abb5793

Kumar, A., & Nayar, R. (2020). COVID 19 and its mental health consequences. *Journal of Mental Health*. https://doi.org/10.1080/09638237.2020.1757052.

Kupferschmidt, K. (2021). New coronavirus variants could cause more reinfections, require updated vaccines. *Science*. https://doi.org/10.1126/science.abg6028

Lavine, J. S., Bjornstad, O. N., & Antia, R. (2021). Immunological characteristics govern the transition of COVID-19 to endemicity. *Science*. https://doi.org/10.1126/science.abe6522

Lawson, M., Piel, M. H., & Simon, M. (2020). Child maltreatment during the COVID-19 pandemic: Consequences of parental job loss on psychological and physical abuse towards children. *Child Abuse and Neglect, 110*, 104709. https://doi.org/10.1016/chiabu.2020.104709

Lechien, J. R., Chiesa-Estomba, C. M., Beckers, E., Mustin, V., Ducarme, M., Journe, F., Marchant, A., Jouffe, L., Barillari, M. R., Cammarota, G., Circiu, M. P., Hans, S., & Saussez,

S. (2021). Prevalence and 6-month recovery of olfactory dysfunction: A multicenter study of 1363 COVID-19 patients. *Journal of Internal Medicine*. https://doi.org/10.1111/joim.13209

Litam, S. D. A., & Balkin, R. S. (2020). Moral injury in health-care workers during the COVID-19 pandemic. *Traumatology*. https://doi.org/10.1037/trm0000290

Logue, J. K., Franko, N. M., McCulloch, D. J., McDonald, D., Magedson, A., Wol, C. R., & Chu, H. Y. (2021). Sequelae in adults at 6 months after COVID-19 infection. *JAMA Network Open, 4*(2), e210830. https://doi.org/10.1001/jamanetworkopen.2021.0830

Maana, N., & Galea, S. (2020). COVID-19 and underinvestment in the health of the US population. *Milbank Quarterly*. https://doi.org/10.1111/1468-0009.12462.

Marchione, M. (2021, February 17). *US life expectancy drops a year in pandemic, most since WWII*. Associated Press. https://apnews.com/article/us-life-expectancy-huge-decline-f4caaf4555563d09e927f1798136a869

Maron, D. F. (2021, August 2). *Wild U.S. deer found with coronavirus antibodies*. National Geographic. https://www.nationalgeographic.com/animals/article/wild-us-deer-found-with-coronavirus-antibodies

Marshall, M. (2020). COVID-19's lasting misery. *Nature, 585*, 339–341. https://doi.org/10.1038/d41586-020-02598-6

Miconi, D., Li, Z. Y., Frounfelker, R. L., Santavicca, T., Cénat, J. M., Venkatesh, V., & Rousseau, C. (2020). Ethno-cultural disparities in mental health during the COVID-19 pandemic: A cross-sectional study on the impact of exposure to the virus and COVID-19-related discrimination and stigma on mental health across ethno-cultural groups in Quebec (Canada). *British Journal of Psychology Open, 7*(1), E14. https://doi.org/10.1192/bjo.2020.146

Miu, A. S., & Moore, J. R. (2021). Behind the masks: Experiences of mental health practitioners of color during the COVID-19 pandemic. *Academic Psychiatry*. https://doi.org/10.1007/s40596-021-01427-w

Moore, J. T., Pilkington, W., & Kumar, D. (2020). Diseases with health disparities as drivers of COVID-19 outcomes. *Journal of Cellular and Molecular Medicine, 24*(19), 11038–11045. https://doi.org/10.1111/jcmm.15599

Morley, J. E. (2020). COVID-19—The long road to recovery. *Journal of Nutrition, Health & Aging, 24*(9), 917–919. https://doi.org/10.1007/s12603-020-1473-6

Nasserie, T., Hittle, M., & Goodman, S. N. (2021). Assessment of the frequency and variety of persistent symptoms among patients with COVID-19: A systematic review. *JAMA Network Open, 4*(5), e2111417. https://doi.org/10.1001/jamanetworkopen.2021.11417

Nauen, D. W., Hooper, J. E., Stewart, C. M., & Solomon, I. H. (2021). Assessing brain capillaries in coronavirus disease 2019. *JAMA Neurology*. https://doi.org/jamaneurol.2021.0225

Nemani, K., Li, C., Offson, M., Blessing, E. M., Razavian, N., Chen, J., Petkova, E., & Goff, D. C. (2021). Association of psychiatric disorders with mortality among patients with COVID-19. *JAMA Psychiatry*. https://doi.org/10.1001/jamapsychiatry.2020.4442

Neumann, E. (2021, September 16). *Overwhelmed with COVID patients, Oregon hospitals postpone surgeries and cancer care*. National Public Radio. https://www.npr.org/sections/health-shots/2021/09/16/1037621883/overwhelmed-with-covid-patients-oregon-hospitals-postpone-surgeries-and-cancer-c

NIH. (2020, August 18). *Immune cells for common cold may recognize SARS-CoV-2*. Author. https://www.nih.gov/news-events/nih-research-matters/immune-cells-common-cold-may-recognize-sars-cov-2

Novacek, D. M., Hampton-Anderson, J. N., Ebor, M. T., Loeb, T. B., & Wyatt, G. E. (2020). Mental health ramifications of the COVID-19 pandemic for Black Americans: Clinical and research recommendations. *Psychological Trauma Theory Research Practice and Policy, 12*(5), 449–451. https://doi.org/10.1037/tra0000796

Nowak, B., Brzóska, P., Piottrowski, J., Sedikides, C., Żemojtel-Piotrowska, M., & Jonason, P. K. (2020). Adaptive and maladaptive behavior during the COVID-19 pandemic: The roles of dark triad traits, narcissism, and health beliefs. *Personality and Individual Differences, 167*, 110232. https://doi.org/10.1016/j.paid.2020.110232

Nyakarahuka, L., Kankya, C., Krontveit, R., Mayer, B., Mwiine, F. N., Lutwama, J., & Skjerve, E. (2016). How severe and prevalent are Ebola and Marburg viruses? A systematic review and meta-analyses of the case fatality rates and seroprevalence. *BMC Infectious Diseases, 16*, 708. https://bmcinfectdis.biomedcentral.com/articles/10.1186/s12879-016-2045-6

Parra, A., Juanes, A., Losada, C. P., Álvarez-Sesmero, S., Santana, V. D., Marti, I., Urricelqui, J., & Rentero, D. (2020). Psychotic symptoms in COVID-19 patients. A retrospective descriptive study. *Psychiatry Research, 291*, 113254. https://doi.org/10.1016/j.psychres.2020.113254

Pearce, C., Honey, J. R., Lovick, R., Creamer, N. Z., Henry, C., Langford, A., Stobert, M., & Barclay, S. (2021). 'A silent epidemic of grief': A survey of bereavement care provision in the UK and Ireland during the COVID-19 pandemic. *BMJ Open, 11*, e046872. https://doi.org/10.1136/bmjopen-2020-046872

Peris, R. H., Ognyanova, K., Santillana, M., Baum, M. A., Lazer, D., Druckman, J., & Volpe, J. D. (2021). Association of acute symptoms of COVID-19 and symptoms of depression in adults. *JAMA Network, 4*(3), e213223. https://doi.org/10.1001/jamanetworkopen.2021.3223

Pew Research Center. (2019, December 17). *1. Views of the major problems facing the country*. Author. https://www.pewresearch.org/politics/2019/12/17/views-of-the-major-problems-facing-the-country/

Pfeifferbaum, B., & North, C. S. (2020). Mental health and the Covid-19 pandemic. *New England Journal of Medicine, 383*(6), 510–512. https://www.nejm.org/

Pollard, M. S., Tucker, J. S., & Green, H. D. (2020). Changes in adult alcohol use and consequences during the COVID-19 pandemic. *JAMA Network Open, 3*(9), e2022942. https://doi.org/10.1001/jamanetworkopen.2020.22942

Price-Haywood, E. G., Burton, J., Fort, D., & Seoane, L. (2020). Hospitalization and mortality among Black patients and White patients with Covid-19. *New England Journal of Medicine, 382*, 2534–2543. https://doi.org/10.1056/NEJMsa2011686

Quinn, S. C., & Kumar, S. (2014). Health inequalities and infectious disease epidemics: A challenge for global health security. *Biosecurity and Bioterrorism: Biodefense Strategy, Practice, and Science, 12*(5), 263–273. https://doi.org/10.1089/bsp.2014.0032

Reuters. (2021, September 17). *COVID-19 victims remembered on Washington's National Mall with 650,000 white flags*. Author. https://www.reuters.com/world/us/covid-19-victims-remembered-washingtons-national-mall-with-650000-white-flags-2021-09-17/

Ridout, K. K., Alavi, M., Ridout, S. J., Koshy, M. T., Harris, B., Dhillon, I., Awsare, S., Weisner, C. M., Campbell, C. I., & Iturralde, E. (2021). Changes in diagnostic and demographic characteristics seeking mental health care during the early COVID-19 pandemic in a large, community-based health care system. *Journal of Clinical Psychiatry, 82*(2), 20m13685. https://doi.org/10.4088/JCP.20m13685

Ritchie, K., Chan, D., & Watermeyer, T. (2020). The cognitive consequences of the COVID-19 epidemic: Collateral damage. *Brain Communications*. https://doi.org/braincomms/fcaa069

Robert Wood Johnson Foundation. (2017, January 11). *Health inequities harm U.S. competitiveness, economic strength, and national security; eliminating them should be a national priority*. Robert Wood Johnson Foundation. https://www.rwjf.org/en/library/articles-and-news/2017/01/health-inequities-harm-u-s-competitiveness-economic-strength-a.html

Roberts, M. (2021, July 11). *Covid: Woman aged 90 died with double variant infection*. BBC. https://www.bbc.com/new/health-57761343

Rossi, R., Socci, V., Talevi, D., Mensi, S., Niolu, C., Pacitti, F., Di Marco, A., Rossi, A., Siracusano, A., & Di Lorenzo, G. (2020). COVID-19 pandemic and lockdown measures impact on mental health among the general population in Italy. *Frontiers in Psychiatry, 11*, 790. https://doi.org/10.3389/fpsyt.2020.00790

Sabino, E. C., Buss, L. F., Carvalho, M. P. S., Prete, C. A., Crispim, M. A. E., Fraiji, N. A., Pereira, R. H. M., Parag, K. V., da Silva Peixoto, P., Kraemer, M. U. G., Oikawa, M. K., Salomon, T., Cucunuba, Z. M., Castro, M. C., Aruska de Souza Santos, A., Nascimento, V. H., Pereira, H. S., Ferguson, N. M., Pybus, O. G., … Faria, N. R. (2021). Resurgence of COVID-19 in

Manaus, Brazil, despite high seroprevalence. *Lancet, 397*, 452–454. https://doi.org/10.1016/S0140-6736(21)00183-5

Sher, L. (2020). The impact of the COVID-19 pandemic on suicide rates. *QJM: An International Journal of Medicine, 113*(10), 707–712. https://doi.org/10.1093/qjmed/hcaa202

Siddiqi, H. K., Libby, P., & Ridker, P. M. (2021). COVID-19—a vascular disease. *Trends in Cardiovascular Medicine, 31*(1), 1–5. https://doi.org/10.1016/j.tcm.2020.10.005

Souilmi, Y., Lauterbur, M. E., Tobler, R., Huber, C. D., Johar, A. S., Moradi, S. V., Johnston, W. A., Krogan, N. J., Alexandrov, K., & Enard, D. (2021). An ancient viral epidemic involving host coronavirus interacting genes more than 20,000 years ago in East Asia. *Current Biology, 31*, e1–e9. https://doi.org/10.1016/j.cub.2021.05.067

Stone, W. (2021, September 5). *A COVID surge is overwhelming U.S. hospitals, raising fears of rationed care*. National Public Radio. https://www.npr.org/sections/health-shots/2021/09/05/1034210487/covid-surge-overwhelming-hospitals-raising-fears-rationed-care

Summers-Gabr, N. M. (2020). Rural-urban mental health disparities in the United States during COVID-19. *Psychological Trauma Theory Research Practice and Policy, 12*(S1), S222–S234. https://doi.org/10.1037/tra0000871

Swedo, E., Idaikkadar, N., Leemis, R., Dias, T., Radhakrishnan, L., Stein, Z., Chen, M., Agathis, N., & Holland, K. (2020). *MMWR, 69*, 1841–1847. https://doi.org/10.15585/mmwr.mm6949a1

Taquet, M., Luciano, S., Geddes, J. R., & Harrison, P. J. (2020). Bidirectional associations between COVID-19 and psychiatric disorder: Retrospective cohort studies of 62354 COVID-19 cases in the USA. *Lancet Psychiatry*. https://doi.org/10.1016/S2215-0366(20)30479-X.

Taquet, M., Geddes, J. R., Husain, M., Luciano, S., & Harrison, P. J. (2021). 6-month neurological and psychiatric outcomes in 236379 survivors of COVID-19: A retrospective cohort study using electronic records. *Lancet Psychiatry* https://doi.org/10.1016/S2215-033(21)00084-5.

Turner-Mesa, J., Ajayi, O., & Kemp, L. (2020). Examining social determinants of health, stigma, and COVID-19 disparities. *Healthcare, 8*, 168. https://doi.org/10.3390/healthcare8020168

van Dorn, A., Cooney, R., & Sabin, M. L. (2020). COVID-19 exacerbating inequalities in the US. *Lancet, 395*, 1243–1244. https://doi.org/10.1016/S0140-6736(20)30893-X

Van Dyke, M. E., Mendoza, M. C. B., Li, W., Parker, E. M., Belay, B., Davis, E. M., Quint, J. J., Penman-Aguilar, A., & Clarke, K. E. N. (2021). Racial and ethnic disparities in COVID-19 incidence by age, sex, and period among persons aged <25 years—16 U.S. jurisdictions, January 1-December 31, 2020. *MMWR, 70*. https://www.cdc.gov/mmwr/volumes/70/wr/mm7011e1.htm

Vera, A., Yan, H., & Holcombe, M. (2021, February 3). *More than 100,000 people have died of Covid-19 in the US since January 1, JHU data shows*. CNN. https://www.cnn.com/2021/02/02/health/us-coronavirus-tuesday/index.html

Vindegaard, N., & Benros, M. E. (2020). COVID-19 pandemic and mental health consequences: Systematic review of current evidence. *Brain, Behavior, and Immunity, 89*, 531–542. https://doi.org/10.1016/j.bbi.2020.05.048

White House. (2021, January 21). *National security memorandum on United States global leadership to strengthen the international COVID-19 response and to advance global health security and biological preparedness*. Author. https://www.whitehouse.gov/briefing-room/statements-releases/2021/01/21/national-security-directive-united-states-global-leadership-to-strengthen-the-international-covid-19-response-and-to-advance-global-health-security-and-biological-preparedness/

WHO. (2008). *Closing the gap in a generation: Health equity through action on the social determinants of health*. Author. https://www.who.int/social_determinants/final_report/csdh_finalreport_2008.pdf

WHO. (2021, August 30). *WHO coronavirus (COVID-19) dashboard*. Author. https://covid19.who.int/

Woolf, S. H., Masters, R. K., & Aron, L. Y. (2021). Effect of the covid-19 pandemic in 2020 on life expectancy across populations in the USA and other high income countries: Simulations of provisional mortality data. *BMJ, 373*, n1343. https://doi.org/10.1136/bmj.n1343

Wu, C-T., Lidsky, P. V., Xiao, Y., Lee, I. T., Cheng, R., Nakayama, T., Jiang, S., Demeter, J., Bevacqua, R. J., Chang, C. A., Whitener, R. L., Stalder, A. K., Zhu, B., Chen, H., Goltsev, Y., Tzankov, A., Nayak, J. V., Nolan, G. P., Matter, M. S., ...Jackson, P. K. (2020). *Cell Metabolism, 33*, 1565–1576.

Young, K. P., Kolcz, D. L., O'Sullivan, D. M., Ferrand, J., Fried, J., & Robinson, K. (2020). Health care workers' mental health and quality of life during COVID-19: Results from a mid-pandemic national survey. *Psychiatric Services* https://doi.org/10.1176/appi.ps.202000424.

Yuan, B., Li, W., Liu, H., Cai, X., Song, S., Zhao, J., Hu, X., Li, Z., Chen, Y., Zhang, K., Liu, Z., Peng, J., Wang, C., Wang, J., & An, Y. (2020). Correlation between immune response and self-reported depression during convalescence from COVID-19. *Brain, Behavior, and Immunity, 88*, 39–43. https://doi.org/10.1016/j.bbi.2020.05.062

Zhou, H., Lu, S., Chen, J., Wei, N., Wang, D., Lyu, H., Shi, C., & Hu, S. (2020). The landscape of cognitive function in recovered COVID-19 patients. *Journal of Psychiatric Research, 129*, 98–102. https://doi.org/10.1016/j.jpsychires.2020.06.022

Zhu, T., Korber, B. T., Nahmias, A. J., Hooper, E., Sharp, P. M., & Ho, D. D. (1998). An African HIV-1 sequence from 1959 and implications for the origin of the epidemic. *Nature, 391*(6667), 594–597. https://doi.org/10.1038/35400

Zimmermann, P., & Curtis, N. (2020). Coronavirus infections in children including COVID-19. *The Pediatric Infectious Disease Journal, 39*(5), 355–368. https://doi.org/10.1097/INF.0000000000002660

Chapter 7
Colonialism, Treatments, and Vaccinations

Abstract Deception, disinformation, and lack of transparency significantly hindered an effective pandemic response, especially in colonial nations with populist-nationalist leaders inclined toward satisfying economic self-interests rather than addressing the well-being of the whole. As a result, effective mitigation measures, such as masking, social distancing, and temporary shutdowns, were controversial and politicized. Misinformation concerning COVID-19 treatments and vaccines were widespread, often fueled by acts of manipulation that risked harm to others. Scientific advances resulted in effective vaccines, new empirically supported treatments, and advanced medical technology that promised to help to control viral spread. However, colonial biases often prevented equal access, appropriate assessment, and quality of care, thwarting positive outcomes and slowing progress significantly. Racial bias, for example, negatively impacted vaccine trials, vaccine access, and the effectiveness of medical technology. Ultimately, vaccine hesitancy proved to be a serious barrier to achieving vaccine-acquired herd immunity in the US, whereas vaccine nationalism and slow production and exportation of vaccines hindered herd immunity globally, leaving the world vulnerable to SARS-CoV-2 variants such as delta. As a result, pandemic response proved to be reactive rather than anticipatory, hindering consistent global progress in restraining the pandemic.

The fall of 2020 was an abysmal time in many parts of the world--tantalizingly close to the availability of vaccines and yet the worst of times for community spread and death. In the US, prior to the fall of 2020, there were mostly localized regional spikes in cases, but by the fall, case numbers were rising to new heights everywhere (Alexander & Siemaszko, 2020). The trend was not localized to the US. Other nations were finding the need to resume lockdowns in October, 2020, (BBC, 2020b; Suliman & Eckardt, 2020; Taylor, 2020), with some lockdowns much stricter than others (BBC, 2021h, 2021j). Europe, which had done a credible job controlling spread in the summer, was in dire straits again by December (Reynolds, 2020). Global death toll from the pandemic exceeded two million by mid-January, and by the end of January, the top 9 death rates per 100,000 citizens were in Europe, and

A. W. Blume, *Colonialism and the COVID-19 Pandemic*, International and Cultural Psychology, https://doi.org/10.1007/978-3-030-92825-4_7

number 10 was the US (Johns Hopkins Coronavirus Center, 2021; Sherman et al., 2021). Perhaps the fall 2020 surge was inevitable due to what is known about pandemic patterns, but its severity was most certainly complicated by acts of colonial deception (remembering Chap. 1). The breadth of deception exacerbated existing distrust in many nations and complicated control of COVID-19 as a result.

Historical Lessons Lost and Found

Alghero, a city in Sardinia, has the distinction of being one of the first communities to utilize a written, comprehensive plan to address a deadly pandemic. No, it was not done during the time of COVID-19 or any of the influenzas of the 20th or 21st centuries, but rather in the sixteenth century to address the plague (Gorvett, 2021). The pandemic intervention manual, *Ectypa Pestilentis Status Allgheriae Sardiniae*, was written by Quinto Tiberio Angelelerio in 1588, a medieval healer who studied the behaviors of his patients and the local citizenry. He arrived at the conclusion that people would do better to keep their distance from one another--that only one designated member of the family should shop at the markets, keeping a two-meter distance between others as measured by a staff. In addition, citizens were encouraged to wash their food, and all commerce with outside communities ceased. Cases were tracked, and the ill were quarantined and their furnishings sanitized by being burned. The result was a much healthier Alghero that did not experience community spread like its neighbors, despite having no idea what caused the plague (Bianucci et al., 2013). However, some citizens were unhappy with the imposed mitigation methods and threatened to kill Angelelerio (Gorvett, 2021). Five hundred years later, death threats were still commonly made against public health officials (see Chap. 9), including Dr. Anthony Fauci, during COVID-19 (Perrett, 2021).

Masks were allegedly used by healers of the plague during the European middle ages, although some dispute this history (Matuschek et al., 2020). Masks were first widely used in medicine when evidence emerged that certain diseases spread through droplets (Matuschek et al., 2020). Face coverings and masks were in wide use during the Spanish Flu pandemic, as were measures of social distancing (Barry, 2018). During the COVID-19 pandemic, both masks and social distancing became controversial topics and a great deal of misinformation followed that discredited the use of either measure. And just like in the 1580s, the closing of commerce and the practices of isolating to prevent community spread were opposed by many citizens, some violently (BBC, 2021h, 2021j; see also Chap. 3). As a result, community spread of the SARS-CoV-2 was not well-contained in many nations and many unnecessary deaths occurred. Widespread skepticism toward the recommendations of public health science to address the pandemic presented significant barriers to adequately respond to the public health threat.

Colonial deception and COVID-19

Deception and disinformation, a widely used practice to divide and keep people off balance to maintain the colonial status quo (Blume, 2020), fueled barriers to appropriate care during the pandemic. The administration of former President Trump, like other populist-nationalist governments, downplayed the risks of the pandemic, suggesting COVID-19 was like a flu that would simply vanish, and that protective measures recommended by health scientists were too extreme or even silly (Wolfe & Dale, 2020; Woodward, 2020). Those acts of deception seriously harmed public health efforts to control significant spread and prevent loss of life. Estimates were that over 50% of infections and mortalities could have been prevented if shutdowns occurred one week earlier in 2020 (Pei et al., 2020).

Mass hospitalizations threatened the capacities of American hospitals. In 2018, hospitals in the US had 924,107 staffed beds, with non-federal administered hospitals having just over 100,000 intensive care beds nationally (American Hospital Association, 2020). Since many citizens believed in the disinformation campaigns and failed to adhere to public health suggestions of masking and social distancing, spread was enormous, sending thousands of people into intensive care. Some US hospitals resorted to using unconventional space such as hallways and parking garages to meet demand (Holcombe et al., 2020; Wilson, 2020). Imagine the financial consequences of all of these hospitalizations to patients and their families due to an unnecessary spread caused by misinformation.

The deception was also extended to possible treatments for COVID-19. In early April, 2020, then US President Trump suggested that hydroxychloroquine would be an effective treatment to prevent and treat COVID-19 although there were absolutely no data to support the assertion. Many political supporters chose to use the drug as suggested, diminishing the supply available for use against lupus and malaria (Mehta et al., 2020), diseases for which the drug is known to be effective. In general, whenever a claim was made during the pandemic that a certain drug might be effective, with or without evidence, it contributed to shortages in those medications, challenging an already fragile supply chain and threatening the health of those who required the drugs for their FDA approved purposes (Schondelmeyer et al., 2020). Even state governments were known to have invested heavily in the possibility that this drug would be effective in treating COVID-19, only to be left with unused stockpiles when empirical data did not support the efficacy for treating COVID-19 (Murphy, 2021a). Unfortunately, one person was known to have died from the advice provided by the president, inadvertently using aquarium cleaner instead of hydroxychloroquine because the names were somewhat similar (Edwards & Hillyard, 2020; Galvan & Cooper, 2020). Later, it was discovered that advocating for the drug may have financially benefitted political allies, donors, and perhaps even the president (Dicker, 2020; Doughton, 2020). The hydroxychloroquine deception is a modern example of a historical colonial practice to deceive people for economic gain and exploitation.

Later in the month of April, former President Trump also speculated about two other prevention and treatment methods for the coronavirus: the use of disinfectant and bright light internally (BBC, 2020a). He first suggested during a news briefing on the pandemic that perhaps disinfectant could be injected or used for a cleaning of lungs (Clark, 2020). The idea was to offer people an opportunity to sanitize from within without any empirical support for the methods that were offered. A large number of people phoned for confirmation that it was recommended to use disinfectant medically, so many that warnings were made against the ingestion of disinfectant by many public health officials including the US Surgeon General (Riechmann & Madhani, 2020). People were likely poisoned as a result of this advice from former President Trump (Gharpure et al., 2020).

The other claim made by former President Trump during the same news briefing was that bright light could be used inside the body to defeat the coronavirus. Dissecting this comment is more complex, because there are uses for ultraviolet light to disinfect surfaces and PPE, and some research examining the use of light to fight diseases and perhaps defeat viruses (Kharkwal et al., 2011; Laulhé et al., 2019; Mackenzie, 2020; Vatansever et al., 2013). However, the use of light in this way with COVID was hypothetical at best. It may have been that the former president was briefed on the hypotheticals of this technology and confused it with a real possibility, or it might have been another act of deception—it is unclear.

Misleading information by government authorities risked the lives of scared and desperate people, many who were minoritized. The sanitizing from within metaphor reflects a certain callousness, especially those who were treated as disposable. It is clear that former President Trump had no intention of using disinfectant himself, yet he was willing to suggest it for the common citizen. The sanitizing from within metaphor calls to mind other examples of colonial leaders treating others as disposable guinea pigs in the face of diseases, the most infamous US example being the Tuskegee experiment. Social media has also been an important vehicle for spreading treatment misinformation, such as the belief that Ivermectin, a deworming drug for animals, was a potential treatment and cure for COVID-19, prompting a warning from the US government concerning the risk of poisoning (CDC, 2021).

Empirical Efforts to Address COVID-19

A variety of other treatment methods were empirically tested, including various antiviral treatments, convalescent plasma, steroids, and anticoagulant medication. The US FDA, for example, used US study findings to approve remdesivir for emergency use treatment of serious cases of COVID-19 (NIH, 2021c; US Food and Drug Administration, October 22, 2020). Transfusing convalescence plasma was a method used historically to try to extend the natural immunity of recovering patients to others when no other treatments were known (such as the flu pandemic; Barry, 2018). Convalescent plasma was also used during the COVID-19 pandemic but the evidence for its effectiveness was sparse (NIH, 2021b; Robbiani et al., 2020).

However, the use of dexamethasone to control the inflammation inherent in robust immune responses showed promise in reducing symptom severity and reduction in mortalities (The RECOVERY Collaborative Group, 2021a), However, dexamethasone's side effect of lowering immune response allowed for opportunistic fungal infections in India during the spring, 2021 surge (Biswas, 2021b). There was some evidence from a UK trial that tocilizumab might also inhibit inflammation to benefit patients (NIH, March 5, 2021c; The RECOVERY Collaborative Group, 2021b). Finally, the use of anticoagulant medication to prevent the cardiovascular consequences of COVID-19 also showed promise (Rentsch et al., 2021).

Much later in the pandemic, progress was made on producing an antiviral specifically targeting SARS-CoV-2 (molnupiravir) associated with reduced hospitalizations and lowered mortality (Herper, October 1, 2021; see also Chap. 11). Interesting research also examined whether SARS-CoV-2 specific nanobody treatment, inspired by llama physiology, might be effective against the virus in humans. Although very exciting and potentially transformative, research had yet to progress to a human trial (Gill, 2021).

The early inability to effectively prevent or treat the SARS-CoV-2 virus made developing effective vaccines even more urgent. As discussed in Chap. 4, vaccines were identified as the most humane and effective path to herd immunity against the virus. The US and other nations opted early in the process to facilitate the research on vaccination, which ultimately was perhaps the wisest course of action taken during the early stages of the pandemic.

Problems with Technology One problem that the US faced was an inability to carry out comprehensive testing and contact tracing when people tested positive. Testing was controversial from the very beginning of the pandemic, with the CDC opting not to use the WHO's test and developing one of its own instead. Unfortunately, the test was found to be rather unreliable (Schneider, 2020), as many other tests were also found to be (Bahreini et al., 2020; Mulchandani et al., 2020; Woloshin et al., 2020). Because of the tardiness of federal and state testing methods in the US, it was hoped that home testing kits might fill the void. However, when a home testing kit was finally released, it ended up being very expensive and unreliable (McLaughlin, 2021). From the very beginning, resources were not provided to enhance virus detection and contact tracing, contributing to widespread community spread in the US (Clark et al., 2020). Despite those limitations to response, scientists demonstrated some creativity to develop alternatives, such as using electronic health records as a proxy for detection and tracing and using statistical modeling to determine risk of spread (Metlay et al., 2021). However, with that bit of scientific ingenuity acknowledged, some nations were highly effective at testing and contact tracing during the pandemic, and those who were proficient seemed to have weathered the pandemic much better than those who took the laissez faire approach to addressing spread.

Medical technology was an important part of identifying and addressing COVID-19. In the early days, the supply chain for medical technology was disrupted as discussed in Chap. 3. Ventilators for example were in short supply during surges, but helpful for addressing critical care when available, although they sometimes left the dilemma of lifetime support for people who remained chronically dependent after COVID-19 for mechanically-assisted breathing (Wunsch, 2021). The supply chain was not the only problem with technology that was revealed during that time. Pulse oximeters were an important tool for signaling hypoxia and respiratory distress in patients with COVID-19. However, pulse oximetry technology was significantly less accurate in accessing blood oxygen of people with darker colored skin when contrasted with white skin, reflecting technological racial bias (Sjoding et al., 2020). The racial biases are not unique to medical technology; racial biases have been identified in self-driving cars that failed to identify dark skinned pedestrians (Wilson et al., 2019). There are also concerns that artificial intelligence, exam proctoring software, facial recognition technology, the Twitter image cropping algorithm, and big data analyses may be subject to racialized programming biases (BBC, 2020c; Bender et al., 2021; Blume, 2020; Collier, 2021; McKenzie, 2021). The Food and Drug Administration acknowledged shortcomings in pulse oximetry technology but did not discuss the evidence that racial bias was to blame for its failure (Brodwin & St. Fleur, 2021). Racial disparities and biases were not only present in important medical technology needed to diagnose respiratory distress related to the COVID-19 disease, they also represented barriers later in vaccination trials and vaccine rollout as discussed subsequently.

The Search for Immunity

Immunity during the pandemic had many meanings in colonial societies. Immunity might mean that one is free from the social responsibilities that burden others, such as the public health suggestions concerning social distancing and wearing of masks. That understanding of immunity implies colonial privilege and is discussed extensively in Chap. 9. Immunity was also referred to liberally when promoting the idea of infection-acquired herd immunity discussed in Chap. 4. Although there was evidence that some long-term immunity from having the COVID-19 disease occurred, it was difficult to know for how long that immunity might last, with research suggesting anywhere from 5–8 months (NIH, 2021a; Rahim, 2021; Ripperger et al., 2020; Roxby, 2020). Antibodies sometimes fell rapidly after having COVID-19 and people were known to be re-infected (Andina Agencia Peruana de Noticias, 2021; Quest, 2020). Interestingly, similar decline in immune response to vaccines was later noted during the delta variant surge, prompting CDC recommendations for boosters between 6–8 months after being fully vaccinated (Levin et al., 2021; O'donnell & Aboulenein, 2021; Tartof et al., 2021).

The type of immunity that was more commonly discussed and considered ideal was vaccination-assisted herd immunity, with the goal being to have 70–85% percent of the population vaccinated during the COVID-19 pandemic (Kaiser Health News, 2021). Unfortunately, in the early stages of the pandemic, colonial tenets associated with concern for proximal outcomes contributed to colonial shortsightedness (Chap. 1) in policies. A focus on economics at expenses of pandemic preparation (Chap. 3) was associated with lost time relevant to vaccine development for SARS-like coronaviruses. In 2012, funding was provided to develop a SARS-coronavirus vaccine (Pathak, 2012), but interests diminished, and funding went away once that epidemic ended. The scientists involved by all accounts were close to a vaccine, but the project was ended with typical colonial shortsightedness due to financial concerns (Allen, 2020; Hixenbaugh, 2020). Fortunately, the preliminary work remained available to help pharmaceuticals save time during 2020, but the execution of a coronavirus vaccine could have been ready before the pandemic started, although it is an open question as to how long it might have taken to adapt a SARS-CoV-1 vaccine for the SARS-CoV-2 virus. Regardless, the stop and start process toward a coronavirus vaccine is an excellent example of how the colonial worldview can be self-defeating for preparing to address pandemics. The lack of continuity in preparation left the US federal government no choice but to pursue vaccine development at warp speed in 2020.

Vaccines and Vaccine Hesitancy

When it because apparent to US policymakers that COVID-19 was not a hoax that would simply dissipate, and that in order to fully reopen the economy a vaccine might be needed, *Operation Warp Speed* was formulated in late April, 2020, and announced on May 15. The goal was to rapidly develop and distribute vaccines against COVID-19 by January, 2021 (US Department of Defense, 2020). Vaccines were introduced and approved before the January, 2021, goal, but unfortunately the rollout of those vaccinations from pharmaceutical producers into the arms of Americans was greatly delayed by logistical barriers in manufacturing and transport not anticipated, problems that Operation Warp Speed attempted to address well after the January, 2021 goal (Howard & Wright, 2021). For example, the splintered health care systems and competition that those systems fostered made coordination, communication, and cooperation difficult (Chen et al., 2021). Operation Warp Speed also reallocated approximately $10 billion set aside to assist hospitals and health care professionals to the vaccine effort (Cohrs, 2021). It is difficult to know how this financial sleight of hand ultimately impacted the pandemic--on the one hand restraining care provision of hospitals and care providers but on the other hand potentially enhancing vaccine development and allotment.

The rapid development of the vaccines through Operation Warp Speed also triggered fears that the production of the vaccines might be haphazard. Additional pressure was applied for rapid development and approval for political reasons (Cohen, 2020b). The political pressures became so pronounced that high-profile scientists expressed concerns that the appearance of meddling might compromise vaccine production and confidence in the process (LaFraniere et al., 2020; Thorp, 2020). Confidence was challenged, including among health care professionals, but those concerns diminished somewhat with time and a change of presidential administrations (Galewitz, 2021; Gharpure et al., 2021; Reinhart, 2020). Minoritized outgroups were understandable skeptical when it came to rapidly produced vaccines (e.g., Fonseca, 2021). General vaccine hesitancy, a problem before the pandemic, was certainly exacerbated by the politicization of vaccines.

Furthermore, SARS-CoV-2 vaccine development trials lacked diverse representation in their samples. The lack of representation in research is a widespread problem in colonial nations that has arisen due to homogenous methodology, neglect or lack of concern for outgroups by ingroup scientists, and distrust in clinical science and practice as a result of that neglect and lack of concern (Blume, 2020). A recent study found that over the last 10 years in the US, vaccine trials for both adults and children had poor ethnic representation, and in many instances did not report breakout of data by ethnicity or race. In addition, for those who did report data by ethnicity and race, over 48% did not report results for Indigenous Americans. For those studies that reported data by ethnicity and race, investigators found that Black, Indigenous, and Latinx participants were underrepresented in vaccine trials whereas White Americans were overrepresented (Flores et al., 2020; St. Fleur, 2021).

Regardless of the reasons, the pharmaceutical companies largely failed once again to have strong representation of the demographic groups most at risk from COVID-19 in their vaccine trials, threatening the validity of the results for certain demographic groups (Chastain et al., 2020). Cultural insensitivity often proves to be a barrier for minoritized group participation, diminishing trust in the process. For example, the Lummi tribe in the US opted to withdraw from the AstraZeneca trial due to inadequate communication with tribal leaders (Bush, 2020), which suggests to this Indigenous scientist that the company was not being culturally sensitive to tribal concerns. The concerns about lack of transparency expressed by the Lummi may have been warranted, since later in the pandemic the company misrepresented efficacy data to the American public (Neergaard & Miller, 2021). Additionally, the outcomes that were tested had significant limitations in how outcomes were evaluated, focused more on proximal and limited outcomes (Doshi, 2020). Plus, there were concerns that public expectations concerning the vaccines were being raised too high and that pharmaceuticals should emphasize that vaccine-assisted herd immunity would take time (Szabo & Allecia, 2020). Pharmaceutical companies are business entities concerned with self-interests, so it is no surprise that they may have presented an overly optimistic and enthusiastic view concerning their products (Cohen, 2020a), raising expectations as well.

Dr. Arthur Evans, the CEO of the American Psychological Association, provided congressional testimony on vaccine hesitancy, suggesting that the distrust of certain minoritized communities could be addressed through empirically supported strategies (Evans, 2021). However, the most important step toward addressing distrust is acknowledging past abuses and neglect and moving forward with transparency and community participation in the present and future. A well-known health psychologist and former NIH official shared that a paternalistic approach to selling vaccine efficacy to the public that avoids full disclosure and transparency is neither honest nor helpful (Kaplan & Frosch, 2020). For minoritized communities, misinformation and lack of transparency is more-of-same, reinforcing a history of distrust and skepticism.

Politics and Vaccine Hesitancy During COVID-19, there was a clear effort to discredit health care experts and politicize public health initiatives. The politicizing of the pandemic in the US also politicized vaccine refusal, with self-identified Republicans more likely to refuse than self-identified Democrats (Hamel et al., 2020; Monmouth University Poll, 2021). Colonial splitting tactics created the remarkable illusion that health care professionals were enemies of common people and that public health recommendations be ignored and opposed (Warren et al., October 28, 2020; Woodward, 2020). The result was confusion and distrust in the messaging of how to appropriately address COVID-19.

The US was not alone in politicizing the response to the pandemic, as several other populist-nationalist colonial governments did likewise (see Table 7.1). In the UK, the belief that the pandemic was a hoax contributed to disregard of public health information and of frontline health care workers and teachers (Smith, 2021a). Brazil President Bolsonaro's administration represented another example of how a populist-nationalistic government engaged in deceptive tactics and actively opposed shutdown responses and other public health measures to contain spread. Regarding COVID-19 vaccinations, President Bolsonaro suggested they may turn people into crocodiles or other gender stereotyped unpleasant side-effects (France24, 2020). When more infectious and lethal variants appeared in the winter of 2021, deceptive anti-science activities left Brazil in dire straits due to significant spikes in hospitalizations and deaths (BBC, 2021e; Savarese & Álvares, 2021). In response to the surge, President Bolsonaro told citizens to quit 'whining' (BBC, 2021i, 2021k).

India was another example of how politics hindered vaccine response, not only nationally, but also globally. The nation, originally with lower cases than expected, apparently became overconfident with its success, with some errantly believing that herd immunity had been achieved despite the lack of empirical support for those assumptions (Kazmin, 2021; Lancet Editorial Board, 2021). There was also extreme confidence in the ability of India, as a significant producer of vaccines in the world, to meet and exceed global and national vaccination demands, including to the COVAX program (Schmali & Singh, 2021).

Table 7.1 SARS-CoV-2 mortality and populist-nationalistic leadership

Nation	Populist-nationalist leader	Official mortality during term as of August, 2021
Brazil	Bolsonaro	~560,000
India	Modi	~410,000
Mexico	Obrador	~240,000
Russia	Putin	~160,000
United Kingdom	Johnson	~150,000
United States	Trump	~400,000 (term ended January 20, 2021)

Note: Official death tallies were often highly politicized during the pandemic. Researchers have projected the official tallies to be unreliably low estimates of actual national mortality. India, for example was projected to have undercounted by millions (see below). Despite the undercounts, these six nations showed mortality disparities to the rest of the world. With 29% of the world's population, they accounted for approximately 45% of accounted deaths by August, 2021

The national government loosened restrictions and many citizens returned to normal activities, resulting in superspreader events related to the national election and a significant religious celebration (Associated Press, 2021b). As a result, India experienced an extremely serious surge beginning in the spring of 2021 due to the delta variant (Biswas, 2021a). The daily death toll during the surge was the highest reported of any nation to that point in the pandemic, resulting in so many cremations that trees were cut in down in city parks for the funeral pyres (Associated Press, 2021a). The government was unable to track deaths, resulting in significant undercounting of COVID-19 incidence and mortality (Johnson, 2021). Excess deaths by summer 2021 were projected to be between 3 to four million (Anand et al., 2021), perhaps doubling the official global mortality rate of COVID-19. There were many fears the health system would collapse, so much so that the US and others received significant pressure to share ventilators, oxygen, and other relevant resources to address the coronavirus (Jha, 2021; White House, 2021). Vaccines for the COVAX program were redirected to national needs, but it was mostly too little too late, with vaccine inequality common (Mehrotra & Saaliq, 2021). The failures of vaccination rollout not only significantly impacted the nation, but also the world, with serious global concerns that extreme spread would create variants for which vaccinations provided no protection (Ghosal & Pathi, 2021; Saaliq & Ghosal, 2021; Thakur, 2021). During the vaccine crisis, the Poonawalla family, who financially controlled vaccine producers, departed India for the UK, perhaps due to death threats (Mascarenhas, 2021). Many in India were left to suffer surge consequences and the vaccine rollout debacle, but not the privileged Poonawalla family.

Twitter was alive with messages blaming the populist-nationalist government for the surge and its consequences, and as a result, the Indian government censored certain tweets uncomplimentary to the government (BBC, 2021g). Misinformation during the surge was also rampant, hindering an empirically informed response (Klepper & Mehrotra, 2021). Some saw the similarities of the failure of the Indian populist-nationalist government and the US populist-nationalist response, one noting that COVID-19 highlighted the fragility of populist-nationalist leadership (Collinson, 2021). Besides significant loss of life, the surge resulted in significant and unexpected election losses for the populist-nationalistic government of Prime Minister Modi (Reuters, 2021a).

Deprioritizing pandemics in the US happened much earlier than the arrival of SARS-CoV-2. Despite protestations by the administration of former President Trump that they were blindsided by the possibility of a pandemic, efforts had been ongoing for many years to prepare and plan for one. A playbook manual for addressing a hypothetical pandemic was passed from the Obama administration to the Trump administration during the transition period before the inauguration (Bowden, 2020; Executive Office of the President of the United States, 2017). President Trump acknowledged on a widely publicized audiotape that the administration had decided to intentionally downplay the threat of the pandemic, despite many briefings that suggested it a national security risk to the US (Lipton et al., 2020; Woodward, 2020).

The reality of the situation is that political strategies were used to discredit efforts to wear masks and social distance because the economics of the pandemic were a higher priority than the public health of the country. In addition, a diffusion of responsibility accompanied by blame of others for perceived failures became common. For example, the former Trump administration delegated responsibility to the states to seek out PPE and implement policies rather than centralize responsibility to the federal government (Siemaszko, 2020).

Diffusion of responsibility and blaming (often by means of colonial splitting) are common strategies from the playbook of colonial institutions, a method for advancing and defending self-interests and certainly not a pathway to assuming social responsibility (Blume, 2020). Distrust in science fostered early in the pandemic to support the economic agenda later extended to distrust in the science related to vaccine production and rollout.

Politics had played a role in vaccine rollouts for many years before SARS-CoV-2. Researchers found that politicizing vaccines tended to enhance vaccine hesitancy. Increased politicization of the HPV vaccine in the 2000s was associated with reduced support of doctors, government, and vaccine programs (Fowler & Gollust, 2015). An anti-science movement (referred to as *antivaxxer*) had grown for many years, driven by misinformation that vaccinations were unsafe—a potential barrier to vaccine-assisted herd immunity.

A survey from France conducted during the lockdown early in 2020 found that people with extreme political views (left or right) or who had neglected to vote at all, were more likely to express hesitancy toward getting a hypothetical COVID-19 vaccine (The COCONEL Group, 2020), likely due to political disinformation and deception. The study scientists suggested it would be critical to depoliticize vaccine information if hesitancy due to political perspectives was to be addressed. Unfortunately, many populist-national governments continued to find value in politicizing pandemic responses for purposes of political self-interests. Experts were concerned that hesitancy might delay vaccine-assisted herd immunity in the US (Kaiser Health News, 2021). Anti-science and antivaxxers are discussed in detail in Chap. 9.

The Rollout The first shipments of the first vaccine approved for emergency use (Pfizer) left the storage facility in Michigan in mid-December, 2020 (Madani, 2020). By February, 2020, there were three vaccines approved for emergency use: The Moderna and Pfizer vaccines used a new messenger RNA process, and the Johnson & Johnson vaccine (and AstraZeneca) used a viral vector adenovirus method to build immunity, a method originally developed for use against Ebola. Moderna and Pfizer utilized a two-vaccination series whereas Johnson & Johnson (and AstraZeneca) used one vaccination (Branswell, 2021).

Interestingly, Pfizer vials were found to contain more doses than advertised, but once they realized the enhanced dosages, they adjusted by reducing the number of vials shipped to fulfill the government contracts. Pfizer suggested that their strategy allowed for more to receive the vaccine but also could be interpreted as a self-interested business decision (Weiland et al., 2021). There was great optimism and pride in producing the vaccines so rapidly, but not every vaccine candidate was successful (Murphy, 2021b). In addition, there were missteps in the supply chain contributing to slow arrival and sometimes wasted doses due to mishandling and unpredictable demand. One county in rural Washington state did not waste a vaccine through late January, attributed to a well-formulated emergency plan established due to re-occurring risks from forest fires and also to county-wide trust in the health officials delivering and administering the vaccines (Zdanowicz, 2021).

The goal was to reach herd immunity with the assistance of these vaccines, but the initial rollout was slow and chaotic. As discussed earlier, the Trump administration left responsibility for vaccinations largely to the states, continuing the policy of diffusion of responsibility. States did not uniformly track data concerning vaccinations, which contributed to confusion (Ramos, 2021). The decentralization of data to the states was a roadblock to developing a national strategy for vaccine rollout after the transition of administrations (Smith, 2021c). In addition, states had different policies concerning who would get vaccinations when, leaving the decisions up to the whims of political forces in charge of those states (Richards, 2020). The initial rollout of vaccines was uneven across US states due to production and supply problems, as well as the splintered policies of 50 splintered states and their splintered health care systems (Horton, 2021). In addition, politicization of vaccines hindered the rollout significantly. State governments were apparently misled about a non-existent federal stockpile of vaccines (Ingram, 2020). A couple of weeks later it was discovered that the Trump administration had opposed providing additional funds to states to fund the vaccine rollout, despite expecting the states to take responsibility for the rollouts within their geographical boundaries (Florko, 2021).

The severe winter weather in February, 2021 (see Chap. 2), also slowed vaccination efforts over much of the US, hindering progress toward vaccination-assisted herd immunity (Ingram & Moschella, 2021). Some scholars expressed the belief that the key to vaccine-assisted immunity in the US was vaccination of children, who risked carrying the virus asymptomatically into homes and schools, but those vaccinations would not become widely available until late 2021 (Moghadas et al., 2021; Velavan et al., 2020). A spokesperson for the WHO indicated that vaccine-assisted global herd immunity was unlikely until 2022 at the earliest (CNN, 2021). Global vaccine-assisted immunity relied upon colonial powers willing to share the vaccines their companies had created is discussed later in this chapter.

There were also concerns that new variants of the SARS-CoV-2 virus might be more resistant to the newly developed vaccinations and perhaps risk reinfections (Callaway, 2021; Joseph, 2021a, 2021b). As evidence of this concern, the spring of 2021 brought more lockdowns in Europe due to the spread of the new variants (Gallagher et al., 2021). However, some vaccines seemed to have some efficacy against the variants (Joseph, 2021b; Moderna, 2021). The overarching concern remained that uncontrolled community spread might enhance the development of variants that could threaten the efficacy of the existing vaccines, so the hope was that existing vaccinations, social distancing, and masks would rein in that spread (American Medical Association, 2021; BBC, 2021d; Yan & Maxouris, 2021).

Vaccination Disparities

Bias and hardened distrust in colonial health care may have contributed to vaccination hesitancy early in the pandemic, but vaccine hesitancy waned in minoritized communities after the Trump administration left office (Huetteman, 2021). Vaccine disparities among minoritized people were largely due to problems with distribution and access in communities and an inequitable system that favored the older White American population (Bass et al., 2021; Lakhani, 2021). As an example of bias in distribution, the state of Florida diverted vaccinations that were meant for African American communities to wealthy White Americans instead (Goldhill, 2021). Data from the CDC regarding early vaccination distribution supported concerns about vaccine distribution disparities (Hughes et al., 2021). Disparities were notable despite the inconsistent nature of tracking vaccinations by race and ethnicity in some states (Ellis & McPhillips, 2021; Johnson et al., 2021; Painter et al., 2020). By late February, 2021, only 4.6% of Latinx and 5.7% of Black Americans had received a single dose of any vaccine (Lakhani, 2021), and testing and vaccine disparities for these groups persisted (McPhillips, 2021b). Indigenous Americans, who struggled between the fears of trusting a colonial system and fears of multiple pandemics over time, chose to vaccinate at higher rates early in the COVID-19 pandemic than one might expect (Morgan, 2021). However, tribes without federal recognition, often victims of racist twentieth Century termination policies meant to assimilate away tribal identities, rights, and sovereignty (Dunbar-Ortiz, 2014), were without federal resources to address pandemic risks and often fell through the cracks (Fernando, 2021).

Later in the pandemic, a study examined the US vaccination rate by counties and found that low SES and limited internet connectivity were associated with low vaccination rates (McPhillips, 2021a). Other demographic groups at risk for being ignored during the pandemic vaccination campaign were older adults and children with disabilities. The online systems that many states offered to schedule vaccinations were difficult to navigate and presented barriers to people who would be considered digital immigrants. Anecdotal evidence suggests that many became frustrated with the process or seeking vaccines, and perhaps resigned not to get one as a result. The risks for neglect increased for older adult living alone and without someone to watch over their welfare during the pandemic (Flaccus et al., 2021). Children with disabilities were considered to be at high risk but were unable to be vaccinated due to the lack of clinical trials for children at that time. Parents were also concerned their children would fall further behind due to the importance of face-to-face instruction to appropriately educate children with special needs (Syed & Siemaszko, 2021). Parents and children were left in educational limbo by circumstances beyond their control. Children were also at risk for missing routine vaccinations for other diseases due to difficulty accessing health care services (Thomas, 2020).

Vaccine Nationalism as a Barrier to Global Vaccination Chapter 1 introduced how a colonial worldview contributes to prioritizing self-interests, including national self-interests, over the interests of the whole. Major colonial powers assumed a sense of ownership over the vaccines created by pharmaceuticals from their own countries, having the financial resources to lock-up vaccine purchases first and thus ensuring the privileged of the world would have first access to vaccines (Smith, 2020b). Rich colonial nations prioritized their own populations first for vaccination in an act referred to as vaccine nationalism (Smith, 2020a). More will be written about this subsequently.

Nationalism creates competition and conflict due to inherent beliefs in the primacy of one country's self-interests over the needs of others, derived from the belief of supremacy of certain peoples and cultures (see Chap. 1). The competition and conflict were visible very early in the vaccine rollout period. In order to compensate for vaccine nationalism and the inequities between rich and poor nations created by colonialism, the UN created a program funded by member nations called *COVAX* to ensure access of poor nations to vaccines (BBC, 2021b). Even with COVAX, it was expected to take months to years for poor nations to fully share in vaccines due to vaccine nationalism (Cheng & Ghosal, 2020). The COVAX program also fell significantly behind because manufacture of vaccines would not match promised delivery, and therefore the program suffered from significant logistical shortcomings that were not helped by vaccine nationalism (Goldhill & Furneaux, 2021).

Several examples make the point concerning the inequities of vaccine nationalism. First, the US originally refused to join the WHO's COVAX program to make vaccine available to countries without the resources, and then later when it joined, the amount contributed to the COVAX fund was miniscule compared to the need and what was spent inside the US to ensure vaccinations (Smith, 2021b). Later, the US opted to recommend booster vaccines to over the protestations from much of the world who had not received even their first vaccination (O'donnell & Aboulenein, 2021). Second, the European Union became very irritated and threatened Pfizer and AstraZeneca over late delivery and unfulfilled vaccinations purchased by the European Union (BBC, 2021a), insisting their investment in the AstraZeneca vaccine entitled them to those shipments immediately (Diaz, 2021). The European Union responded by blocking the shipment of any AstraZeneca vaccine produced in the union as their claimed property even if "owned" by another country, which was called out as unfair by the WHO (BBC, 2021c). Later in the year, Australia complained to the European Union that Italy was interfering with an export shipment of the AstraZeneca vaccine (BBC, 2021i, 2021k). A third example was Israel, who widely vaccinated its citizens and was held up as a model of success in terms of vaccination rollout (Jeffay, 2021). However, Israelis were only vaccinating Israelis--not sharing vaccines with Palestinians in areas controlled by Israel (UN, 2021). Vaccination decisions were well-aligned to Israel's self-interests, but not well-aligned with the interests of the whole. And a final example was India, who in the spring of 2021 halted exports of the AstraZeneca vaccine to address a surge of cases in its own country (BBC, 2021f). Vaccine nationalism and other inequitable struggles to address the pandemic resulted in deep seated anger and frustration between nations, driving wedges in international relationships, especially within the European Union (McGee, 2021).

Use of vaccine nationalistic tactics was not just limited to rich national governments. When negotiating with Latin American nations for sales and distribution of vaccines, Pfizer insisted that purchases be backed by national collateral such as government office buildings, military installations, and other national resources that would be forfeited to Pfizer if payment did not occur. Pfizer also insisted the agreements be confidential (Davies et al., 2021). Rich nations opposed a UN effort to waive patents on vaccinations in order to allow poorer nations to make and distribute the vaccines more quickly (Cheng & Hinnant, 2021; Reuters, 2021b). Opposition to waiving patents was an effort to protect the national business interests of rich colonial nations. Advancing business self-interests during COVID-19 were as obvious as efforts to advance national self-interests.

In response to vaccine nationalism, the UN has persistently chided rich colonial nations to share rather than hoard vaccines (Hallam, 2021). Director-General Tedros Ghebreyesus of the WHO insisted that acting with only national self-interests in vaccine distribution left the world vulnerable to COVID-19 (Li, 2020). Later, he wrote an op-ed suggesting that placing national interests first in vaccination efforts would not effectively stop the pandemic, referring to it as a 'me first' approach (Ghebreyesus, 2021). Africa was significantly impacted by the lack of equity in vaccine distribution, leaving the continent far behind the rich colonial nations that practiced vaccine nationalism (Imray, 2021). Contrast Africa's need with reports that the US had likely wasted over a million vaccine doses by during that same period of time (Levin, 2021).

From an Indigenous psychological perspective, Director-General Ghebreyesus presented a realistic appraisal of the circumstances of a pandemic in an interdependent world, a world that is only as strong as its most vulnerable members. Acting only with me-first self-interests ignores the realities of the natural world, but colonial societies are often blinded to those realities by their proximal foci on self and individuals. A legitimate concern was that vaccine nationalism would prolong the pandemic globally. As suggested by Dr. Larry Brilliant, a scientist heavily involved in the eradication of smallpox, 'until everyone in the world is safe, no one is safe' (as quoted in Ramgopal et al., 2021).

Impatience and Defiance The vaccination rollout was accompanied by relaxation of public health prevention strategies, such as reopening at-risk businesses (e.g., indoor dining) and relaxing social distancing and masking requirements that had been associated with reduced virus spread (Fitzsimons, 2021; Stobbe, 2021). The vaccines gave a false sense of security in the face of a new wave driven by virus variants. Vaccines were also used as an excuse to advance political agendas—all against the collective advice of health scientists (Leonhardt, 2021; Siemaszko, 2021; Weber & Webber, 2021). Impatience is also a function of colonial privilege when people expect to have their needs and desires accommodated upon demand. People without privilege typically do not have those expectations, and in fact, often expect the opposite outcome. In addition, many people experienced "pandemic fatigue," a risk predicted several years earlier in a comprehensive report to the World Bank on pandemic threats (Jonas, 2013). Many frontline health care professionals were angry and discouraged by the relaxation of safety measures when vaccinations offered optimism about lowering spread hospitalizations (Rahim et al., 2021). A UK study suggested vaccinations alone were insufficient to end the pandemic and relaxing social distancing, masking, and other mitigations was unwise (Moore et al., 2021).

Anticipating Rather than Reacting: An Indigenous Interpretation

Many pandemic mitigation measures had been known for centuries, yet that knowledge appeared to be forgotten, perhaps due to the proximal thinking of colonial nations. In addition, mitigation methods had always faced opposition by those who wished to assert colonial libertarianism and pursue self-interests at the risk of the whole. Misinformation and deception were widely used during the COVID-19 pandemic to oppose mitigation measures, including by populist-nationalist politicians in ways that fostered widespread skepticism and distrust in the COVID-19 science. Vaccines were projected to have saved hundreds of thousands of lives and prevented perhaps more than a million hospitalizations (Galvani et al., 2021), but their successes were undercut by widespread misinformation. Treated unvaccinated people in June to July 2021 was estimated to cost over $5,000,000,000, with average costs for COVID-19 hospitalization at around $20,000 per individual, with significantly greater costs for treating severe illness (Amin & Cox, 2021). Vaccine hesitancy was driven by politicized disinformation and deception. Politicians also used diffusion of responsibility as a way to avoid social responsibility by blaming others for failures to control virus spread. Divisiveness and deception enhanced distrust and skepticism in methods to curb COVID-19.

The splintered US colonial health care system responded poorly given the inability to have a unified collective vision and mission. Thousands of independent systems and institutions operated with their own local interests that enhanced competition and limited cooperation and collaboration across state, county, and even municipalities. Some locales would tighten mitigation measures when surges spiked whereas their neighbors would not. The result was a chaos and mass confusion as policies and vaccine rollout varied greatly across governmental entities under the errant colonial belief that artificial boundaries created safety.

National and business self-interests were advanced during the pandemic through vaccine nationalism. True to colonial values, nations and businesses claimed ownership over life-saving vaccines, hindering the global response to control an end to the pandemic.

The continued defiance toward social distancing and masking cost many people their lives in colonial nations governed by populist-nationalist leaders even after vaccines became available. Despite the efforts of public health sciences, the pandemic rollout became an exercise in colonial privilege that favored rich nations over poor and rich Americans over minoritized others. Vaccine nationalism seriously hindered a global response to end of the pandemic that risked virus mutations that might be immune to existing vaccinations. Colonial racial biases were exposed in medical technology and treatment, and in vaccine clinical trials rollouts.

An IAPP perspective would interpret these events as self-interests run amok in such a way that pandemic response was thwarted. Hierarchical thinking contributed to the idea of acceptable risks to the vulnerable in order to favor the liberties of the privileged. Colonial perspectives of proximal linear time made for impatience with the mitigation process, prioritizing a return to proximal liberties for self at the expense of distal protections for the whole. Many people never warmed up to the idea of slowing down to help others, even when vaccinations promised an end-in-sight to the pandemic. The result was more spread and risk due to the impatience to get back to a colonial normal.

Reacting rather than anticipating is a foundational problem of colonialism. Colonial worldviews focus on the proximal to the detriment of the long view—focus on the self and individual to the detriment of the whole. Proximal, self-oriented views contributed to reacting after the fact to COVID-19. Reacting negated preparation because it reflects a here and now focus. A long-view of time, and a broad rather than local view of impact, helps to anticipate what is needed to both prepare for and address the next pandemic. A long-view would have promoted patience in the process as well (Blume, 2020). An egalitarian perspective would negate the perspective of privilege that impatiently demands that the needs and desires of the one should be met immediately. Unfortunately, the colonial world is stuck in the moment and on itself in such a way that does not bode well for future pandemic preparation. A transformed perspective toward collective anticipations appears to be a necessary step toward wellness.

References

Alexander, P., & Siemaszko, C. (2020, November 17). Covid-19 cases are on the rise in all 50 states, NBC news data shows. NBC News. https://www.nbcnews.com/news/us-news/covid-19-cases-are-rise-all-50-states-nbc-news-n1248006.

Allen, A. (2020, January 31). How the feds missed their chance at a coronavirus vaccine. Politico. https://www.politico.com/news/2020/01/31/coronavirus-vaccine-missed-chance-109709.

American Hospital Association. (2020). 2020 AHA hospital statistics. Author. https://www.aha.org/statistics/fast-facts-us-hospitals.

American Medical Association (2021, February 15). Peter Hotez, MD, PhD, on his 10 years of work on coronavirus. Author. https://www.ama-assn.org/delivering-care/public-health/peter-hotez-md-phd-his-10-years-work-coronavirus.

Amin, K., & Cox, C. (2021, September 14). Unvaccinated COVID-19 hospitalizations cost billions of dollars. Peterson Center/Kaiser Family Foundation. https://www.healthsystemtracker.org/brief/unvaccinated-covid-patients-cost-the-u-s-health-system-billions-of-dollars/.

Anand, A., Sandefur, J., & Subramanian, A. (2021). Three new estimates of India's all-cause excess mortality during the COVID-19 pandemic. Center for Global Development. https://www.cgdev.org/sites/default/files/three-new-estimates-indias-all-cause-excess-mortality-during-covid-19-pandemic.pdf.

Andina Agencia Peruana de Noticias. (2021, February 12). What is known about COVID-19 reinfection cases in Peru?: Author. https://andina.pe/ingles/noticia-what-is-known-so-far-about-covid19-reinfection-cases-in-peru-833533.aspx.

Associated Press. (2021a, April 25). Mass funeral pyres reflect India's COVID crisis. Author. https://apnews.com/article/health-india-coronavirus-8788a4dadc2103ec30f40111dec92f15.

Associated Press. (2021b, April 28). India's deadly virus surge follows crowded events. Author. https://apnews.come/article/health-india-coronavirus-4b105300bbf93cc844ef9b44a462c.

Bahreini, F., Najafi, R., Amini, R., Khazaei, S., & Bashirian, S. (2020). Reducing false negatives PCR test for COVID-19. *International Journal of Maternal and Child Health and AIDS, 9*(3), 408–410. https://doi.org/10.21106/ijma421

Barry, J. M. (2018). The great influenza: The story of the deadliest pandemic in history. Penguin Books.

Bass, K., Morial, M., & Grills, C. (2021, March 9). Opinion: Vaccine hesitancy is not the problem among people of color. It's vaccine access. Washington Post. https://www.washingtonpost.com/opinions/2021/03/09/vaccine-hesitancy-is-not-problem-among-people-color-its-vaccine-access/.

BBC. (2020a, April 24). Coronavirus: Trump's disinfectant and sunlight claims fact-checked. BBC. https://www.bbc.com/news/world-us-canada-52399464.

BBC. (2020b, November 1) Covid-19: English lockdown may last beyond 2 Dec, says Gove. Author. https://www.bbc.com/news/uk-54767118.

BBC. (2020c, December 20). Facial recognition fails on race, government study says. BBC. https://www.bbc.com/news/technology-50865437.

BBC. (2021a, January 23). Coronavirus: EU vaccine woes mount as new delays emerge. Author. https://www.bbc.com/new/world-europe-55771223.

BBC. (2021b, January 27). Covax: How will Covid vaccines be shared with poorer countries. Author. https://www.bbc.com/news/world-55795297.

BBC. (2021c, January 30). Coronavirus: WHO criticizes EU over vaccine export controls. Author. https://www.bbc.com/news/world-europe-55860540.

BBC. (2021d, March 2). Covid-19 variants pose 'real threat' to vaccine progress, CDC warns. Author. https://www.bbc.com/news/world-us-canada-56247656.

BBC. (2021e, March 10). Covid: Brazil experts issue warning as hospitals 'close to collapse. Author. https://www.bbc.com/new/world-latin-america-56342303.

BBC. (2021f, March 24). Coronavirus: Indian temporarily halts Oxford-AstraZeneca vaccine exports. BBC. https://www.bbc.com/news/world-asia-india-56513371.

BBC. (2021g, April 26). Indian Covid: Anger as twitter ordered to remove critical virus posts. Author. https://www.bbc.com/new/world-asia-56883483

BBC. (2021h, January 25). Lebanon's coronavirus lockdown: 'We can't leave our homes day or night. Author. https:///www.bbc.com/news/world-middle-east-55717523.

BBC. (2021i, March 5). Covid: Bolsonaro tells Brazilians to 'stop whining' as deaths spike. Author. https://www.bbc.news/news/world-latin-america-56288548.

BBC. (2021j, January 25). Covid: Dutch PM mark Rutte condemns curfew riots as 'criminal violence.' Author. https://www.bbc.com/news/world-europe-55796126.

BBC. (2021k, March 5). Covid-19: Australia asks European Commission to review Italy's vaccine block. Author. https://www.bbc.com/news/world-australia-56290226

Bender, E. M., Gebru, T., McMillan-Major, A., & Shmitchell, S. (2021). On the dangers of stochastic parrots: Can language models be too big? FAccT 21. https://doi.org/10.1145/3442188.3445922.

Bianucci, R., Benedictow, O. J., Fornaciari, G., & Giuffra, V (2013). Quinto Tiberio Angeleiro and new measures for controlling plague in 16th-century Alghero, Sardinia. *Emerging Infectious Diseases, 19*(9), 1–8. https://doi.org/10.3201/eid1909.120311

Biswas, S. (2021a, April 22).What is the India Covid variant and will vaccines work? BBC. https://www.bbc.com/news/world-asia-india-56844925

Biswas, S. (2021b, May 9). Mucormycosis: The 'black fungus' maiming Covid patients in India. BBC. https://www.bbc.com/news/world-asia-india-57027829.

Blume, A. W. (2020). A new psychology based on community, equality, and care of the earth: An indigenous American perspective. ABC-CLIO/Praeger.
Bowden, J. (2020, July 29). Susan Rice: Obama admin gave Trump 'pandemic for dummies playbook'. The Hill. https://www.thehill.ocm/homenews/administration/509592-susan-rice-obama-admin-gave-trump-pandemic-for-dummie-playbook
Branswell, H. (2021, February 2). Comparing the Covid-19 vaccines developed by Pfizer, Moderna, and Johnson & Johnson. STAT News. https://www.statnews.com/2021/02/02/comparing-the-covid-19-vaccines-developed-by-pfizer-moderna-and-johnson-johnson/
Brodwin, E., & St. Fleur, N. (2021, February 19) FDA issues alert on 'limitations' of pulse oximeters, without explicit mention of racial bias. STAT News. https://www.statnews.com/2021/02/19/fda-issues-alert-on-limitations-of-pulse-oximeters-without-explicit-mention-of-racial-bi/
Bush, E. (2020, October 15) Lummi nation withdraws from AstraZeneca COVID-19 vaccine trial. Seattle Times. https://www.seattletimes.com/seattle-news/health/lummi-nation-withdraws-from-astrazeneca-covid-19-vaccine-trial/
Callaway, E. (2021, January 21). Fast-spreading COVID variant can elude immune responses. Nature. https://www.nature.com/articles/d41586-021-00121-z
CDC. (2021, August 26). Rapid increase in Ivermectin prescriptions and reports of severe illness associated with use of products containing Ivermectin to prevent or treat COVID-19. Author. https://emergency.cdc.gov/han/2021/pdf/CDC_HAN_449.pdf
Chastain, D. B., Osae, S. P., Henao-Martínez, A. F., Franco-Paredes, C., Chastain, J. S., & Young, H. N. (2020). Racial disproportionality in Covid clinical trials. *New England Journal of Medicine, 383*(9), e59. https://www.nejm.org/.
Chen, C., Arnsdorf, I., & Gabrielson, R. (2021, January 19) How operation warp speed created vaccination chaos. ProPublica. https://www.propublica.org/article/how-operation-warp-speed-created-vaccination-chaos
Cheng, M., & Ghosal, A. (2020, December 14) Poor countries face long wait for vaccines despite promises. Associated Press. https://apnews.com/article/poorer-countires-coronavirus-vaccine-0980fa905b6e1ce2f14a149cd2c438cd
Cheng, M., & Hinnant, L. (2021, March 1). Countries urge drug companies to share vaccine know-how. Associated Press. https://apnews.com/article/drug-companies-called-shre-vaccine-info-22d92afbc3ea9ed519be007f8887bcf6
Clark, D. (2020, April 23). Trump suggests 'injection' of disinfectant to beat coronavirus and 'clean' the lungs. NBC News. https://www.nbcnews.com/politics/donald-trump/trump-suggests-injection-disinfectant-beat-coronavirus-clean-lings-n1191216
Clark, E., Chiao, E. Y., & Amerian, E. S. (2020). Why contact tracing efforts have failed to curb coronavirus disease 2019 (COVID-19) transmission in much of the United States. *Clinical Infectious Diseases*. https://doi.org/10.1093/cid/ciaa1155
CNN. (2021, January 12). WHO warns that herd immunity won't happen in 2021, even with vaccines. Author. https://www.cnn.com/wolrd/live-news/coronavirus-pandemic-vaccine-updates-01-12-21/h_13f615c58ad6f0febd860d514e36fc99
Cohen, E. (2020a, October 30) Already, pharmaceutical companies' predictions about Covid-19 vaccines haven't come true. CNN. https://www.cnn.com/2020/10/30/health/covid-19-vaccine-predictions-pharmaceutical-companies/index.html
Cohen, J. (2020b). Here's how the U.S. could release a COVID-19 vaccine before the election—And why that scares some. Science https://doi.org/10.1126/science.abe5150.
Cohrs, R. (2021, March 2). The Trump administration quietly spent billions in hospital funds on operation warp speed. Stat News. https://www.statnews.com/2021/03/02/trump-administration-quietly-spent-billions-in-hospital-funds-on-operation-warp-speed/
Collier, K. (2021, August 9). Twitter's racist algorithm is also ageist, ableist, and Islamaphobic, researchers find. NBC News. https://www.nbcnews.com/tech/tech-news/twitters-racist-algorithm-also-ageist-ableist-islamaphobic-researchers-rcna1632
Collinson, S. (2021, April 26). Covid-19 exposed populist leaders like Modi and Trump. CNN. https://www.cnn.com/2021/04/26/world/meanwhile-in-america-populism/index.html

Davies, M., Furneaux, R., Ruiz, I., & Langlois, J. (2021, February 23). 'Held to ransom': Pfizer demands governments gamble with state assets to secure vaccine deal. The Bureau of Investigative Journalism. https://www.thebureauinvestigates.com/stories/2021-02-23/held-to-ransom-pfizer-demands-governments-gamble-with-state-assets-to-secure-vaccine-deal

Diaz, J. (2021, January 26). European Union warns AstraZeneca over reduction in vaccine shipments. National Public Radio. https://www.npr.org/sections/coronavirus-live-updates/2021/01/26/960642692/european-union-warns-astrazeneca-over-reduction-in-vaccine-shipments

Dicker, R. (2020, April 7). Donald Trump has stake in hydroxychloroquine drugmaker: Report. Huffington Post. https://www.huffpost.com/entry/donld-trump-stake-company-hydroxychloroquine_n_5e8c41d7c5b6e1d10a696280

Doshi, P. (2020). Will covid-19 vaccines save lives? Current trials aren't designed to tell us. BMJ, 371, m4037. https://doi.org/10.1136/bmj.m4037.

Doughton, S. (2020, October 24) Gates-funded UW study shows hydroxychloroquine doesn't prevent COVID-19. Seattle Times. https://www.seattletimes.com/seattle-news/health/big-uw-study-shows-hydroxychloroquine-doesnt-prevent-covid-19/

Dunbar-Ortiz, R. (2014). An indigenous peoples' history of the United States. Beacon Press.

Edwards, E., & Hillyard, V. (2020, March 23). Man dies after taking chloroquine in an attempt to prevent coronavirus. NBC News. https://www.nbcnews.com/health/health-news/man-dies-after-ingesting-chrloroquine-attemtp-prevent-coronavirus-n1167166

Ellis, N. T., & McPhillips, D. (2021, January 26). White people are getting vaccinated at higher rates than black or Latino Americans. CNN. https://www.cnn.com/2021/01/26/us/vaccination-disparities-rollout/index.html

Evans, A. C. (2021, February 3). Written testimony of the American Psychological Association. Hearing: On road to recovery: Ramping up COVID-19 vaccines, testing, and medical supply chain. 117th US Congress.

Executive Office of the President of the United States. (2017). Playbook for early response to high-consequence emerging infectious disease threats and biological incidents. Author. https://assets.documentcloud.org/documents/6819268/Pandemic-Playbook.pdf.

Fernando, C. (2021, February 27). Pandemic leaves tribes without US recognition at higher risk. Associated Press. https://apnews.com/article/pandemics-tribal-governments-united-states-coronavirus-pandemic-9eb1a8218c602d80385f2fce89625147

Fitzsimons, T. (2021, March 2). Texas and Mississippi to lift mask mandates and roll back Covid restrictions. NBC News. https://www.nbcnews.com/news/us-news/gov-greg-abbott-lift-teaxas-mask-mandate-open-state-100-n1259329

Flaccus, G., Hollingsworth, H., & Bynum, R. (2021, March 4). Falling through cracks': Vaccine bypasses some older adults. Associated Press. https://apnews.com/article/coronavirus-vaccine-bypass-some-older-adults-374da36856dd9428643db2c3e85564da

Flores, L. E., Frontera, W. R., Andrasik, M. P., del Rio, C., Mondriguez-González, P., Krantz, E. M., Pergam, S. A., & Silver, J. K. (2020). Assessment of the inclusion of racial/ethnic minority, female, and older individuals in clinical trials. *JAMA Network Open, 4*(2), e2037640. https://doi.org/10.1001/jamanetworkopen.2020.37640

Florko, N. (2021, January 31). Trump officials actively lobbied to deny states money for vaccine rollout last fall. STAT News. https://www.statnews.com/2021/01/31/trump-officials-lobbied-to-deny-states-money-for-vaccine-rollout/

Fonseca, F. (2021, January 4). Fast rollout of virus vaccine trials reveals tribal distrust. Associated Press. https://apnews.com/article/us-news-flagstaff-arizona-clinical-trials-coronavirus-pandemic-712d482a83cb49464745fca7f8b93692

Fowler, E. F., & Gollust, S. E. (2015). The content and effect of politicized health controversies. *The Annals of the American Academy of Political and Social Science, 658*, 155–171. https://doi.org/10.1177/0002716214555505

France24. (2020, December 18). Brazil's Bolsonaro warns virus vaccine can turn people into 'crocodiles'. Author. https://www.france24.com/en/live-news/20201218-brazil-s-bolsonaro-warns-virus-vaccine-can-turn-people-into-crocodiles

Galewitz, P. (2021, January 27). Poll: Nearly half of American adults now want the Covid vaccine—ASAP. Kaiser Health Network. https://khn.org/news/article/poll-nearly-half-of-american-adults-now-want-the-covid-vaccine-asap/

Gallagher, D., Di Donato, V., & Fox, K. (2021, March 13). Italy prepares for an Easter lockdown as Covid-19 cases grow exponentially. CNN. https://www.cnn.com/2021/03/13/europes/italy-coronavirus-national-lockdown-intl/index.html

Galvan, A., & Cooper, J. J. (2020, March 24). Arizona death prompts warning against self-medication. Associated Press. https://apnews.com/article/1c8219c0d586317ae3432 5d1276ae4f

Galvani, A., Moghadas, S. M., & Schneider, E. C. (2021, July 7). *Deaths and hospitalizations averted by rapid U. S. vaccination rollout.* Commonwealth Fund. https://www.commonwealthfund.org/publications/issue-briefs/2021/jul/deaths-and-hospitalizations-averted-rapid-us-vaccination-rollout

Gharpure, R., Guo, A., Bishnoi, C. K., Patel, U., Gifford, D., Tippins, A., Jaffe, A., Shulman, E., Stone, N., Mungai, E., Bagchi, S., Bell, J., Srinivasan, A., Patel, A., & Link-Gelles, R. (2021). Early COVID-19 first-dose vaccination coverage among residents and staff members of skilled nursing facilities participating in the pharmacy partnership for long-term care program—United States, December 2020-January 2021. *MMWR, 70*, 178–182. https://www.cdc.gov/mmwr/volumes/70/wr/mm7005e2.htm?s_cid+mm7005e2_w

Gharpure, R., Hunter, C. M., Schnall, A. H., Barrett, C. E., Kirby, A. E., Kunz, J., Berling, K., Mercante, J. W., Murphy, J. L., & Garcia-Williams, A. G. (2020). Knowledge and practices regarding safe household cleaning and disinfection for COVID-19 prevention—United States, May 2020. MMWR, 69(23), 705–709. https://doi.org/10.15585/mmwr.mm6923e2.

Ghebreyesus, T. A. (2021, March 5). A 'me first' approach to vaccination won't defeat Covid. The Guardian. https://www.theguardian.com/commentisfree/2021/mar/05/vaccination-covid-vaccines-rich-nations

Ghosal, A., & Pathi, K. (2021, May 12). Scientists race to study variants in India as cases explode. Associated Press. https://apnews.com/article/europe-india-coronavirus-pandemic-science-health-fab2f1d6d08fd2442acf6a7e737866c4

Gill, V. (2021, September 22). Covid: Immune therapy from llamas shows promise. BBC. https://www.bbc.com/news/science-environment-58628689

Goldhill, O. (2021, March 4). In Palm Beach, Covid-19 vaccines intended for rural Black communities are instead going to wealthy Floridians. STAT News. https://www.statnews.com/2021/03/04/covid19-vaccines-for-rural-black-communities-going-to-wealthy-white-floridians/

Goldhill, O., & Furneaux, R. (2021, October 8). 'Naively ambitious': How COVAX failed on its promise to vaccinate the world. STAT News. https://www.statnews.com/2021/10/08/how-covax-failed-on-its-promise-to-vaccinate-the-world/

Gorvett, Z. (2021, January 8). The 432-year-old manual on social distancing. BBC. https://www.bbc.com/future/article/20210107-the-432-year-old-manual-on-social-distancing

Hallam, J. (2021, February 17). UN secretary general calls on wealthy nations to ensure vaccines are distributed fairly across the globe. CNN. https://www.cnn.com/world/live-news/coronavirus-pandemic-vaccine-updates-02-17-21/h_f2b0c513026201483ff7e911b54f2b4a

Hamel, L., Kirzinger, A., Muñana, C., & Brodie, M. (2020). KFF COVID-19 vaccine monitor: December 2020. Kaiser Family Foundation. https://www.kff.org/coronavirus-covid-19/report/kff-covid-19-vaccine-monitor-december-2020/.

Hixenbaugh, M. (2020, March 5). Scientists were close to a coronavirus vaccine years ago. Then the money dried up. NBC News. https://www.nbcnews.com/health/health-care/scientists-were-close-coronavirus-vaccine-years-ago-then-money-dried-n1150091

Holcombe, M., Sidner, S., & Jones, J. (2020, December 11). It took 10 days for a Ren hospital to turn a parking garage into a wing for Covid patients. Now it has 700 beds. CNN. https://www.cnn.com/2020/12/10/us/reno-hospital-covid-parking-garage/index.html

Horton, J. (2021, January 26). Covid-19: Was vaccine rollout a 'dismal failure' under Trump? BBC. https://www.bbc.com/news/world-us-canda-55721437

Howard, K. L., & Wright, C. N. (2021, February 11). Operation warp speed: Accelerated COVID-19 vaccine development status and efforts to address manufacturing challenges. US Government Accounting Office. https://www.gao.gov/products/gao-21-319

Huetteman, E. (2021, March 30). Covid vaccine hesitancy drops among all Americans, new survey shows. Kaiser Health News. https://khn.org/news/article/covid-vaccine-hesitancy-drops-among-americans-new-kff-survey-shows/

Hughes, M. M., Wang, A., Grossman, M. K., Pun, E., Whiteman, A., Deng, L., Hallisey, E., Sharpe, J. D., Ussery, E. N., Stokley, S., Musial, T., Weller, D. L., Murthy, B. P., Reynolds, L., Gibbs-Scharf, L., Harris, L. T., Ritchey, M. D., & Toblin, R. L. (2021). County-level COVID-19 vaccination coverage and social vulnerability—United States, December 14, 2020-March 1, 2021. *MMWR, 70*(12), 431–436. https://doi.org/10.15585/mmwr.mm7012e1externalicon

Imray, G. (2021, June 9). 'This is INSANE': Africa desperately short of COVID vaccine. Associated Press. https://apnews.com/article/uganda-south-africa-cape-town-africa-coronavirsu-pandemic-c5d7c2b0f927c8bd4d8d91fbfcda1ea

Ingram, D. (2020, January 15). No stockpile? Governors hit Washington as vaccine chokepoints pile up. NBC News. https://www.nbcnews.com/news/us-news/no-stockpile-governors-hit-washington-vaccine-chokepoints-pile-n1254442

Ingram, D., & Moschella, M. (2021, February 17). Extreme weather may delay reaching herd immunity, experts warn. NBC News. https://www.nbcnews.com/science/science-news/extreme-weather-may-delay-reaching-herd-immunity-experts-warn-rcna288

Jeffay, N. (2021, January, 24). Israel sees 60% drop in hospitalizations for age 60-plus 3 weeks after 1st shot. Times of Israel. https://www.timesofirael.com/israel-sees-60-drop-in-hospitalizations-for-over-60s-in-weeks-after-vaccination/

Jha, A. K. (2021, April 24). Opinion: India's coronavirus surge could collapse it health system. The U.S. can help. Washington Post. https://www.washingtonpost.com/opinions/2021/04/24/indias-coronavirus-surge-could-collapse-its-health-system-us-can-help/

Johns Hopkins Coronavirus Resource Center. (2021, January 27). Mortality analyses. Author. https://coronavirus.jhu.edu/data/mortality

Johnson, C. K. (2021, May 2). EXPLAINER: Why India's pandemic data is vastly undercounted. Associated Press. https://apnews.com/article/canada-business-pandemics-science-health-9a5edad508f63b05e4465fdffa61bcb8

Johnson, C. K., Kastanis, A., & Stafford, K. (2021, January 30). AP analysis: Racial disparity seen in US vaccination drive. Associated Press. https://apnews.com/article/race-and-ethnicity-health-coronavirus-pandemic-hispanics-d0746b028cf56231dbcdeda0fba24314

Jonas, O. B. (2013). Pandemic risk. World Bank. https://www.worldbank.org/content/dam/Worldbank/document/HDN/Health/WDR14_bp_Pandemic_Risk_Jonas.pdf.

Joseph, A. (2021a, January 28). South Carolina identifies the first U.S. case of coronavirus variant first seen in South Africa. STAT News. https://www.statnews.com/2021/01/28/south-carolina-first-cases-of-south-africa-variant/

Joseph, A. (2021b, February 5). The good and the (potentially) bad: What scientists know about variants and Covid-19 vaccines. STAT News. https://www.statnews.com/2021/02/05/what-scientists-know-variants-covid-19-vaccines/

Kaiser Health News. (2021, February 11). Vaccine resistance may delay herd immunity goals until end of year. Author. https://khn.org/morning-breakout/vaccine-resistance-may-delay-herd-immunity-goals-until-end-of-year/

Kaplan, R. M., & Frosch, D. L. (2020, December 28). Honesty is the best policy in selling vaccines. Wall Street Journal. https://www.wsj.com/articles/honesty-is-the-best-policy-in-selling-vaccines-11609196433

Kazmin, A. (2021, February 5). With millions of cases, has India achieved herd immunity? National Post. https://nationalpost.com/news/world/with-millions-of-case-has-india-acheived-herd-immunity/wcm/e69d5cd0-0eae-4ff4-8d3d-e3fc691fb590/amp/

Kharkwal, G. B., Sharma, S. K., Huang, Y.-Y., Dai, T., & Hamblin, M. R. (2011). Photodynamic therapy for infections: Clinical applications. *Lasers in Surgery and Medicine, 43*(7), 755–767. https://doi.org/10.1002/lsm21080

Klepper, D. & Mehrotra, N. (2021, May 13). Misinformation surges amid India's COVID-19 calamity. Associated Press. https://apnews.com/article/misinformation-surges-india-covid-c52d04de1c3b2332d572736ee069a495

LaFraniere, S., Thomas, K., Weiland, N., Baker, P., & Karni, A. (2020, August 2). Scientists worry about political influence over coronavirus vaccine project. New York Times. https://www.nytimes.com/2020/08/02/us/politics/coronavirus-vaccine.html

Lakhani, N. (2021, February 25). US racial inequities in vaccination raise risk of new Covid hotspots and variants. The Guardian. https://www.theguardian.com/us-news/2021/feb/25/coronavirus-vaccination-us-latino-black-americans-race

Lancet Editorial Board. (2021). India's COVID-19 emergency. *Lancet, 397*, 1683. https://doi.org/10.1016/S0140-6736(21)01052-7

Laulhé, M., Lefebvre, S., Le Broc-Ryckewaert, D., Pierre, M., Ferry, A., & Delorme, B. (2019). A standardized methodological approach to characterize the influence of key parameters on the in vitro efficacy of extracorporeal photopheresis. *PLoS One, 14*(3), e0212835. https://doi.org/10.1371/journal.pone.0212835

Leonhardt, D. (2021, March 3). Good morning. States are lifting pandemic restrictions before health experts think is wise. New York Times. https://messaging-custom-newsletters.nytimes.com/template/oakv2

Levin, D. (2021, August 1). The U.S. is wasting vaccine doses, even as cases rise and other countries suffer shortages. New York Times. https://www.nytimes.com/2021/08/01/us/covid-us-vaccine-wasted.html

Levin, E. G., Lustig, Y., Cohen, C., Fluss, R., Indenbaum, V., Amit, S., Doolman, R., Asraf, K., Mendelson, E., Ziv, A., Rubin, C., Freedman, L., Kreiss, Y., & Regev-Yochay, G. (2021). Waning immune humoral response to BNT162b2 Covid-19 vaccine over 6 months. *New England Journal of Medicine*. https://doi.org/10.1056/NEJMoa2114583

Li, D. K. (2020, August 6). WHO chief calls on governments to reject 'vaccine nationalism' and share plans globally. NBC News. https://www.nbcnews.com/news/world/who-chief-calls-governments-reject-vaccine-nationalism-share-plans-globally-n1236006

Lipton, E., Sanger, D. E., Haberman, M., Shear, M. D., Mazzetti, M., & Barnes, J. E. (2020, April 11). He could have seen what was coming: Behind Trump's failure on the virus. New York Times. https://www.nytimes.com/2020/04/11/us/politics/coronavirus-trump-response.html

Mackenzie, D. (2020). Ultraviolet light fights new virus. *Engineering, 6*, 851–853. https://doi.org/10.1016/j.emg.2020.06.009

Madani, D. (2020, December 13). First trucks with Covid-19 vaccine roll out of Pfizer plant in Michigan. NBC News. https://www.nbcnews.com/news/us-news/first-trucks-covid-19-vaccine-roll-out-pfizer-plant-michigan-n1251037

Mascarenhas, A. (2021, May 16). Adar's father Cyrus joins family in London, 'looking at units in Europe.' Indian Express. https://indianexpress.com/article/india/cyrus-poonawalla-sii-vaccine-production-7316769/lite/

Matuschek, C., Moll, F., Fangerau, H., Fischer, J. C., Zänker, K., van Griensven, M., Schneider, M., Kindgen-Milles, D., Knoefel, W. T., Lichtenberg, A., Tamaskovics, B., Djieepmo-Njanang, F. J., Budach, W., Corradini, S., Häussinger, D., Feldt, T., Jensen, B., Pelka, R., & Orth, K.,…Haussmann, J. (2020). The history and value of face masks. *European Journal of Medical Research, 25*, 23. https://doi.org/10.1186/s40001-20-00423-4

McGee, L. (2021, March 27). The pandemic is stirring deep resentments in Europe. They may not be quick to heal. CNN. https://www.cnn.com/2021/03/27/europe/europe-is-angry-with-itself-intl-analysis-cmd/index.html

McKenzie, L. (2021, April 6). Proctoring tool failed to recognize dark skin, students say. Inside Higher Ed. https://www.insidehighered.com/quicktakes/2021/04/06/proctoring-tools-failed-recognize-dark-skin-students-say

McLaughlin, K. (2021, February 5). 'A waste of money': The home Covid-19 test funded by the Biden administration is too costly and complex, critics say. STAT News. https://www.statnews.com/2021/02/05/a-waste-of-money-the-home-covid-19-test-funded-by-the-biden-administration-is-too-costly-and-complex-critics-say

McPhillips, D. (2021a, May 28). Disparities in Covid-19 vaccination rates among US counties fall among digital and economic divide. CNN. https://www.cnn.com/2021/05/28/health/disparities-covid-19-vaccine-divide/index.html

McPhillips, D. (2021b, September 14). Black, Hispanic people miss out on Covid-19 testing and vaccinations. CNN. https://www.cnn.com/2021/09/14/health/jhu-covid-data-disparities/index.html

Mehrotra, N. & Saaliq, S. (2021, May 26). Vaccine inequality in India sends many falling through gaps. AssociatedPress.https://apnews.com/article/india-technology-coronavirus-pandemic-business-health-9fc262598b4a6e1fc5ff223fdd748cea

Mehta, B., Salmon, J., & Ibrahim, S. (2020). Potential shortages of hydroxychloroquine for patients with lupus during the coronavirus disease 2019. JAMA Health Forum https://jamanetwork.com/channels/health-forum/fullarticle/2764607.

Metlay, J. P., Haas, J. S., Soltoff, A. E., & Armstrong, K. A. (2021). Household transmission of SARS-CoV-2. *JAMA Open, 4*(2), e210304. https://doi.org/10.1001/jamanetworkopen.2021.0304

Moderna. (2021, January 25). Moderna COVID-19 vaccine retains neutralizing activity against emerging variants first identified in the U.K. and the Republic of South Africa. Author.

Moghadas, S. M., Fitzpatrick, M. C., Shoukat, A., Zhang, K., & Galvani, A. P. (2021). Simulated identification of silent COVID-19 infections among children and estimated future infection rates with vaccination. *JAMA Network Open, 4*(4), e217097. https://doi.org/10.1001/jamanetworkopen.2021.7097

Monmouth University Poll. (2021, February 3). National: 1 in 4 say 'no thanks' to vaccine. Monmouth University. https://www.monmouth.edu/polling

Moore, S., Hill, E. M., Tildesley, M. J., Dyson, L., & Keeling, M. J. (2021). Vaccination and non-pharmaceutical interventions for COVID-19: A mathematical modelling study. *Lancet Infection*. https://doi.org/10.1016/S1473-3099(21)00143-2

Morgan, S. B. (2021, February 17). Native Americans embrace vaccine, virus containment measures. Associate Press. https://apnews.com/article/native-americans-coronavirus-vaccine-9b3101d306442fbc5198333017b4737d

Mulchandani, R., Jones, H. E., Taylor-Phillips, S., Shute, J., Perry, K., Jamarani, S., Brooks, T., Charlett, A., Hickman, M., Oliver, I., Kaptoge, S., Danesh, J., Di Angelantonio, E., Ades, A. E., & Wyllie, D. H. (2020). Accuracy of UK Rapid Test Consortium (UK-RTC) "AbC-19 Rapid Test" for detection of previous SARS-CoV-2 infection in key workers: Test accuracy study. *BMJ, 371*, m4262. https://doi.org/10.1136/mbj.m4262

Murphy, S. (2021a, January 27). Oklahoma seeking to return $2M worth of hydroxychloroquine. Associated Press. https://apnews.com/article/donald-trum-malaria-coronavirus-pandemic-oklahoma-09e33f4db37dda112ecec70d780bc964d

Murphy, T. (2021b, January 25). Merck ends development of two potential COVID-19 vaccines. Associated Press. https://apnews.com/article/coronavirus-pandemic-5e0de4fdbceea5b2517afc7846aff5c

Neergaard, L., & Miller, Z. (2021, March 23). AstraZeneca accused of cherry-picking vaccine study data. Associated Press. https://apnews.com/article/astrazeneca-may-have-used-outdated-info-vaccine-trial-a98ef616f4e861a4b7568891d06b7da8

NIH. (2021a, January 26). Lasting immunity found after recovery from COVID-19. Author. https://www.nih.gov/news-events/nih-research-matters/lasting-immunity-found-after-recovery-covid-19

NIH. (2021b, March 2). NIH halts trial of COVID-19 convalescent plasma in emergency department patients with mild symptoms. Author. https://www.nih.gov/news-events/news-releases/nih-halts-trial-covid-19-convalescent-plasma-emergency-department-patients-mild-symptoms

NIH. (2021c, March 5). *What's new in the* guidelines. Author. https://www.covid19treatmentguidelines.nih.gov/whats-new/

O'donnell, C., & Aboulenein, A. (2021, August 18). U.S. to begin offering COVID-19 vaccine booster shots in September. Reuters. https://www.reuters.com/world/us/us-start-offering-covid-19-vaccine-booster-doses-september-2021-08-18/

Painter, E. M., Ussery, E. N., Patel, A., Hughes, M. M., Zell, E. R., Moulin, D. L., Scharff, L. G., Lynch, M., Ritchey, M. D., Toblin, R. L., Murthy, B. P., Harris, L. T. Q., Wasley, A., Rose, D. A., Cohn, A., & Messonnier, N. E. (2020). Demographic characteristics of persons vaccinated during the first month of the COVID-19 vaccination program—United States, December 14, 2020-January 14, 2021. *MMWR*, 70. https://www.cdc.gov/mmrw/volumes/70/wr/mm7005e1

Pathak, D. (2012, May 22). Baylor College of Medicine receives over $6 million from NIH to develop SARS vaccine. Baylor College of Medicine. https://www.bcm.edu/news/bcm-receives-6-million-develop-sars-vaccine

Pei, S., Kandula, S., & Shaman, J. (2020). Different effects of intervention timing on COVID-19 spread in the United States. *Science Advances, 6*(49), eabd6370. https://doi.org/10.1126/sciadv.abd6370

Perrett, C. (2021, January 24). As he faced death threats, Fauci said he once opened an envelope that contained a 'puff of powder' he feared was anthrax or ricin. Business Insider. https://www.businessinsider.com/fauci-opened-envelope-containing-mystery-powder-during-trump-admin-2021-1

Quest, R. (2020, October 14) Richard Quest: After recovering from COVID-19, I thought I was safe. Now my antibodies are waning. CNN. https://www.cnn.com/2020/10/14/health/quest-covid-recovery-antibodies-intl/index.html

Rahim, Z. (2021, January 14). Covid-19 infection grants immunity for five months, UK study suggests. CNN. https://www.cnn.com/2021/01/14/health/covid-immunity-antibodies-intl/index.html

Rahim, Z., Khadder, K., Strange, H., & Yeung, J. (2021, March 3). The latest on the coronavirus pandemic and vaccines. CNN. https://www.cnn.com/world/live-news/coronavirus-pandemic-vaccine-updates-03-03-21/h_93c18ad7cd7aed3e5d171682e84b304d

Ramgopal, K., Romo, C., & McFadden, C. (2021, January 23). How 'vaccine nationalism' could prolong the Covid-19 pandemic. NBC News. https://www.nbcnews.com/news/us-news/how-vaccine-nationalism-could-prolong-covid-19-pandemic-n1255417

Ramos, E. (2021, January 15). States want to vaccinate more people. But data on who has received a shot is lacking. NBC News. https://www.nbcnews.com/news/us-news/states-want-vaccinate-more-people-data-who-has-received-shot-n1254449

Reinhart, R. J. (2020, November 17). More Americans now willing to get COVID-19 vaccine. Gallup. https://news.gallup.com/poll/325208/americans-willing-covid-vaccine.aspx

Rentsch, C. T., Beckman, J. A., Tomlinson, L., Gellad, W. F., Alcorn, C., Kidwai-Khan, F., Skanderson, M., Brittain, E., King, J. T., Ho, Y.-L., Eden, S., Kundu, S., Lann, M. F., Greevy, R. A., Ho, P. M., Heidenreich, P. A., Jacobson, D. A., Douglas, I. J., Tate, J. P., … Freiberg, M. S. (2021). Early initiation of prophylactic anticoagulation for prevention of coronavirus disease 2019 mortality in patients admitted to hospital in the United States: Cohort study. *BMJ, 372*, n311. https://doi.org/10.1136/bmj.n311

Reuters (2021a, May 2). Prime minister Modi's ruling party losses crucial Indian state election. Author. https://www.reuters.com/world/india/vote-count-five-indian-states-begin-amid-pandemic-2021-05-02/

Reuters. (2021b, March 10). Rich, developing nations wrangle over COVID vaccine patents. Author. https://www.reuters.com/article/us-health-coronavirus-wto/rich-developing-nations-wrangle-over-covid-vaccine-patents-idUSKBN2B21V9

Reynolds, E. (2020, December 11) Europe in meltdown as Covid death tolls soar and progress unravels. CNN. https://www.cnn.com/2020/12/11/europe/europe-covid-cases-restrictions-intl/index.html

Richards, S. E. (2020, December 11) Who is really 'first in line' for the vaccine? It depends on your state. National Geographic. https://www.nationageographic.com/science/2020/12/who-is-really-first-in-line-coronavirus-vaccine-states-not-guaranteed/

Riechmann, D., & Madhani, A. (2020, April 26). No, don't inject disinfectant: Outcry over Trump's musing. Associated Press. https://apnews.com/article/697d9ecef7f89cf5e9abb3b008c7faa7

Ripperger, T. J., Uhrlaub, J. L., Watanabe, M., Wong, R., Castaneda, Y., Pizzato, H. A., Thompson, M. R., Bradshaw, C., Weinkauf, C. C., Bime, C., Erickson, H. L., Knox, K., Bixby, B., Parthasarathy, S., Chaudhary, S., Natt, B., Cristan, E., El Aini, T., Rischard, F., … Bhattacharya, D. (2020). Orthogonal SARS-CoV-2 serological assays enable surveillance of low prevalence communities and reveal durable humoral immunity. *Immunity*. https://doi.org/10.1016/j.immuni.2020.10.004

Robbiani, D. F., Gaebler, C., Muecksch, F., Morenzi, J. C. C., Wang, Z., Cho, A., Agudelo, M., Barnes, C. O., Gazumyan, A., Finkin, S., Hägglöf, T., Oliveira, T. Y., Viant, C., Hurley, A., Hoffman, H.-H., Millard, K. G., Kost, R. G., Cipolla, M., & Gordon, K.,…Nussenzeig, M. C. (2020). Convergent antibody responses to SARS-CoV-2 in convalescent individuals. *Nature, 584*, 437–442. https://doi.org/10.1038/s41586-020-2456-9

Roxby, P. (2020, November 3) T-cell response 'lasts six months after Covid infection.' BBC. https://www.bbc.com/news/health-54781496

Saaliq, S., & Ghosal, A. (2021, April 13). India reels amid virus surge, affecting world vaccine supply. Associated Press. https://apnews.com/article/india-coronavirus-surge-vaccine-supply-55b7313c688b9a4c05a68a9c13e499da

Savarese, M., & Álvares, D. (2021, March 25). Bolsonaro under fire as Brazil hits 300,000 virus deaths. Associated Press. https://apnews.com/article/brazil-jair-bolsanaro-coronavirus-pandemic-9eeadec9835665c5937ffac507a42b9a

Schmali, E., & Singh, K. D. (2021, May 7). India and its vaccine maker stumble over their pandemic promises. New York Times. https://www.nytimes.com/2021/05/07/world/india-serum-institute-covid19.html

Schneider, E. C. (2020). Failing the test—The tragic data gap undermining the U.S. pandemic response. *New England Journal of Medicine, 383*(4), 299–302. https://www.nejm.org/

Schondelmeyer, S. W., Seifert, J., Margraf, D. J., Mueller, M., Williamson, I., Dickson, C., Dasararaju, D., Caschetta, C., Senne, N., & Osterholm, M. T. (2020, October 21) COVID-19: The CIDRAP viewpoint. Part 6: Ensuring a resilient US prescription drug supply. University of Minnesota. https://www.cidrap.umn.edu/covid-19/covid-19-cidrap-viewpoint

Sherman, C., Cheng, M., Leicester, J., & Goodman, J. (2021, January 15). 'This is not a game': Global virus death toll hits 2 million. Associated Press. https://apnews.com/article/global-death-toll-coronavirus-2-million-19c7f4611df0a8535ebb83f833c7b89f

Siemaszko, C. (2020, October 28). Top Trump health official warns of 'draconian measures' if America doesn't mask up. NBC News. https://www.nbcnews.com/news/us-news/top-trump-health-official-warns-draconian-measures-if-america-doesn-n1245116

Siemaszko, C. (2021, March 3). Texas doctors say Gov. Greg Abbott's decision to scrap mask mandate could result in another Covid-19 surge. NBC News. https://www.nbcnews.com/news/us-news/texas-doctors-say-gov-greg-abbott-s-decision-scrap-mask-n1259513

Sjoding, M. W., Dickson, R. P., Iwashyna, T. J., Gay, S. E. & Valley, T. S. (2020). Racial bias in pulse oximetry measurement. *New England Journal of Medicine, 383*(25), 2477–2478. https://doi.org/10.1056/NEJMc2029240

Smith, Ale. (2020a, May 16). Wave of 'vaccine nationalism' hinders global efforts to halt coronavirus. NBC News. https://www.nbcnews.com/news/world/wave-vaccine-nationalsim-hinders-global-efforts-halt-coronavirus-n1207846

Smith, Ale. (2020b, December 16). Covid-19 vaccines are being hoarded by rich countries — Poor ones are missing out. NBC News. https://www.nbcnews.com/news/world/covid-19-vaccines-are-being-hoarded-rich-countries-poor-ones-n1251351

Smith, Ale. (2021a, January 18). Covid misinformation takes its toll on British doctors, teachers. NBC News. https://www.nbcnews.com/news/world/covid-misinformation-takes-its-toll-british-doctors-teachers-n1254568

Smith, Ale. (2021b, February 26). COVAX: Why Biden's billions won't fix Covid vaccine inequality worldwide. NBC News. https://www.nbcnews.com/news/world/covax-why-biden-s-billions-won-t-fix-covid-vaccine-n1258816

Smith, All. (2021c, January 24). New CDC director said Biden administration is struggling with lack of vaccine data. NBC News. https://www.nbcnews.com/politics/white-house/new-cdc-director-said-biden-administration-struggling-lack-vaccine-data-n1255455

St. Fleur, N. (2021, February 19). 'A massive gap in information': Most vaccine clinical trials fail to report data on participants' ethnicity or race. STAT News. https://www.statnews.com/2021/02/19/a-massivmost-vaccine-clinical-trials-fail-to-report-data-on-participants-ethnicity-or-race/

Stobbe, M. (2021, March 5). Study finds mask mandates, dining out influence virus spread. Associated Press. https://apnews.com/article/rochelle-walensky-coronavirus-pandemic-fe2e65c19506b99ebdb8f1e0badc846b

Suliman, A., & Eckardt, A. (2020, November 7). Record number of coronavirus cases reported in several European countries amid lockdowns. NBC News. https://www.nbcnews.com/news/world/record-number-coronavirus-cases-reported-several-european-countries-amid-lockdowns-n1246898

Syed, M., & Siemaszko, C. (2021, February 26). Parents desperate to get their disabled kids vaccinated face big hurdle: CDC guidelines. NBC News. https://www.nbcnews.com/news/us-news/parents-deperate-get-their-disabled-kids-vaccinated-face-big-hrudle-n1258881

Szabo, L., & Allecia, J. N. (2020, October 28) Scientists debate how much to lower the bar on Covid-19 vaccine potential. NBC News. https://www.nbcnews.com/health/health-news/scientists-debate-how-much-lower-bar-covid-19-vaccine-potential-n1244956

Tartof, S. Y., Slezak, J. M., Fischer, H., Hong, V., Ackerson, B. K., Ranasinghe, O. N., Frankland, T. B., Ogun, O. A., Zamparo, J. M., Gray, S., Valluri, S. R., Pan, K., Angulo, F. J., Jodar, L., & McLaughlin, J. M. (2021). Effectiveness of mRNA BNT162b2 COVID-19 vaccine up to 6 months in a large integrated health system in the USA: A retrospective cohort study. *Lancet*. https://doi.org/10.1016/S0140-6736(21)02183-8

Taylor, A. (2020, October 22). Why countries are resorting to pandemic lockdowns again. Washington Post. https://www.washingtonpost.com/world/2020/10/22/second-lockdown-ireland-europe-coronavirus/

Thakur, D. (2021, May 5). India is suffering immensely under the weight of Covid. Now its failures are threatening much of the world. STAT News. https://www.statnews.com/2021/05/05/india-vaccine-heist-shoddy-regulatory-oversight-imperil-global-vaccine-access/

The COCONEL Group. (2020). A future vaccination campaign against COVID-19 at risk of vaccine hesitancy and politicization. *Lancet Infection, 20*, 769–770. https://doi.org/10.1016/S1473-3099(20)30426-6

The RECOVERY Collaborative Group. (2021a). Dexamethasone in hospitalized patients with Covid-19. *New England Journal of Medicine, 384*, 693–704. https://doi.org/10.1056/NEJMoa2021436

The RECOVERY Collaborative Group. (2021b). Tocilizumab in patients admitted to hospital with COVID-19 (RECOVERY): Preliminary results of a randomized, controlled, open-label, platform trial. https://www.medrxiv.org/content/10.1101/2021.02.11.21249258v1.

Thomas, N. (2020, November 18) Millions of children have missed routine vaccinations during the pandemic, insurance data shows. CNN. https://www.cnn.com/world/live-news/coronavirus-pandemic-11-18-20-intl/h_b7e731a059f69fe0ecee6a08cb0dd30b

Thorp, H. H. (2020). Not throwing away our shot. *Science, 370*(6514), 266. https://doi.org/10.1126/science.abf2306

UN. (2021, January 14). Israel: Ensure equal COVID-19 vaccine access to Palestinians—UN independent experts. UN News. https://news.un.org/en/story/2021/01/1082152

US Department of Defense. (2020). Coronavirus: Operation warp speed. Author. https://www.defense.gov/Explore/Spotlight/Coronavirus/Operation-Warp-Speed/.

US Food and Drug Administration. (2020, October 22). Frequently asked questions for Veklury (remdesivir). Author. https://www.fda.gov/media/137574/download#:~:text=On%20October%2022%2C%202020%2C%20FDA,of%20COVID%2D19%20requiring%20hospitalization.

Vatansever, F., Ferraresi, C., Pires de Sousa, M. V., Yin, R., Rineh, A., Sharma, S. K., & Hamblin, M. R. (2013). Can biowarfare agents be defeated with light? *Virulence, 4*(8), 796–825. https://doi.org/10.4161/viru.26475

Velavan, T. P., Pollard, A. J., & Kremsner, P. G. (2020). Herd immunity and vaccination of children for COVID-19. *International Journal of Infectious Diseases, 98*, 14–15. https://doi.org/10.1016/j.ijid.2020.06.065

Weber, P. J., & Webber, T. (2021, March 3). Texas and other states ease COVID-19 rules despite warnings. Associated Press. https://apnews.com/article/texas-other-states-ease-covid-19-restrictions-af9fc21469O270fe617864abc772ecce

Weiland, N., Thomas, K., & LaFraniere, S. (2021, January 22). Pfizer will ship fewer vaccine vials to account for 'extra' doses. New York Times. https://www.nytimes.com/2021/01/22/health/pfizer-vaccine.html

White House. (2021, April 25). Statement by NSC spokesperson Emily Horne on National Security Advisor Jake Sullivan's call with National Security Advisor Ajit Doval of India. Author. https://www.whitehouse.gov/briefing-room/statements-releases/2021/04/25/statement-by-nsc-spokeperson-emily-horne-on-national-security-advisor-jake-sullivan-s-call-with-national-security-advisor-ajit-doval-of-india

Wilson, B., Hoffman, J., & Morgenstern, J. (2019). Predictive inequity in object detection. *arXiv.1902*.11097. https://arxiv.org/abs/1902.11097

Wilson, S. (2020, December 18) Overwhelmed. Washington Post. https://www.washingtonpost.com/graphics/2020/national/california-hospital-covid-capacity/

Wolfe, D., & Dale, D. (2020, October 28). 'It's going to disappear': A timeline of Trump's claims that Covid-19 will vanish. CNN. https://www.cnn.com/interactive/2020/10/politics/covid-disappearing-trump-comment-tracker/index.html

Woloshin, S., Patel, N., & Kesselheim, A. S. (2020). False negative tests for SARS-CoV-2 infection—Challenges and implications. *New England Journal of Medicine, 383*, e38. https://doi.org/10.1056/NEJMp2015897

Woodward, B. (2020). Rage. Simon & Schuster.

Wunsch, H. (2021, August 20). That 'damn machine': The dark side of mechanical ventilators in the ICU. STAT News. https://www.statnews.com/2021/08/20/that-damn-machine-the-dark-side-of-mechanical-ventilators-in-the-icu/

Yan, H., & Maxouris, C. (2021, March 1). All our recent progress with Covid-19 could be wiped out by variants, CDC director says. 'Please stay strong.' CNN. https://www.cnn.com/2021/03/01/health/us-coronavirus-monday/index.html

Zdanowicz, C. (2021, January 25). A rural county in Washington state hasn't wasted a single Covid-19 vaccine dose. Here's the secret. CNN. https://www.cnn.com/2021/01/25/health/kittitas-county-washington-covid-19-vaccine-trnd/index.html

Chapter 8
Colonial Suffrage

Abstract Politicizing the COVID-19 pandemic significantly hampered a consistent and scientifically grounded response to prevent and control the spread of sickness. Populist-nationalist leaders used the COVID-19 pandemic to consolidate power and maintain the status quo of their inequitable societies through divisive means. Colonial forces have historically controlled and restricted the privilege of voting to maintain the status quo of the nation. Disinformation was consistently wielded to enhance anger, fear, and social divisions for political gain. The 2020 US pandemic election was a textbook example of colonial hierarchical processes and privilege at work. Political events and voter barriers contributed greatly to SARS-CoV-2 viral spread, risking exposure of vulnerable minoritized people to COVID-19, and resulting in inequitable treatment. Colonial proponents made every effort to protect hierarchical self-interests, privilege, and white supremacy through intimidation, voting barriers, and challenging results. Indigenous psychology is used to examine these events with an eye toward the healing the inherent divisions inherent in colonial social orders. True democracy, like health equity, is incompatible with artificial colonial social hierarchies. Psychological stability and well-being would be better served by egalitarian governance with an interdependent vision that thrives on consensus rather than hierarchy and privilege.

Astute readers may be wondering why a chapter on politics and voting is included in a book on colonialism and COVID-19. The reason is this: The 2020 US election presented an excellent example of how colonial divisiveness destroys coordinated efforts to solve collective health problems. The election was exacerbated by the stressors of the pandemic—what I colloquially called the background noise of the COVID-19 era--where normal stressors and tensions became extraordinarily magnified under the conditions of the pandemic. The 2020 US election was pathologically impacted by SARS-CoV-19 and the spread of SARS-CoV-19 was pathologically impacted by the election—a symbiotic relationship that demonstrated the toxicity of colonialism on the modern era. The circumstances were a reminder that colonialism must be retired, or painful historical events will repeat themselves again and again.

A. W. Blume, *Colonialism and the COVID-19 Pandemic*, International and Cultural Psychology, https://doi.org/10.1007/978-3-030-92825-4_8

The Politics of COVID

The politicization of the disease has been discussed off and on throughout this book, such as the politicization of the vaccine. In this section, the attention is turned to the source of COVID politicization, which was pursuit of political power and advantage. The national fight concerning how to appropriately address COVID-19 represented a symptom of much larger problems embracing colonial nations. The struggle during the 2020 US election was not only about COVID-19 and its consequences, it was a battle over the worldview and the culture of the nation. US President Joseph Biden got it partly right when he described the election as a struggle for the soul of the nation (Cummings, 2020). What he did not fully understand, or address, was that the soul being struggled over was the colonial soul of the nation. The voters who sided with former President Donald Trump were fighting for its colonial soul, hoping for a return to the old days of America. The voters of President Joseph Biden split between those who wanted to return to covert colonialism as it was represented just prior to Mr. Trump's administration (back to "normal") and those who wanted something different than "normal" colonialism. Many minoritized voters wanted to retire colonialism and its damage and saw the election skeptically as a very small step away from overt colonialism of the populist-nationalist administration. Minoritized voters have seen many elections but very little movement away from colonial inequities over the centuries, hence the skepticism.

The political strategy of Former President Donald Trump Former President Donald Trump was an outstanding colonial strategist in winning the 2016 election, using blame, colonial deception tactics, blame, and colonial splitting in highly effective ways. His 2020 campaign believed those methods would also be a winning strategy. Examples follow for each of the three tactics.

First, from the very inception of the COVID-19 pandemic, Mr. Trump and many of his allies used deception to downplay COVID-19 (Woodward, 2020). Between February and October, 2020, he suggested the virus and the pandemic would one day simply vanish way, including after his hospitalization for the disease (Wolfe & Dale, 2020). His suggestions that the virus was inconsequential and the pandemic a hoax would continue to circulate among his supporters even after the election. The campaign also used deception to justify ignoring social distancing and masking, against the advice of scientists. Large crowds were encouraged at campaign events with little consideration for consequences. An excellent example was the indoor rally first scheduled for Juneteenth, a sacred day (and subsequently a federal holiday) among Black Americans celebrating liberation from slavery. The rally was to be held in Tulsa, Oklahoma, the site of the infamous massacre of hundreds of Black Americans by White Americans in 1921 that destroyed the economic livelihood of one of the most economically successful Black neighborhoods of the Jim Crow era (Brown, 2016; Fain, 2017). After public pressure, the rally was rescheduled but not cancelled. When the rally occurred, many contracted COVID-19 in a super-spreader event (Stanish, 2020). One of the attendees was Herman Cain, a former Black

Republican candidate for president, who passed away from COVID-19 not long after the event (Wagner, 2020). The Trump campaign was aware of the potential health risks of a large indoor event, requiring attendees to sign a waiver of legal responsibility prior to attending, which many did (Perper, 2020).

In-person campaign rallies continued throughout the campaign, despite warnings from health officials that the events risked high levels of virus spread--warnings that proved to be true. One study found that 14 of 17 counties hosting in-person campaign rallies had increased rates of COVID-19 within a month of those rallies (Kounang, 2020). Another study by econometricians projected approximately 30,000 additional SARS-CoV-2 infections and 700 additional deaths from the 18 in-person rallies from June to September, 2020 (Bernheim et al., 2020). Maskless rallies continued after the 2020 election, contributing to more illness within the Republican party (Peiser, 2021).

Second, Mr. Trump use blame as a tactic in a spirit reminiscent of colonial leaders of the past. Some of Mr. Trump's blame targeted China, capitalizing on colonial xenophobia to energize supporters. The Chinese government was not forthcoming about the history and nature of the virus, which gave energy to the blaming strategies of the Trump administration. The virus seemed to have spread much more rapidly and earlier than was initially reported (Walsh, 2021). In fact, when the WHO research team arrived to investigate the origins of the virus, the Chinese government was not fully cooperative (BBC, 2021), enhancing percolating suspicions. Regardless of the reason, the blaming by Trump energized many in the US with racist and xenophobic tendencies as discussed in Chap. 4.

Simultaneously, other nations blamed the US military for the pandemic (Kinetz, 2021), contributing to a global colonial blame-fest. The use of colonial deception tactics by a formerly colonized China may be a surprise. However, the Chinese government has internalized colonialism to expand its territory and influence, so a position of non-disclosure would be justified by its colonial self-interests. Since China was colonized, it has great distrust toward other colonial powers. As an emerging colonial power itself, the Chinese government likely thought it had everything under control, which hints at colonial arrogance.

Thirdly, Mr. Trump capitalized on the consequences of colonial splitting over the centuries—he used wedge politics to fire up his supporters with fear messages and divisiveness that referenced existing colonial stereotypes. One principal strategy was to appeal to existing prejudices by stoking racial fears among White Americans, linking people of color to anarchists and socialists, an interesting comparison since anarchists and socialists have completely different political agendas--the former typically favoring no government at all and the latter typically favoring strong centralized government. The speech that former President Trump gave before the insurrection on January 6, 2021, suggested that it might be the last chance to take back the country from those who threatened it (Associated Press, 2021)--not so subtly hinting that anarchists, socialists, and minoritized outgroups were a threat to supporters.

The messaging by the former president also had racialized overtones, linking the 2020 Black Lives Matter (BLM) protests occurring in response to police shootings of unarmed Black Americans to anarchy and racialized fears. During the campaign, former President Trump took ample opportunity to pit his followers against the perceived threat of BLM protesters using racialized messages of anger and fear. One high profile media event occurred when national guard troops were used by the administration to clear a path through a crowd of peaceful protestors from the White House to St. John's Church. Mr. Trump was photographed holding a Bible in front of the church, outraging the church's bishop that peaceful protestors were placed at risk and the church was used without consent (Colvin & Superville, 2020; Gjelten, 2020). Some unfairly described Trump's divisive political tactics as "tribal" (Babatunde, 2021), using a racialized colonial stereotype of aggressiveness assigned to Indigenous people. As an Indigenous psychologist, I can say with no doubt that the libertarian privilege exhibited by populist-nationalistic leaders in the 2020 election was anything but tribal.

Colonial splitting capitalizes on an us-versus-them mentality. The us-versus-them messaging of Mr. Trump was so successful that unsubstantiated social media rumors emerged that anarchists were going to rural communities to stir-up trouble. Counter-protests by Trump supporters spontaneously sprung up to oppose perceived threats from anarchists, socialists, and people of color. White supremacy was obvious during the counter-protests--profanity and racialized slurs common, some captured on video (e.g., NBC Montana, 2020).

Rural residents seemed to be scanning the environment for evidence of anarchists entering their communities, preparing a coordinated militia-like defense in case of an "invasion." In Klamath Falls, Oregon, in June, 2020, a large crowd of Trump supporters gathered to repel an antifa "invasion," and then when it did not materialize, claimed they had beaten antifa by preventing the invasion (Zadrozny & Collins, 2020). In Forks, Washington, a group of armed militia-types harassed a multiracial family on vacation they accused of being anarchists. When the family set up their campsite, the militia-types felled several trees using chainsaws to entrap the vacationing family in the camping area. Fortunately, others came to their rescue (Toropin & Maxouris, 2020). The Forks event not only demonstrates the consequences of racialized colonial splitting, but also how bullying and intimidation are important features of colonial splitting tactics. As a result of the former President's messaging, racists armed themselves in response to perceived racialized threats, very much how White vigilante mobs have acted across colonial history. In this way, the president's colonial splitting strategy succeeded by energizing supporters with pre-existing biases and racialized fears.

Campaign messaging inflamed supporters of the president to counter protest against the BLM protestors, often contributing to violence. An area of prolonged conflict occurred very near where this book was drafted: Portland, Oregon. One extreme event was spearheaded by Trump supporters driving into Portland in a caravan of trucks, spraying BLM protesters with mace, bear spray, and paintballs as they drove by. One Trump protester was killed (Olmos et al., 2020; Wilson, 2020). Racialized conflicts continued for many nights, previewing what happened in Washington, DC, on January 6, 2021.

Trump supporters also harassed the campaign of candidate Biden and other democrats. On a Texas highway, Trump supporters were videoed literally surrounding and weaving towards a Biden campaign bus with intent to intimidate and disrupt the campaign. The intimidation worked, and the event was cancelled (Bradner et al., 2020). Many wielded weapons during protests in a dare to others to start a fight. Weapons and violence had become so worrisome that at least one state opted to ban them from polling places during the election (Grayer, 2020). Colonial splitting stirred up hard feelings during the campaign, feelings that also hindered effective responses to address COVID-19.

The adept use of colonial splitting to claim victimization The president also used "us vs. them" colonial splitting effectively to suggest that he and his allies ("us") were being victimized by anarchists, socialists, and people of color ("them"), thereby justifying a defensive response by he and his allies ("us"). An appeal of victimization has been used frequently by colonial ingroups as a pretext to justify violence against outgroups. Trump's victimization claim was to "righteously justify" use of force against a mythic threat while arguing absolution of blame for the outcomes. Note that only privileged people could get away with such a strategy, since it relies on the high probability of prevailing against the perceived threat without being held accountable. The Trump administration masterfully fostered the public perception of being unjustly victimized while deceptively orchestrating great harm through its divisive activities.

Before former President Trump won the election, there was a strong belief by "conservatives" that "the media" was biased against them and their political perspectives. Some of this sensitivity by "conservatives" was likely a result of the media fact-checking the talking points, many which deviated from scientific evidence and verifiable facts. Trends toward wide-spread beliefs in conspiracy theories and anti-science perspectives, elaborated upon in Chap. 9 of this book, have certainly made it easy for the media to challenge such assertions. In order to test the assertion by "conservatives" of political bias, a research study was conducted to ascertain if the claims by "conservatives" that social media censored their political messages were supported by data. The study found no evidence to support the claim that social media entities were unfairly targeting "conservative" messages (Barrett & Sims, 2021).

The reader will note that in this section I am using quotation marks about the words "conservative," "liberal," and "the media" to highlight the us-versus-them distinction through use of absolute labels—a classic representation of colonial splitting tactics. These terms say nothing about reality of colonialism. Colonialism remains colonialism whether it is "conservative" or "liberal." The labels are false representations of the surreality of colonialism. The terms invite people to choose a side, and when choosing a side, they invoke the perceived superiority of that side—classic colonial thinking.

Psychological research suggests that humans selectively attend to information that supports a pre-existing point of view through confirmation bias and through cognitive dissonance ignore evidence that contradicts that point of view. Perception of the world tends to be filtered through the lenses of pre-existing points of view and their particular biases, similar to what has been found in research investigating implicit biases. Researchers have found that "liberals" were much more likely to find weaknesses in conservative political arguments and "conservatives" much more likely to find weaknesses in "liberal" political arguments (Gampa et al., 2019), suggesting that people can be effective critics of other points of view but not so effective on critiquing their own points of view.

One tool utilized by the Trump administration to effectively divide and confuse the public was the use of what some called *fake news*. Use of falsehoods to one's own advantage is not a new strategy in politics or colonial social orders, but the sheer number of falsehoods that were documented during the Trump area was astonishing (Kessler et al., 2021). Many *alternative facts* were generated from conspiracy theories and anti-science campaigns. It is a steep and slippery slope downward into the mire of distrust and poor choices once one begins to dispute empirical evidence. Research suggests that those who are exposed to greater levels of misinformation distrust the media more but are more likely to trust a government that aligns with one's own personal beliefs (Ognyanova et al., 2020). The research suggests political confirmation biases that may explain why so many supporters of Donald Trump dismissed scientific evidence in favor of *alternative facts*. Alternative facts seemed to contribute to distrust and poor choices during COVID-19 that cost many lives and left many people even more wounded by colonialism post-pandemic.

Psychological science and other social sciences have investigated the phenomenon surrounding fake news and alternative facts recently as a result of the trends. Such behaviors run contrary to the basic tenets of science, therefore they represent an existential threat to science and scientific advancement, and threaten technological progress in many arenas of societies, including health care. Researchers have noted the rise of fake news and alternative facts with the expansion of media and social media in societies (Lazer et al., 2020). There have always been movements against science, hence the beliefs even today of a flat earth by some. But what is different today is the rapidity in which ideas without empirical support can be messaged. With shutdowns and easy access to social media during COVID-19, people spread disinformation on both politics and SARS-CoV-19 unwittingly, easily, and rapidly--with older adults and members of the Republican party more likely to share links to disinformation than other demographic groups (Baptista & Gradim, 2020; Lazer et al., 2020). Researchers have also found that fake news with shock value and exaggerated messaging that elicit strong emotional responses were more likely to be consumed and shared on social media (Baptista & Gradim, 2020). Interestingly, other researchers have found that lower analytic skills may be associated with greater acceptance of misinformation and that people may have blind spots to misinformation when they overestimate their knowledge in a given area and have an openness toward accepting "pseudo-profound bullshit" (Pennycook & Rand, 2018, p. 197). The authors go on to suggest that people vulnerable to misinformation campaigns may be initially open to new information but do not necessarily take time to reflect on the veracity of the claims. In another assessment of misinformation, when study participants were allowed time to rationally consider the veracity of the claims rather than settle for a knee-jerk response to the message, they were often able to debunk the claims by deliberative processes (Bago & Pennycook, 2020).

There are a couple of ideas that need unpacking in the context of the research on vulnerability to fake news and alternative facts. First, the messengers of fake news and alternative facts are intentionally trying to manipulate people who they know are vulnerable to those types of messages. Agendas are being pushed by misinformation, and those messages often use methods to encourage colonial splitting to divide people with us versus them messages. Second, knee-jerk responses are important to spreading misinformation. When people take time to evaluate the messages rationally or empirically, the misinformation often seem to lose its power over the individual. The scholarship of psychologist Daniel Kahneman is also important to consider here, which speaks to two cognitive processing systems--one that is fast and automatic (knee-jerk), prone to misinterpretations and often linked to fear and anger (amygdala) cognitive system (fast thinking), and our more deliberate and slow processing higher order cognitive system that is much more rational (slow thinking; Kahneman, 2011). Fast thinking in some appears to be linked to acceptance of fake news and alternative facts.

Fast thinking seemed to be associated with poor public health responses during COVID-19, which in turn complicated the US election. Colonial splitting and deception were used to minimize the risk of SARS CoV-2, to discourage social distancing and mask wearing, and to encourage reopening the economy. All were done with the election in mind. The disinformation campaign focused the US on its divisions and fears, and perpetuated beliefs of us versus them. Slow thinking would have saved a great deal of suffering but was not encouraged politically.

Self-Interests Above All

Senator Bernie Sanders indicated that he saw the current Republican party as "kind of a cult of the Individual, that individual being Donald Trump" (CNN, 2020). Aside from his inherent political biases, Mr. Sander's assertion concerning the "cult of the individual" introduces an interesting point to consider when psychologically critiquing colonial America's response to pandemics. First, referring to an organization as a cult of the individual implies that some Americans willingly surrendered their slow thinking processes to manipulative forces that contributed to great national harm. The cult-like suspension of reality over the last few years illustrates how incompatible self-orientation is with a collective process such as addressing a pandemic. Self-centeredness dooms the colonial cult of the individual to holistic failure.

Secondly, the colonial cult of the individual is also incompatible with democracy, a lesson accentuated by the insurrection of January 6, 2021 (see also Chap. 9). Modern democracy, coopted from Indigenous people that dwelled in the land before American settlers (Stubben, 2000), is a system of government based upon egalitarianism. Democracy is inherently incompatible with colonial hierarchy. Therefore, it is no surprise that a cult of the individual might resort to self-interested tactics to control the vote and its outcome.

Voting Rights for the Privileged

Many people appeal to the US constitution as the authority for ensuring civil rights. It is obvious that many of the people who make this appeal have not read the document or hope that the rest of us do not read it. In looking at suffrage rights alone, it is clear that the original constitution protected the voting rights of a very few White male citizens when first drafted. Many people were not granted the privilege to vote by law in the US until the twentieth Century (see Table 8.1), and even today, many have not been granted the privilege to vote without harassment. Voting has never been a guaranteed right in the US—only a privilege.

Many states interfered with mail-in voting in every possible way, afraid that mail-in voting would enhance the number of votes from minoritized communities who were fed up with racialized mistreatment. One strategy was to tamper with the US mail service, with the goal of slowing delivery of ballots to and from voters (Bogage & Ingraham, 2020; Goodkind, 2020). Some states opted not to allow voters to use absentee ballots to avoid virus exposure, despite concern for community spread of SARS-CoV-2 related to in-person voting (Kamarck et al., 2020; National Conference of State Legislators, 2020a). Many states reduced or restricted the number of ballot collection sites (drop boxes) or restricted hours for early voting (National Conference of State Legislators, 2020b; Schneider, 2020). The lines for voting, especially in minoritized communities, were epic (Fowler, 2020). Not so coincidentally, the tactics discussed above were often carried out by the same states that discouraged social distancing and masking, confounding voter suppression efforts with pandemic risks.

Daily assaults by COVID-19 and political conflict left Americans extremely stressed when election day arrived, much more than previous elections (APA, 2020; Seitz-Wald, 2020). The political stress and its mental health consequences compounded pre-existing mental health inequities experienced by minoritized people,

Table 8.1 Examples of when certain groups gained the right to vote in the U.S.

Demographic group	Year voting rights were extended
White Males Who Owned Property	1787
White Male non-Christians	1828
White Males Without Property Requirement	1856
Black Males	1868 (1965[a])
White and Black Females	1920 (1965[a])
Indigenous Americans	1924 (1955)[b]
Asian Americans	1952
Adults aged 18–21	1971

Notes: [a]Although rights were theoretically extended to Black males and females earlier in history, it took the 1965 Voting Rights Act to enforce those rights. However, since that time, the authority of the 1965 Voting Rights Act has been diminished by court cases and legislation

[b]Although voting rights were theoretically extended to Indigenous Americans earlier, states resisted those rights until 1955

but also challenged White citizens unused to political chaos and national uncertainty. Stress was collectively harmful, experienced across political persuasions. Many hoped for resolution when votes were tallied.

Despite efforts by some states to suppress the vote at every turn, President Trump lost the election, which he later blamed on dead voters, judges, immigrants, and Indigenous Americans (MSNBC, 2021). Trump supporters immediately rejected results (Miller, 2020), continuing to espouse conspiracies that the election was stolen due to widespread fraud (see Chap. 9), recurring claims never supported by evidence set in motion by the former president at the very beginning of his term (Cottrell et al., 2018; Villeneuve, August 3, 2020). Conspiracy theories brought armed supporters to where ballots were being counted in Philadelphia (Hanna et al., 2020).

The election was legally challenged by supporters again and again. One consistent strategy was to call into question the legitimacy of votes cast in racial and ethnic communities, with supporters offering many reasons to toss ballots except for the most plausible reason: racism (e.g., Grayer & Cohn, 2020). Multiple efforts to prove fraud were unsuccessful due to lack of evidence. Dozens of court cases filed by the Trump campaign and allies of the president were lost or not heard due to lack of evidence or lack of standing in court, including four appeals to the "conservative" US Supreme Court--one rejected three months into the Biden presidency (De Vogue & Janfaza, 2021; Shamsian & Sheth, 2021). Evidence emerged late in 2021 that the former president's legal time even went so far as to develop a strategy for how Former Vice President Mike Pence could systematically overturn the election results during the congressional certification process on January 6, 2021 (Gangel & Herb, 2021). All these activities occurred despite overwhelming evidence that widespread election fraud had not occurred, including from Trump's Attorney General William Barr (Balsamo, 2020; Tucker & Bajak, 2020).

Allegations of fraud were so outrageous, widespread, and without evidential support that Republican colleagues chastised conspiracy-minded Republicans for their efforts to overturn or decertify the election (Parks, 2021). Threats were even made upon the lives of poll workers in certain states with baseless allegations of fraud and conspiracy (Brumback & Joffe-Block, 2020). Later, when a Trump lawyer was sued for defamation by a voting machine company after the election, the attorney suggested that her claims of fraud should not have been believed by rational people, acknowledging her fraud claims were fictious legal tactics rather than fact (McCarthy, 2021). Later, the Trump lawyers were sanctioned for their misbehavior by a federal judge in Michigan (White, 2021). The colonial splitting tactics that ensured a splintered nation also ensured a splintered Republican party. The social climate became so volatile during and after the insurrection that a "conservative" media owner told his radio commentators to stop the hateful and conspiracy laden rhetoric (Farhi, 2021). Unfortunately, this was not the end of the politicization of voting during the pandemic. Matthew Dowd, a former White House official and Republican strategist at the time, later referred to the colonial splitting and misinformation campaign within the party as akin to black mold infestation in a house (Dowd, 2021).

Democracy vs. Hierarch-racy

The Republican party attempted to codify voting suppression in almost every state through passing new voting restrictions and barriers, even after losing in court (Wolf, 2021). The lieutenant governor of Georgia at the time linked the wave of new voter suppression legislation to deceptive voter fraud charges by the former Trump administration (Murray & Morris, 2021). The voting restrictions imposed after the 2020 election were so obviously hypocritical that the point was made that gun buying was easier than voting in several states (Bump, 2021). The renewed activities to suppress voting do raise important questions concerning the future of democracy in the US as a colonial nation, questions were complicated by the insurrection of January 6, 2020 (discussed in Chap. 9). The changes also make it more likely that voting could be even more difficult in a future pandemic.

What the American public is left with are a series of questions rather than answers. First, will true democracy ever be possible in a hierarchical colonial society that protects supremacy and maintains inequities? Second, if a sizeable number of citizens are not interested in protecting voting rights for all Americans, doesn't that also help us to understand why they were not interested in protecting the rights of Americans to be safe from COVID-19? Third, after 160 years of racialized conflict and death, when will the US Civil War truly be resolved?

Other challenges to representation The US constitution was never meant to protect the rights of everyone, even with the appended Bill of Rights (Echo-Hawk, 2013). The US constitution was a document of compromises designed to get all 13 colonies on board with signing it. The 13 colonies did everything they could to protect their self-interests, including slavery. One key feature of American governance is the principle of protecting *state rights* that begun with protecting the autonomous rights of the original 13 colonies (Cohen, 2019; Constitutional Rights Foundation, 2021). American election processes are still oriented toward protecting individual state rights with policies that echo from slavery (Perea, 2018).

An example is the Electoral College (West, 2020), a process by which electors rather than citizens vote for the president of the US. Citizen votes are used to guide the selection of the electors. States have their own rules concerning electors, and they also seem to have the capacity to arbitrarily change those rules from one election cycle to another. One can count on an election mechanism originally used to maintain slavery and Jim Crow to also maintain voting inequity and injustices. The US Electoral College must be retired to advance voting equity.

Many of us also discovered during the 2020 election that congress has the ability to challenge electoral votes (Bomboy, 2020). Through a complicated process, representatives and senators have the opportunity to dismiss the electoral results of states and return the voting authority for new electors to the state legislative bodies rather than the voters. The legislative oversight and authority threaten to disenfranchise voters, and happens occasionally when a vote is disputed or close; the vote in 2020 was not close. The voting results of several states were challenged on January

6, 2021. Representatives and senators had the gall to try to overrule the election after an insurrection by supporters (Beaumont & Salter, 2021; Fram & Taylor, 2021), despite dozens of failed court cases where evidence of fraud could have been provided but never produced (Shamsian & Sheth, 2021).

Colonial processes inherent in elections and governance in the US are meant to protect the status quo of privilege rather than protect the needs of the whole. The senate procedural maneuver referred to as a filibuster is another example of a colonial tactic designed to slow or stall systemic change. The filibuster, not codified into the constitution as some might believe, became an important obstructive tool during the Jim Crow era to prevent civil rights legislation. Today, it continues to be used to stall any meaningful social change, including change relevant to protecting civil, human, and voting rights for outgroups (Robinson, 2021). There are some in the senate who discuss ending the filibuster, but many want to retain it as a weapon they might use in the future to prevent social change. The filibuster and election machinery in the US are reminders that those who have benefitted from colonial hierarchies want those benefits preserved. These long-standing colonial legal barriers also hinder improving pandemic preparation since they will likely be used by colonial proponents to block needed social change.

Searching for the Council Tree: An Indigenous Interpretation

Voting as a privilege rather than a right is symbolic of the exclusive nature of colonial societies--filled with deceptive practices by colonial proponents and white supremacists to protect the status quo. Challenges with 2020 voting went hand-in-hand with COVID-19 spread—those favoring voting privileges for the few were often the ones who rejected COVID-19 science, demonstrating a common theme of disrespect toward sacred others in society.

The US government in 2020 proved to be a completely unreliable source of protection for people, not only contributing to election violence and chaos, but also contributing to thousands of needless deaths from the pandemic and harming the health, mental health, and psychological well-being of citizens for years to come. Colonial divisiveness was so profound during the pandemic that the US government threatened its own national security by being complicit with activities that nearly toppled a nation. The symbiosis between pandemic and politics in the US was undeniable—denial of the pandemic drove the politics of privilege (a central focus of Chap. 9). But the US was not alone, because many populist-nationalistic leaders brought death and ruin upon their nations during the pandemic (e.g., Brazil, India, Mexico, the Phillipines, in addition to the US; Santoshini et al., 2021). Divisiveness and deception inevitably led to distrust and chaos. As a hierarchical nation, the US has not fully embraced democracy since its foundational roots are not egalitarian.

The coronavirus revealed on a daily basis how poorly prepared and equipped colonial governments were to protect all their people. Perhaps the lack of preparedness was because the founding covenants within those nations never intended to protect all the people, instilling basic distrust in the system. A new social order is needed, rooted in equity and trust and dwelling within the realities of an interdependent and closed natural order. In order to be better prepare for future pandemics and other global crises, governments will need to become less colonial and more Creation-centered to function effectively in an interdependent world.

The tradition of some Indigenous communities is to have difficult and important collective discussions under a large tree, often referred to a council tree. The people would come together as friends or enemies, but always as equals. Everyone under the tree would be heard and everyone contributed to the democratic resolutions that followed. The tree would shelter the proceedings, representing a safe place of refuge for all that would gather under its crown. Council trees were often elder trees with impressive sizes that invoked humility in those who stood in their presence. Council trees are sacred--a place where collective wisdom emerged and right relationships restored. Acts of consensus, compromise, reconciliation, and shared visions of peace occurred under the protection of council trees. They presided over acts of reconciliation for decades, perhaps even centuries depending upon tree longevity. The council tree was a reminder of human connectivity to the whole of Creation and connectivity to ancestors who used the tree before and to grandchildren who would use the tree thereafter.

Council trees provide lessons to conflicted peoples during difficult times. Council trees also provide a model for how to how to have difficult dialogues in safety, and how to move from divisiveness to unity of purpose and vision as egalitarian people. Colonial nations would greatly benefit from coming together in humility--engaging in reflection, conversation, shared wisdom, and restoration under the safety of a metaphorical council tree--seeking the collective peace with its citizenry needs to address future crises such as pandemics as one people.

References

APA. (2020, October 7). *2020 presidential election a source of significant stress for more Americans that 2016 presidential race*. Author. https://www.apa.org/news/press/releases/2020/10/election-stress

Associated Press. (2021, January 13). *Transcript of Trump's speech at rally before US Capitol riot*. Author. https://apnews.com/article/election-2020-joe-biden-donald-trump-capitol-siege-media-e79eb5164613d6718e9f4502eb471f27

Babatunde, M. (2021, March 25). *Trump's partisan presidency was a lot of things. 'Tribal' doesn't need to be one of them*. NBC News. https://www.nbcnews.com/think/opinion/trump-s-partisan-presidency-was-lot-things-tribal-doesn-t-ncna1261992

Bago, B., & Pennycook, G. (2020). Fake news, fast and slow: Deliberation reduces belief in false (but not true) news headlines. *Journal of Experimental Psychology: General, 149*(8), 1608–1613. https://doi.org/10.1037/xge0000729

Balsamo, M. (2020, December 1). *Disputing Trump, Barr says no widespread election fraud*. Associated Press. https://apnews.com/article/barr-no-widespread-election-fraud-b1f1488796c9a98c4b1a9061a6c7f49d

Baptista, J. P., & Gradim, A. (2020). Understanding fake news consumption: A review. *Social Sciences, 9*, 185. https://doi.org/10.3390/socsci9100185

Barrett, P. M., & Sims, J. G. (2021). *False accusation: The unfounded claim that social media companies censor conservatives*. New York University Center for Business and Human Rights. https://bhr.stern.nyu.edu/blogs/2021/1/29/report-false-accusation-the-unfounded-claim-that-social-media-companies-censor-conservatives

BBC. (2021, February 14). *Covid-19 pandemic: China 'refused to give data' to WHO team*. Author. https://www.bbc.com/news/world-asia-china-56054468

Beaumont, T., & Salter, J. (2021, January 8). *'Great damage': Republicans recoil from Missouri Sen. Hawley*. Associated press. https://apnews.com/article/donald-trump-josh-hawley-electoral-college-michael-brown-3eddeb6d0ed114999ea074c9e70380cf

Bernheim, B. D., Buchmann, N., Freitas-Groff, Z., & Otero, S. (2020, 18 December). The effects of large group meetings on the spread of COVID-19: The case of Trump rallies. *SSRN*. https://papers.ssrn.com/sol3/papers.cfm?abstract_id=3722299

Bogage, J., & Ingraham, C. (2020, October 30). *Swing-state voters face major mail delays in returning ballots on time, USPS data shows*. Washington Post. https://www.washingtonpost.com/business/2020/10/30/postal-service-absentee-ballots-2020-election/

Bomboy, S. (2020, December 15). *Explaining how congress settles electoral college disputes*. National Constitution Center. https://constitutioncenter.org/blog/explaining-how-congress-settles-electoral-college-disputes

Bradner, E., Mucha, S., & Holmes, K. (2020, October 31). *Biden campaign cancels Texas event after trump supporters surround bus on interstate*. CNN. https://www.cnn.com/2020/10/31/politics/biden-bus-2020-campaign-texas-trump-supporters/index.html

Brown, L. (2016, June 17). *The story of Juneteenth*. JSTOR. https://daily.jstor.org/the-story-of-juneteenth/

Brumback, K., & Joffe-Block, J. (2020, November 7). *Georgia poll worker in hiding after false claims online*. Associated Press. https://apnews.com.article/election-2020-georgia-media-social-media-elections-aa0f256ec21de96fd5a41da703c4b443

Bump, P. (2021, March 18). *Which is easier in your state: Buying a rifle or voting?* Washington Post. https://www.washingtonpost.com/politics/2021/03/18/which-is-easier-your-state-buying-rifle-or-voting/

CNN. (2020, December 2). *Transcripts*. CNN. https://transcripts.cnn.com/TRASCRIPTS/2012/02/acd.01.html

Cohen, A. (2019, September 17). *Constitution's biggest flaw? Protecting slavery*. UC Berkeley Law. https://news.berkeley.edu/2019/09/17/constitutions-biggest-flaw-protecting-slavery/

Colvin, J., & Superville, D. (2020, June 1). *Tear gas, threats for protesters before Trump visits church*. Associated Press. https://apnews.com/article/15be4e293cdebe72c10304fe0ec668e4

Constitutional Rights Foundation. (2021). *The constitution and slavery*. Author. https://crblog.org/

Cottrell, D., Herron, M. C., & Westwood, S. J. (2018). An exploration of Donald Trump's allegations of massive voter fraud in the 2016 general election. *Electoral Studies, 51*, 123–142. https://doi.org/10.1016/j.electstud.2017.09.002

Cummings, W. (2020, August 13). *'Battle for the soul of the nation': Before they were running mates, Joe Biden and Kamala Harris both used the slogan*. USA Today. https://www.usatoday.com/story/news/politics/elections/2020/08/13/biden-and-harris-both-see-election-fight-soul-nation/3355971001/

De Vogue, A., & Janfaza, R. (2021, April 19). Supreme Court tosses out another Republican 2020 election challenge. CNN. https://www.cnn.com/2021/04/19/politics/supreme-court-tosses-gop-2020-election-challenge/index.html

Dowd, M. (2021, May 11). *America as a mold problem*. https://mdowd-97828.medium.com/america-has-a-mold-problem-1989cd7f1b03

Echo-Hawk, W. R. (2013). *In the light of justice: The rise of human rights in native America*. Fulcrum.

Fain, K. (2017, July 5). *The devastation of Black Wall Street*. JSTOR. https://daily.jstor.org/the-devastation-of-black-wall-street/

Farhi, P. (2021, January 11). *Talk-radio owner orders conservative hosts to temper election fraud rhetoric*. Washington Post. https://www.washingtonpost.com/lifestyle/media/cumulus-radio-conservative-election-fraud/2021/01/11/e12ec46e-537c-11eb-a817-e5e7f8a406d6_story.html

Fowler, S. (2020, October 17). *Why do nonwhite Georgia voters have to wait in line for hours? Too few polling places*. National Public Radio. https://www.npr.org/2020/10/17/924527679/why-do-nonwhite-georgia-voters-have-to-wait-in-line-for-hours-too-few-polling-pl

Fram, A., & Taylor, A. (2021, January 6). *Senate GOP leader: Challenging Biden win threatens republic*. Associated Press. https://apnews.com/article/election-2020-joe-biden-donald-trump-elections-electoraul-college-ec338e17920f0390d93128230b30beb6

Gampa, A., Wojcik, S. P., Motyl, M., Nosek, B. A., & Ditto, P. H. (2019). (Ideo)Logical reasoning: Ideology impairs sound reasoning. *Social Psychological and Personality Science, 10*(8), 1075–1083. https://doi.org/10.1177/1948550619829059

Gangel, J., & Herb, J. (2021, September 21). *Memo shows Trump lawyer's six-step plan for Pence to overturn the election*. CNN. https://www.cnn.com/2021/09/20/politics/trump-pence-election-memo/index.html

Gjelten, T. (2020, June 1). *Peaceful protesters tear-gassed to clear way for Trump church photo-op*. National Public Radio. https://www.npr.org/2020/06/01/867532070/trumps-unannounced-church-visit-angers-church-officials

Goodkind, N. (2020, July 24). *Trump-backed postmaster general plans to slow mail delivery*. Fortune Magazine. https://fortune.com/2020/07/24/usps-mail-delivery-postmaster-general-louis-dejoy-us-postal-service/

Grayer, A. (2020, October 16). *Michigan bans open carrying of guns at polling sites on election day*. CNN. https://www.cnn.com/2020/10/16/politicis/michigan-bans-open-carry-of-guns-at-polling-sites/index.html

Grayer, A., & Cohn, M. (2020, November 18). *Michigan's largest county certifies election results after Republicans earlier blocked certification*. CNN. https://www.cnn.com/2020/11/17/politics/michigan-detroit-election-results/index.html

Hanna, J., Frehse, R., & Moghe, S. (2020, November 7). *Armed men arrested in Philadelphia may have believed fake ballots were being counted, Philadelphia DA office says*. CNN. https://www.cnn.com/2020/11/07/us/pennsylvania-convention-center-arrests/index.html

Kahneman, D. (2011). *Thinking, fast and slow*. Farrar, Strauss, and Giroux.

Kamarck, E., Ibreak, Y., Powers, A., & Stewart, C. (2020, November 3). *Voting by mail in a pandemic: A state-by-state scorecard*. Brookings Institute. https://www.brookings.edu/research/voting-by-mail-in-a-pandemic-a-state-by-state-scorecard/

Kessler, G., Rizzo, S., & Kelly, M. (2021, January 24). *Trump's false or misleading claims total 30,573 over 4 years*. Washington Post. https://www.washingtonpost.com/politics/2021/01/24/trumps-false-or-misleading-claims-total-30573-over-four-years/

Kinetz, E. (2021, February 14). *Anatomy of a conspiracy: With COVID, China took leading role*. Associated Press. https://apnews.com/article/pandemics-beijing-only-on-ap-epidemics-media-122b73e134b780919cc1808f3f6f16e8

Kounang, N. (2020, October 29). *Many counties that hosted Trump rallies had a significant increase in Covid-19 cases*. CNN. https://www.cnn.com/2020/10/29/health/covid-trump-rallies-counties-cases/index.html

Lazer, D., Ruck, D. J., Quintana, A., Shugars, S., Joseph, K., Grinberg, N., Gallagher, R. J., Horgan, L., Gitomer, A., Bajak, A., Baum, M. A., Ognyanova, K. Qu, H., Hobbs, W. R., McCabe, S., & Green, J. (2020). *The state of the nation: A 50-state COVID-19 survey report #18: COVID-19 fake news on twitter*. Northeastern University Network Science Institute. https://www.covidstates.org/

McCarthy, T. (2021, March 23). *Pro-Trump lawyer says 'no reasonable person' would believe her election lies*. The Guardian. https://www.theguardian.com/us-news/2021/mar/23/sidney-powell-trump-election-fraud-claims

Miller, S. (2020, November 7). *'It's not over': Trump supporters flock to state capitols after Biden victory is announced*. USA Today. https://www.usatoday.com/story/news/nation/2020/11/07/election-protests-updates-trump-supporters-state-capitols-biden-win/6203271002/

MSNBC. (2021, July 22). *Trump blames 2020 loss on bad judges and Indians paid to vote*. Author. https://msnbc.com/msnbc/amp-video/mmvo117158981785

Murray, S., & Morris, J. (2021, April 8). *Georgia's GOP lieutenant governor says Guiliani's false fraud claims helped lead to restrictive voting laws*. CNN. https://www.cnn.com/2021/04/07/politics/geoff-duncan-voter-fraud-cnntv/index.html

National Conference of State Legislators. (2020a, November 3). *Absentee and mail voting policies in effect for the 2020 election*. Author. https://www.ncls.org/research/elections-and-campaigns/absentee-and-mail-voting-policies-in-effect-for-the-2020-election.aspx

National Conference of State Legislators. (2020b, November 3). *State laws governing early voting*. Author. https://www.ncsl.org/research/elections-and-campaigns/early-voting-in-state-elections.aspx#Early%20Voting%20Law%20Table

NBC Montana. (2020, June 4). *Whitefish protest video*. Author. https://nbcmontana.com/news/local/whitefish-man-charged-after-protest-confrontation

Ognyanova, K., Lazer, D., Robertson, R. E., & Wilson, C. (2020). Misinformation in action: Fake news exposure is linked to lower trust in media, higher trust in government when your side is in power. *Harvard Kennedy School Misinformation Review, 1*(4), 024. https://doi.org/10.37016/mr-2020-024

Olmos, S., Levinson, J., Parks, B. W., & Freda, K. (2020, August 30). *Person shot and killed during pro-Trump car caravan through downtown Portland*. Oregon Public Radio. https://www.opb.org/article/2020/08/30/portland-trump-cruis-rally-protest-rogue-river-pendleton/

Parks, M. (2021, January 4). *Georgia election official: Don't let misinformation 'suppress your own vote.'* National Public Radio. https://www.npr.org/2021/01/04/953321408/georgia-election-official-dont-let-misinformation-suppress-your-own-vote

Peiser, J. (2021, April 16). *Michigan GOP official blames maskless colleagues for his covid-19: 'Masks and vaccines shouldn't be political.'* Washington Post. https://www.washingtonpost.com/nation/2021/04/16/michigan-gop-jason-watts-covid/

Pennycook, G., & Rand, D. G. (2018). Who falls for fake news? The roles of bullshit receptivity, overclaiming, familiarity, and analytic thinking. *Journal of Personality, 88*, 185–200. https://doi.org/10.1111/jopy.12476

Perea, J. (2018). Echoes of slavery II: How slavery's legacy distorts democracy. *University of California, Davis, Law Review, 51*, 1081–1103.

Perper, R. (2020, June 11). *Trump is making rally attendees sign a waiver so if they catch the coronavirus, it's on them not him*. Business Insider. https://www.businessinsider.com/trump-campaign-requiring-people-to-signpcoronavirus-waiver-tulsa-rally-2020-6

Robinson, R. (2021, March 1). *The senate filibuster has a racist past and present. End it so America can move forward*. USA Today. https://www.usatoday.com/story/opinion/2021/03/01/end-filibuster-make-progress-race-voting-guns-health-care-column/6779720002/

Santoshini, S., Ionova, A., & Llana, S. M. (2021, April 30). *Global populism: Big promises, poor pandemic results*. Christian Science Monitor. https://www.csmonitor.com/World/2021/0430/Global-populism-Big-promises-poor-pandemic-results

Schneider, A. (2020, October 2). *Texas governor plans to limit number of ballot drop boxes to 1 per county*. National Public Radio. https://www.npr.org/2020/10/02/919658842/texas-governor-plans-to-limit-number-of-ballot-drop-boxes-to-1-per-county

Seitz-Wald, A. (2020, November 2). *One election eve, this country is just unbelievably stressed out*. NBC News. https://www.nbcnews.com/politics/2020-election/election-eve-country-just-unbelievably-stressed-out-n1245841

Shamsian, J., & Sheth, S. (2021, February 22). *Trump and his allies filed more than 40 lawsuits challenging the 2020 election results. All of them failed*. Business Insider. https://www.businessinsider.com/trump-cmpaign-lawsuits-election-results-2020-11

Stanish, E. (2020, June 20). *Large crowd gathers in Tulsa for 'Make America Great Again' rally*. Fox News. https://okcfox.com/news/local/large-crowd-gathers-in-tulsa-for-make-america-great-again-rally

Stubben, J. D. (2000). The indigenous influence theory of American democracy. *Social Science Quarterly, 81*(3), 716–731. https://www.jstor.org/stable/42863999

Toropin, K., & Maxouris, C. (2020, June 9). *A family suspected of being Antifa protesters was trapped on a road near their campsite, police say*. CNN. https://www.cnn.com/2020/06/09/us/wahsington-family-accused-antifa/index.html

Tucker, E., & Bajak, F. (2020, November 13). *Repudiating Trump, officials say election 'most secure.'* Associated Press. https://apnews.com/article/top-officials-elections-most-secure-66f9361084ccbc461e3bbf42861057a5

Villeneuve, M. (2020, August 3). *Report: Trump commission did not find widespread voter fraud*. Associated Press. https://apnews.com/article/f5f6a73b2af546ee97816bb35e82c18d

Wagner, L. J. A. (2020, July 30). *Former GOP presidential hopeful Herman Cain dies of COVID-19*. Associated press. https://apnews.com/8173fe14f7c7095ced3b55fdc65581e

Walsh, N. P. (2021, February 15). *CNN exclusive: WHO Wuhan mission finds possible signs of wider original outbreak in 2019*. CNN. https://www.cnn.com/2021/02/14/health/who-mission-china-intl/index.html

West, D. M. (2020). *It's time to abolish the Electoral College*. Brookings Institute. https://www.brookings.edu/policy2020

White, E. (2021, August 26). *Lawyers allied with Trump penalized over Michigan lawsuit*. Associated Press. https://apnews.com/article/lawsuits-michigan-ed328f20f55944164a68bc6003206c90

Wilson, J. (2020, September 3). *Breadth of rightwing Portland network reveals energized Trump base*. The Guardian. https://www.theguardian.com/us-news/2020/sep/03/how-the-rightwing-portland-protest-organizers-represent

Wolf, Z. B. (2021, March 23). *At least 45 states have seen bills aimed at voter suppression. Here's why*. CNN. https://www.cnn.com/2021/03/16/politics/voting-rights-debates-by-state/index.html

Wolfe, D., & Dale, D. (2020, October 28). *'It's going to disappear': A timeline of Trump's claims that Covid-19 will vanish*. CNN. https://www.cnn.com/interactive/2020/10/politics/covid-disappearing-trump-comment-tracker/index.html

Woodward, B. (2020). *Rage*. Simon & Schuster.

Zadrozny, B., & Collins, B. (2020, June 6). *In Klamath Falls, Oregon, victory declared over antifa, which never showed up*. NBC News. https://www.nbcnews/com/tech/social-media/klamath-falls-oregon-victory-declared-over-antifa-which-never-showed-n1226681

Chapter 9
Colonial Privilege and COVID-19

Abstract Privilege exists because of colonial hierarchy that encourages inequity and supremacy over others. Colonial privilege has proved to be self-defeating for societies, discouraging prosocial behavior and promoting conflict, division, and a narcissistic orientation that significantly hindered pandemic preparation and response—contributing to needless suffering and deaths. Communication privilege during the pandemic was often wielded to manipulate others and promote self-interests. Economic privilege allowed some to prosper when others were suffering. Health care privilege allowed some to access quality pandemic care and vaccines when others could not. Personal privilege allowed some to manipulate and exercise control over others for self-benefit, to bend the truth and extend misinformation to manipulate others, and to exercise liberties without concerns for social responsibility. As an example, racists and white supremacists exercised strong influences on election processes in 2020, eventually contributing to the first attempted coup in US history. Indigenous psychology offers an interdependent and egalitarian perspective on how to challenge hierarchy and therefore retire privilege to reduce the consequences of relational psychopathology. Equitable societies devoid of privilege would be psychologically healthier and better prepared to meet the challenges of the next global crisis.

Christian Theologian Reinhold Niebuhr accurately captured a snapshot of colonial privilege when he wrote, "The moral attitudes of dominant and privileged groups are characterized by universal self-deception and hypocrisy" (Niebuhr, 1960, p. 117). Colonialists have been able to convince themselves over time that as the "superior" people and culture in social orders they hold the moral high ground, regardless of what they say and do–not only with deceiving others they deem inferior but also themselves in their fallacious beliefs concerning hierarchy. Niebuhr goes on to suggest in that same paragraph that those of privilege rely upon inventing plausible truths to support their claims that are in fact misinformation. However, those deceptive practices failed miserably because a tiny virus does not respect privilege. The pandemic has exposed that colonial self-deception and hypocrisy are self-defeating for colonial societies in ways that harm the well-being of the whole.

A. W. Blume, *Colonialism and the COVID-19 Pandemic*, International and Cultural Psychology, https://doi.org/10.1007/978-3-030-92825-4_9

The consequences of colonial privilege were very apparent during COVID-19 due to the extreme inequities and disparities in education, health, income, and wealth. Colonial privilege results from intergenerational social hierarchies contributing to differential treatment within those societies (Blume, 2020). Privilege developed over the centuries due to inherent benefits and protections granted to certain groups in colonial societies, benefits that other groups have not shared (Bonds & Inwood, 2015; McIntosh, 1989). The -isms discussed in Chap. 4 constitute the constructs colonial nations use to define hierarchies that contribute to privilege for some groups but not to others. Privilege operates implicitly when the cultural benefits of colonialism are taken for granted—many people do not have the privilege to access to those very same benefits, such as groups where intergenerational poverty is commonplace.

Privilege was an important contributor to the progression of the COVID-19 pandemic (see Table 9.1). First, privilege contributed to inherent inequities and disparities, contributing to pre-existing vulnerabilities to a pandemic. Second, privilege had a tremendous impact on the spread of COVID-19 through the libertarian expressions of interpersonal behavior during pandemic. From the very early days of the pandemic, it was clear that some embraced public health recommendations such as masking to protect others from SARS-CoV-2 (CDC, 2020), and it was equally clear that some rejected those same recommendations as contrary to their self-interests. Communication was also used in manipulative ways to advance self-interested agendas. Third, privilege hindered global accessibility to prevention and treatment methods essential to addressing and recovering from the pandemic. Vaccine accessibility were an example of colonial privilege that interfered with global progress on mitigating the pandemic—when some people were getting third booster vaccinations when much of the world's population had yet to receive one vaccination (WHO, 2021).

Privilege is revealed when one feels safe to choose self-interests over the interests of others. Exercising the freedom to ignore the public good is inherently privileged—some people assume the privilege to do what they want regardless of risk to others, whereas others in colonial societies do not share that privilege. However, as one might expect in an interdependent world, following self-interests often lead to self-inflicted consequences, such as observed among the many who exercised personal freedom and became ill as a result. Chap. 9 provides examples of how privileged choices during the pandemic threatened the well-being of the whole, therefore harming the well-being of individuals including the privileged.

The Privilege of Opposing Science

Scientific inquiry can be helpful for developing public health policy because it provides evidence of what may be the best course of action to remain healthy and well. However, many have ignored or actively opposed heeding scientific evidence during the pandemic to the detriment of the whole, defiantly resisting any suggestions for prosocial behavior that might have mitigated community spread. The acts of

Table 9.1 Colonial privilege observed during the COVID-19 pandemic

Type of privilege	Expressions of that privilege
Communication privilege	"Alternative facts" Being an influencer Colonial splitting Manipulating with disinformation Media businesses
Economic privilege	Defrauding vulnerable people with miracle cures Inequitable taxation policies benefitting wealthy Profiting while others suffer Stimulus to large corporations and cronies Telework vs. face-to-face work or unemployment Wealth building activities
Educational privilege	Access to state-of-the-art technology Well-resourced schools and school districts Private education
Health care privilege	Access to well-funded health care systems Access to treatment unavailable to all Access without racialized biases Insurance and other financial support Lifetime access to state-of-the-art care Technology that favors light colored skin
Personal privilege	Advocating for fraudulent pseudoscience Benefitting from social hierarchies Conspiracy generation Exercising liberties without social responsibility Immune from laws and rules imposed on others Opposition to science White supremacy
Vaccine privilege	Booster shots when others had none Cheating/paying to get vaccines early Prioritizing supporters/donors for vaccines Vaccine nationalism Vaccine tourism
Voting privilege	Creating barriers to reduce voters Empowered to declare fraud without evidence Populist-nationalism opposing democracy Questioning the right of others to vote

defiance in the face of a globally threatening illness were some of the most privileged activities I have observed in my lifetime.

Many examples of the defiance toward US public health policies occurred. States could never agree on a coordinated public health response to address community spread, with some embracing recommended public health mitigation measures and others actively opposing those same measures. As the 2020 winter holidays approached, many defiant states were at high risk for US travel (Kelleher, 2020). When some governors attempted to instill mitigation measures, their state legislatures reversed enactment of the measures or undermined governor orders (Kaplan, 2020). Some state governments intended to ignore public health mitigation recommendations from the onset and experienced out of control virus spread as a result (Cilizza, 2020; Levenson, 2020). South Dakota allowed a large motorcycle rally despite recommendations against large crowds—a rally that resulted in a national superspreader event. The following year, the annual event was held despite the delta variant surge with essentially the same results (Kesslen & Murphy, 2021). North Dakota allowed health care providers with COVID-19 to continue working due to an overwhelming surge of patients with COVID-19 (Maxouris & Levenson, 2020).

The privilege of defiance was stimulated by political activities using colonial splitting strategies, often instigated by representatives of the Trump administration who downplayed the risks of SARS-CoV-2 and advocated for policies linked to infection-acquired herd immunity (Erdman et al., 2020–see also Chaps. 4 and 8). One medical spokesperson of the administration, in an interview with a Russian state media outlet, suggested that mitigation measures should be defied since be believed they were harming the mental health of younger Americans (Treisman, 2020). Supporters of former President Donald Trump were incited to defy public health recommendations. By autumn 2020, counties in which the majority voted for the former president were also the counties with the greatest SARS-CoV-2 spread (Johnson et al., 2020).

Some Americans were particularly defiant about wearing face coverings or masks during the pandemic. Then President Trump consistently refused to wear a face cover. Other defiant Americans saw masking as a sign of weakness, an infringement on rights, and some even suggested it was sacrilegious for Christians. One particularly defiant act was the use of a Ku Klux Klan (KKK) mask in public (Lithwick, 2020), naturally conflating beliefs of racial superiority with non-masking privilege. Some scholars suggested that American individualism was to blame for the defiance against masking (Vargas & Sanchez, 2020). Radical individualism as interpreted by an IAPP is an extreme expression of individualism oriented toward narcissistic goals. Radical individualism is expressed through acts of privilege that do not consider the welfare of others. However, individualism does not need to be a radical expression of privilege if conducted with egalitarian intent (Blume, 2020). Many of the acts of defiance were not carried out with egalitarian intent, as suggested by the KKK mask.

Privilege that opposed public health mitigation measures was noteworthy because it suggested a high level of cultural certainty in self-reliance and invulnerability to SARS-CoV-2, despite scientific evidence to the contrary—a strong sense of superiority over those who followed the public health recommendations. To an Indigenous psychologist, the proponents of defiance likely represented the true believers of colonialism, and their defiance represented unwillingness to compromise on their colonial principles. The culture war often discussed in US politics and media appears to be a war in defense of American colonialism, and the COVID-19 pandemic was one of its most visible frontlines.

Colonial masculinity and resistance to science Defiance against masking seems to be a function of hypermasculinity, where people hold stereotypes of strength and the perception of invincibility rather than collective vulnerability (Gupta, 2020a). Former President Trump capitalized on manipulating the culture of masculinity inherent in colonial America, creating a loyally defiant group to the public health mitigation measures suggested by health scientists (Kurtzleben, 2020). It became a badge of honor and a symbol of unity among supporters of Mr. Trump to refuse social distancing and masking. Interestingly, US states with women as governors experienced lower numbers of COVID-19 fatalities than states with male governors (Sergent & Stajkovic, 2020).

Males in the US society have lower life expectancies, largely due to a large number of gender-based health and mental health disparities. The preponderance of research suggests that hypermasculity norms have been associated with poor health outcomes (APA Working Group on Health Disparities in Boys and Men, 2018). A large study examining the relationship of masculinity with attitudes toward COVID-19 found that sexist norms were significantly associated with engaging in fewer COVID-related precautions and a greater likelihood of becoming sick from SARS-CoV-2 (Reny, 2020). Sexism is one of the -isms (Chap. 4) utilized in colonial societies to dehumanize groups of people. Masculinity in colonial societies has been wielded as privilege, but the reality was, from an Indigenous perspective, that masculinity made all of us vulnerable during the COVID-19 pandemic.

Colonial masculinity and global defiance The global extent of colonialism (see Chap. 1) has contributed to inherent colonial values globally, so colonial defiance of COVID-19 mitigation recommendations occurred around the planet as a result. Many populist-nationalistic governments were not supportive of the recommendations of science, especially if they were perceived to hinder commerce. Many populist-nationalistic political leaders became sick (e.g., Collins et al., 2020; Sherman, 2021; Stargardter & Paraguassu, 2020), and some passed away from COVID-19 (e.g., Foran & Wilson, 2021). Colonial privilege generated masculine self-defeating pride suggesting invulnerability to the virus. One high profile example was the country of Tanzania, which as a policy denied the existence of COVID-19 within its borders, resulting in harm to citizens and barriers to assistance from the WHO. Many government officials succumbed to COVID-19, including the president (BBC, 2021c; Odula & Muhumuza, 2021)

Many citizens in colonial nations defied shutdowns and other mitigation measures during times of surging spread (e.g., BBC, 2020; Bradley et al., 2020). The WHO saw this defiance as a threat to global health and formulated alternative methods to control the spread of virus when lockdown orders were not heeded (Payne, 2020). Some citizens embraced misinformation such as the pandemic was a hoax, often shared by conspiracy theorists on social media, to support their defiance against mitigation policies (Specia, 2020). However, there seemed to be tipping points where pandemic pain prompted citizens to turn on their populist-nationalist leaders despite the deception campaigns (Stargardter, 2021). Conspiracy theories and their relationships to privilege and health will be discussed later in this chapter.

Self-defeating defiance Rural America was among the most defiant demographic toward public health mitigation strategies, so physicians understood that rural patients might not be willing to seek vaccinations. Local rural doctors modelled receiving the vaccination publicly in hopes of encouraging vaccination compliance (McCausland, 2020). The anger from those who resisted and defied public health mitigation strategies often translated into threats against public health officials. In rural America, public health officials were publicly harassed, verbally abused, and physically threatened (Smith et al., 2020). The harassment, abuse, and threats took a toll on those who were only attempting to keep their neighbors safe. By late 2020, the mistreatment in rural locales prompted a mass migration of public health servants away from counties and states where such harassment occurred (King, 2020), leaving already vulnerable rural locales even more vulnerable without local health officials. The consequences of rural harassment were an excellent example of how colonial privilege proved to be self-defeating for perpetrators. Harassment also occurred nationally: Dr. Anthony Fauci disclosed that he, too, had been threatened by mystery powder sent through the mail that he feared was poisonous (Perrett, 2021).

Anti-science and pandemics Populist-nationalism also resulted in another form of defiance—a complete disregard for scientific evidence by many people on how to address the pandemic (Meitzner, 2020). The results of ignoring or rebelling against the recommendations of scientists was profound. Many did not understand how self-defeating their defiance of science could be, including media accounts of COVID-19 patients on their death beds continuing to believe they could not be dying from a "hoax" (e.g., Elliot, 2020). Since many people have little understanding of science, they also did not understand that vast community spread encouraged new variants that may have lengthened the duration of the COVID-19 pandemic (WHO, 2020). With a sizeable number of populist-nationalistic citizens opposing the recommendations of health scientists, many societies suffered unnecessary losses during the COVID-19 pandemic.

Recent years have brought a backlash against science and anti-intellectualism threatening harm to social and technological progress, including in medicine (Hotez, 2020; Parker, 2017). The anti-science sentiment of the US today is so far removed from the race-to-the-moon era that the differences seem baffling. There is a growing sentiment that self-perceptions and self-interpretations are to be trusted over scientific findings, resulting in a great deal of misinformation. Social media and sensation-oriented news has perpetuated ideas not supported by scientific evidence and inquiry, including conspiracy theories and cult-like behavior addressed subsequently.

Research has found that three types of belief systems may be associated with a propensity toward anti-science perspectives (Gauchat, 2008). The first belief system involves fear of science due to a lack of science literacy. Science literacy concerns one's level of understanding and familiarity of science, which can of course vary across different sciences. The less one understands science, the more likely one will oppose science. The second belief system emerges from religious fundamentalism that fosters beliefs that oppose science, making believers more likely to reject science on the basis of faith. The third belief system is referred to as social embeddedness, which accounts for beliefs that reject the modern world and progress, with people who are disengaged from modern society more likely to have anti-science beliefs. The common theme across each of these models appears to be envisioning science as a personal threat rather than as a gateway to knowledge or a means for personal growth.

Opposition to new medical treatment or vaccines in the US is not new (Hotez, 2021a). Today, however, it is clear that anti-science attitudes toward medicine and health care have contributed to misinformation and medical non-compliance resulting in needless loss of life (Hotez, 2021b), including among many antivaxxer "conservative" talk radio hosts who passed during the delta variant surge (Alonso, 2021). The contemporary anti-science movement against medicine and health care may have its roots in what has been called the *antivaxxer movement*. A research paper published in the 1990s fraudulently reported that vaccinations were linked to autism. The investigator was found to have falsified data and the paper was withdrawn, but the damage persists due to the fear and paranoia the paper generated toward vaccinations. Even though there is no evidence to support the link of vaccines to autism, antivaxxer interest groups and high-profile celebrities continue to perpetuate that cultural myth today despite falsification by science (Flaherty, 2011). Scientists have privilege in that they wield power through data and ideas. When scientists engage in fraud, that privilege generates misinformation that may harm people—similar to perpetrators of deception who generate alternative facts and disinformation. The antivaxxer movement is an excellent example of what happens when scientists conduct fraud and consumers are uneducated about science. When a movement is united by groupthink to a shared belief system with little to no basis in reality, the result is a cult-like phenomenon that psychologically harms participants and their families (Wexler, 1995).

Predictably, those with antivaxxer attitudes have strongly opposed vaccinations to address COVID-19, protesting at vaccine sites to persuade or prevent people from getting vaccinations (BBC, 2021b). Many resisted efforts to prevent exposure to the unvaccinated in public places where exposure was likely. As an example, New York City restricted indoor dining to those who could show proof of vaccination during the delta variant surge. When asked to show that proof at a New York restaurant before being seated, a group of customers attacked the maître d' (Smith & Chirbas, 2021). Antivaxxers went so far as to bully other antivaxxers from seeking health care when sick with COVID-19 during the delta variant surge (Collins, 2021). Public health scientists were rightfully concerned that antivaxxing campaigns would enhance vaccine hesitancy in an already frightened populace, thwarting efforts to achieve vaccine-assisted herd immunity (Ashton, 2021; Hotez, 2021a). Misinformation played a significant role in vaccine hesitancy. For example, 73% of parents of unvaccinated adolescents cited worries that their children would have their fertility compromised by the vaccination (Hamel et al., 2021), misinformation from a vaccine disinformation campaign. Another misinformed idea was that vaccines would turn people into zombies, a social media disinformation campaign against the COVID-19 vaccinations developed from the misinterpretation of the plot of the Hollywood movie, *I am legend* (Lee, 2021).

Also predictably, scientists have a growing interest in addressing anti-science and anti-vaccination attitudes since they tend to undermine advancement of well-being and health. One study examining anti-vaccination attitudes found that interventions may help to prevent the development of such attitudes, but it is much more difficult to overcome those attitudes once they have become engrained (Jolley & Douglas, 2017). Transparency and open communication may help to instill a level of trust in seeking vaccines (Desmon, 2021). The APA recommended community engagement as a way to foster trust in vaccinations, especially among minoritized communities that have many reasons to distrust colonial government and health care systems (APA, 2020). Anti-vaccination and anti-science attitudes presented significant barriers to mitigating the COVID-19 pandemic, frustrating medical professionals (Gupta, 2020b). However, requirements for vaccinations (such as mandated by employers) were found to be effective in coercing compliance among those who fundamentally opposed vaccinations (Kirzinger et al., 2021). The National Football League used a similar tactic to coerce vaccine compliance when they formulated a policy to punish teams with forfeited losses rather than rescheduling games due to illness among unvaccinated players (Patra, 2021). Movement toward nationally mandated vaccinations in the US occurred when President Biden ordered all federal employees and federal contractors to be vaccinated (Ogrysko, 2021). Canada mandated that all employees on planes, trains, and marine vessels be vaccinated (Government of Canada, 2021), all governmental employees be vaccinated, and that all travelers on planes, trains, and cruise ships be vaccinated (Gillies, 2021). United Airlines demonstrated that businesses can coerce high vaccination rates with very effective results—over 99% of their employees appeared to comply with the mandates showing how powerful these methods can be to mitigate virus spread (Schaper, 2021). Alternatively, Delta Airlines encouraged compliance by charging unvaccinated employees $200 more per month in insurance premiums and no longer extending pay protection benefits to cover COVID-19 sickness (Koenig, 2021). However, a month after the announcement, Delta reported only an 82% employee vaccination rate as a result of their policy changes (Reuters, 2021). Anti-science and anti-vaccination sentiments remain barriers to preventing and addressing future pandemics, but coerced compliance can be helpful and effective to overcome those barriers. Mitigation methods focused on the needs of the collective will be much more effective toward addressing the next pandemic than simply counting on individual compliance by choice.

The reversal The CDC (2021) in the spring of 2021 abruptly changed course and eliminated masking mandates for those who were fully vaccinated. On its surface, the decision seemed designed to reward those who had chosen to be vaccinated and perhaps to encourage others to follow suit. The reaction to this reversal of policy was interesting, with some who were fully vaccinated dropping their masks but with many others continuing to use them anyway, presumably to protect the unvaccinated including most children. The reversal of policy was found the be unenforceable for those who had not been vaccinated, who were expected to continue on their honor masking but able to anonymously non-comply with those recommendations. The result was some who were fully vaccinated and many who opposed masking in the first place were unmasking in most public places.

One can understand how the colonial cultural reasoning of such a policy, which was meant to reward individuals who had complied with medical advice in a country that could not fully enforce mandates. One can also see the flaws in the logic, since masking was always considered a method for protecting self *and others*. The protection of others was poorly considered when lifting the masking mandate for the vaccinated. It was exceedingly obvious that those who defiantly opposed masking would take advantage of the reversal of policy.

But deeper than that, the reversal of masking policy illustrated how liberty can be wielded in ways that impose harm on others—that the harms from acts of liberty without social responsibility can impact all. Although it was less than obvious with the policy change, the relaxation of masking mandates was an act of throwing those who had opposed vaccinations under the proverbial bus of society—they were suddenly placed in the position of being among the disposable people of colonial America. Originally during the pandemic, it was the non-compliant and socially irresponsible in society that threated those who were compliant with pandemic guidelines for mitigation. After the policy change, those who opposed masking had less protection without the masking mandates than before and more exposure due to their insistence on exercising personal liberties. Ironically, the unmasked who are fully vaccinated now hypothetically may be the source of spread to the unvaccinated and unmasked, with both groups exercising liberties that risk harms to others. For example, Dr. Anthony Fauci revealed less than 2 months later that over 99% of deaths were occurring among the unvaccinated at that time (Miller & Culver, 2021), highlighted risks to the unvaccinated in an unmasked society.

The reversal of policy was an abysmal public health failure, lasting less than 3 months due to spiking infection rates from the extremely contagious delta variant (Joseph, 2021), including among children who were not yet cleared for vaccination access. In fact, children accounted for about 29% of new US cases by the second week of September, 2021 (American Academy of Pediatrics, 2021), and pediatric COVID-19 hospitalizations spiked by August (Ramos, 2021). Unvaccinated people often expressed regret about not being vaccinated, with some reportedly pleading to be vaccinated just prior to being placed on a ventilator, illustrating a clear lack of understanding of how vaccinations work (Holcombe & Kaye, 2021). One unvaccinated person who later passed away from COVID-19 reportedly texted his partner that he wished he had received the vaccine (CNN, 2021a). Although viral spread was primarily experienced by the unvaccinated, some of the vaccinated were viral spreaders (Brown et al., 2021), prompting a return to indoor masking guidelines for all and recommendations for booster vaccines due to waning immunity in the face of the delta variant (O'donnell & Aboulenein, 2021). In many respects, the decision to unmask the vaccinated reflected the same colonial thoughtlessness as the libertarian non-compliance with masking and social distancing before the reversal.

Reversing CDC guidelines was an illustration of how colonial acts of justice often implicitly involve an element of retribution (see Chap. 11).

The reversal of the CDC masking policy also made it even more difficult to encourage those who opposed masking in the first place to return to masking during the delta variant surge. Some communities restored masking mandates, only to find those mandates challenged by public officials in their state. An example was when Attorney General Eric Schmitt of Missouri legally challenged the reinstated St. Louis City masking mandate in July of 2021 (Hollingsworth & Salter, 2021), once again illustrating the self-defeating libertarianism of colonialism. During that same period of time, the Governor of Arkansas Asa Hutchinson expressed regret that his state had banned mask mandates when the surge was out of control in his state (LeBlanc, 2021).

Misinformation concerning COVID-19 Disinformation social media campaigns helped to spread pseudoscience babble and other unscientific information globally compounded public health officials' attempts to address COVID-19 (Islam et al., 2020). Misinformation about possible virus treatments, cures and conspiracies were particularly troublesome, resulting in fraud and manipulation that increased pandemic risks (Islam et al., 2020; Roozenbeek et al., 2020). Even some media outlets were documented to have promoted misinformation to the detriment of the public good (Meade, 2021). International agencies concerned about public harm from disinformation campaigns issued a joint statement highlighting the problem and proposing methods to combat misinformation (WHO et al., 2020). The WHO set up a way to report misinformation online so that they could take steps to address it (WHO, 2020b). With consideration for a future pandemic, plans to control for misinformation would be helpful to prevent unnecessary sicknesses and deaths (Taylor, 2019).

Sometimes we do not know what we do not know Social psychologists have found an interesting phenomenon concerning the self-perception of personal competence in wielding knowledge in certain topic areas, such as science, referred to as the *Dunning-Krueger Effect* (Krueger & Dunning, 1999). The Dunning-Krueger Effect is a cognitive bias in which people who have low levels of knowledge about a particular topic tend to overestimate their knowledge when compared to others, whereas people with high levels of knowledge on a specific topic tend to underestimate their knowledge when compared to others. The Dunning-Krueger Effect helps to understand the complicated relationships that scientists have with some non-scientists. Scientists, on the one hand, may assume that non-scientists have a greater capacity to understand the science than they do in reality, and therefore assume the public understands some of the basics of the science when they likely do not. On the other hand, non-scientists may believe they know more about the science than they do, contributing to assumptions about the science that are simply unsupported and the perceptions they know more on the topic than the scientist. The Dunning-Krueger Effect suggests non-scientists may know less about science than they think they do and that both scientists and non-scientists may have poor perceptions about the size of the chasm of knowledge between them. One solution may be better lay communication by scientists to non-scientists while simultaneously engaging non-scientists in better education about science.

As a scientist, it is clear to me that many non-scientists assume a couple of things about science that are not true. One is that science involves the production of facts or alternative facts depending upon one's perspective, when in reality science is interested in testing whether hypotheses are falsifiable rather than provable. Science does not create facts, but rather is a process that generates a body of evidence that either supports or refutes hypotheses or theories. A second assumption by non-scientists is that scientists have agendas, usually political agendas, that disagree with what the non-scientist believes. Scientists typically do not have agendas, but rather have predictions developed from pre-existing data concerning hypotheses. Since scientists study reality, sometimes they discover evidence about reality that is uncomfortable and may challenge conventional wisdom. Scientists may be the messengers, but they did not create the messages that data suggest. Scientists are not creating fake news, but the collected data may be falsifying what others thought was news. Simplistically speaking, science exposes fake news about reality rather than creates it. Some people do not like it when ideas are falsified, but scientists are only the messengers rather than the opponents.

One more thing that is true about science—since scientists are human creatures, it is not and never has been fully objective. However, it is not a political agenda that typically drives scientific subjectivity as some anti-science people believe and fear—implicit cultural biases drive science. Scientists as human beings are subject to the same cultural implicit biases to which all people have been subject–so to categorically assume that science is objective is unrealistic. Implicit cultural biases shape ideas and theoretical assumptions, the focus of research, research methods and measures, and the populations being studied (or not studied) as discussed in Chap. 6. If colonial science is guilty of anything, it is the vast exclusion of diverse peoples and ideas in the development and expansion of scientific education, inquiry, and research—exclusions that have been extremely damaging to minoritized groups within those societies (Blume, 2020). In fact, homogenous, non-diverse science may be one reason why people are less trusting of its products. Diversifying science helps instill trust in its methods and results, producing an inclusive enterprise that might be embraced by diverse peoples.

Earlier in this section I referred to the privilege of scientists, but those who wield misinformation also are exercising privilege. Rejecting science is privilege because misinformation has power to manipulate those who are vulnerable to its influence–those who wield that power are typically aware of what they are doing. Those who reject science are able to do so because of their self-interested privilege allows them to make that choice, but by so doing they may threaten others. During the pandemic, the privilege of exercising defiance and misinformation contributed to needless deaths due to poor choices and lack of adherence to recommended public safety measures. People may exercise the liberty to disagree oppose science, but once they used that liberty to spread COVID-19 or evangelize their positions opposing science to the detriment of others, they have crossed an ethical line from personal liberties to irresponsibly weaponizing misinformation. An IAPP perspective would view such activities as an expression of relational psychopathology by exercising liberties and self-interests at the expense of social responsibility (Blume, 2020).

Wielding Privilege During the COVID-19 Pandemic

Vaccine nationalism was an excellent example of colonial privilege exercised during pandemic, but there were many other examples of privilege driven by colonial self-interests that harmed others. Some high-profile sports figures and celebrities acted in risky ways that perpetuated spread, almost as if they were invulnerable and certainly oblivious of the risk to others. For example, in an unusual major league baseball season marked by periodic disruptions due to COVID-19 infections of players, there was no mystery to why the world champion Los Angeles Dodgers would have several players test positive for COVID-19 immediately after the celebration of winning the 2020 World Series (Gauk-Roger & Martin, 2020). Another example was the behavior of the first family in 2020. One family member violated masking rules at a children's hospital when visiting young patients (Klein, 2020). Another example discussed in Chap. 5 was when a school where three grandchildren of former President Trump attended expressed concerns about family members not practicing pandemic safety precautions (Bennett, 2020a). Ordinary citizens also engaged in activities that suggested pursuing self-interests with an utter lack of concern toward others as well. One couple who knew they had COVID-19 boarded a plane with their child despite the risks to the child and others on the plane (Griffith, 2020b).

Exercising privilege was flagrant during the pandemic, exhibiting callousness towards others during a time of great pain and vulnerability. Former White House Chief of Staff Mark Meadows, who frequently refused to social distance and mask himself in public, suggested at one point that it was unreasonable to try to control the pandemic (Smith, 2020). Testing for COVID-19 was often a luxury during the pandemic. When reflecting upon concerns that the wealthy and well-connected were being routinely tested whereas others were not, President Trump suggested that was just the way things are in life (Griffith, 2020a). Another Trump family member pursued construction of an expensive White House tennis pavilion when millions were unemployed and hungry (Bennett, 2020b). Frustrated by the privilege of defying social distancing and masking, the governor of Tennessee reportedly suggested that vaccines would not overcome selfishness (Burnside, 2021).

Many colonial politicians refused to support public health recommendations during the pandemic, but often engage in hypocrisy that suggested manipulation. For example, Senator Rand Paul, an ophthalmologist by trade, was quite vocal in opposition to many mitigation measures suggested by public health officials to control the spread of COVID-19 throughout the pandemic, However, during the summer of 2021, it was revealed that Senator Paul's wife had purchased a significant amount of stock in the company that produces remdesivir (see Chap. 7) in February, 2020 (Fox & LeBlanc, 2021). The revelation certainly suggested hypocrisy and deception, and an implied conflict of interest. The privilege of Senator Paul to be associated with such a purchase while voicing disbelief in the potency of the virus and opposition to public health mitigation measures may seem astonishing to some, but perhaps not astonishing when examined in the context of his colonial libertarian worldview.

Some of the most callous examples of exercised privilege during the COVID-19 pandemic involved abuses in vaccine administration and distribution. For example, several hospitals were found to have offered vaccines to their board of directors and donors, rewarding them for giving to the hospitals, at a time when the vaccines were only being directed toward those at highest risk (Budryk, 2021; Bynum et al., 2021). In Wisconsin, a 33-year old man from a billionaire family announced on social media that he was able to get the vaccination during a time when very few had the same opportunity (Richmond, 2021). In Florida, vaccines were being delivered to wealthy citizens that were meant for Black communities (Goldhill, 2021b; Murphy et al., 2021). One high profile abuse of privilege made vaccines available to one of the wealthiest communities in the state of Florida as a political favor to supporters. When Governor DeSantis was confronted by a county official from his own party about the poor optics and favoritism, he threated to take vaccines away from the county entirely (Toropin, 2021). Others fraudulently offered "treatments" for COVID-19 for personal economic gain, leveraging the desperation and fear of people that was predicted pre-pandemic (Taylor, 2019). One example was a state legislator from the state of Missouri who sold fake treatments under the guise they were created from stem cells (Madani, 2021; Stafford, 2021).

Vaccine privilege was not a uniquely American phenomenon, however. In Brazil, some wealthy citizens paid to be vaccinated before others (Savarese, 2021). One high profile act of privilege was reported in Canada where a millionaire couple chartered a plane and traveled to the Yukon to get vaccinations intended for First Nations citizens. In the process, they violated government pandemic rules related to safe travel, placing others selfishly at risk (Associated Press, 2021a). Globally, a new type of travel package emerged for the privileged: *vaccine tourism*. Many people who could afford to do so traveled to other nations, including the US, to get vaccinations well before their fellow citizens received them. Tour companies organized the vaccine tours (Siemaszko, 2021).

Contrast all these acts of privilege with those who had no privilege. For example, African health care workers faced the pandemic with little PPE, minimal hospital resources, and mostly unvaccinated due to vaccine nationalism (Kupferschmidt, 2021). In the US, vaccine disparities favored the privileged in US society, who were typically not the most vulnerable to the pandemic (Goldhill, 2021a). The BBC (, 2021a) made the notation early in the vaccination campaign that the increase of wealth to the world's ten richest men during pandemic wealth building (see also Chap. 3) would have provided enough money to buy vaccines for the entire world. Eventually, the consequences of vaccine nationalism became obvious with wealthier colonial nations reopening and poorer nations struggling (Mueller, 2021). When it was clear that the needs of the rich colonial nations were being met, those nations began to discuss how to address the needs of other nations during the G-7 meeting of 2021. The photos of several male leaders making those commitments from a posh beach resort spoke volumes about colonial privilege (Lawless et al., 2021).

President Trump's illness: A case study of colonial privilege Mr. Trump flaunted social distancing and masking routinely during his tenure as American president, acting with the defiance and certainty of invulnerability that privilege often imbues. As discussed earlier, his many campaign rallies were associated with the spread of COVID-19 (Bernheim et al., 2020; Kounang, 2020). Eventually the Trump administration's defiant policies toward protecting others from COVID-19 contributed to Trump family members and aides becoming ill from the disease (Westcott et al., 2020). Although details were very sketchy at the time of his illness and hospitalization, continuing a pattern of understating the threat of the illness, it eventually became clear that the former president had been quite ill (Collins & Acosta, 2021). However, as president of the US, he was afforded health care privileges that most citizens of the world would never receive. During his illness, he was provided with every available option of treatment, including experimental treatments such as regeneron, a monoclonal antibody treatment that had been tested on the cells of fetal tissue—research methods actively opposed by the administration and many of its followers (Kaiser Health News, 2020). Mr. Trump recovered but, in the process, engaged in another act of privilege by downplaying the illness without acknowledging the privilege of his recovery as a function of accessing the highest quality of health care available on the planet. Mr. Trump exercised his colonial privilege when he asked his secret service detail to chauffeur him around the hospital in a motorcade, placing agents at risk for exposure (Sprunt, 2020). Mr. Trump allegedly held stock in the producers of regeneron and remdesivir and benefitted from a privileged relationship with the regeneron producer CEO (La Monica, 2020).

Almost a year later, Governor Greg Abbott of Texas was found to be positive for COVID-19 and was immediately placed on regeneron despite apparently having mild symptoms. Not only was it discovered that he was receiving regeneron for mild symptoms, it was also disclosed that the governor was being tested daily for COVID-19 at a time that he was legally preventing mask mandates in Texas schools during the delta variant surge (Office of the Texas Governor, 2021). Having access to both regeneron and testing at a time when children were not being protected is a particularly callous example of personal privilege during the pandemic.

Privilege is power that results from colonial hierarchies and divisiveness. Those who wield their privilege often do so with self-interests that victimize others. Privilege is often wielded without consideration of the consequences on others, such as what might happen from a motorcade for a sick president. The figure head of American colonialism is the office of the president of the US, a position of great international power and influence that may be wielded to advance or oppress others. In the context of hierarchical colonialism, those who hold the office of the president are afforded privilege that many global citizens will never experience.

Conspiracies and Privilege

From its inception, colonialism has been a conspiracy by the privileged. A small group of people of privilege made agreements to explore and conquer people who were considered inferior–lands were considered to be there for the taking. Since its beginning, colonial conspiracies have protected the status quo of privilege and been used to disempower outgroups in society. Sometimes, colonial conspiracies were meant to be covert activities to undermine some peoples for the benefit of others and at other times the conspiracy activities were exceedingly obvious. The COVID-19 pandemic and its consequential instability offered fertile ground for the re-emergence of colonial conspiracy themes.

Listening to public radio in 2019 before an election, I heard a candidate for mayor for the city of Spokane, Washington, say, among other things, that "perception is reality" (Spokane Public Radio, 2019). As a psychologist, I was so struck by the comment that I wrote it down with the idea of discussing its implications in an article or a book at some point. Psychologists know from research that our minds play tricks on us–that both our perceptions and our interpretations of those perceptions can lead our conclusions astray, so in reality our perceptions are not entirely to be trusted. As an Indigenous psychologist, I also accept there is much that we perceive that we do not understand–there are incomprehensible perceptions that tend to be more spiritual in nature than from the material world.

The conspiracy theories featured prominently today are great examples of the "perception is reality" vision of the world. However, as a psychologist, those perceptions are suspect without further confirmation and data to support the assertions. They are like the alternative facts and fake news discussed earlier in that they tend to lack empirical evidence. As an Indigenous psychologist, the conspiracy theories of today are not spiritual experiences, but rather distrustful narratives about others that tend to divide people including families. Although Indigenous people enjoy good stories, enjoyable stories require a positive lesson about life to be valuable, and the conspiracy theories that were circulating during the pandemic did not provide positive lessons. In that way, contemporary conspiracy theories are most closely aligned with colonial deception tactics such as colonial splitting. The consequences of conspiracy theories have not been psychologically helpful to the whole, therefore they are also an expression of relational psychopathology rooted in distrust of others.

Conspiracy thinking and theories were especially toxic during the COVID-19 pandemic, creating barriers to working collectively to address virus spread (Kramer, 2021; Romer & Jamieson, 2020). Conspiracies have been a common phenomenon associated with pandemics (Taylor, 2019), and they were highly influential during COVID-19. The evidence of the destructiveness of conspiracy thinking and misinformation could be seen globally. Hundreds of health care professionals during a global pandemic were threatened by people who believed in various conspiracies related to COVID-19 (Devi, 2020). In Britain it was reported that 5G wireless towers were set afire due to baseless conspiracies linking the technology to the pandemic (Satariano & Alba, 2020). In Nashville, Tennessee, a person who believed in conspiracies bombed the central district of the city due to concerns that lizard people were taking over the country and the planet (Parramore, 2021). The depth of belief in conspiracy theories was so profound that some believers acted in contradictory ways depending upon the most recent misinformation. One example featured conspiracy theorists that initially resisted masking and social distancing for what they considered a pandemic hoax, but later reconsidered—masking up and socially distancing when another round of misinformation suggested that being around the vaccinated was harmful to human reproductivity (Lamoureux, 2021). West Virginia Governor Jim Justice appeared so annoyed by low state vaccination rates due to misinformation that he chided citizens publicly about the absurdity of the conspiracy theories on camera (CNN, 2021b). Some believers may be vulnerable to conspiracy theories due to mental health issues, some may be searching for meaning and identity in fantastic untruths, and others are simply manipulating the vulnerable.

Conspiracy theories, from my perspective as an Indigenous psychologist, are fueled by the injustices of colonial societies. The conspiracy generators are using disinformation to drive an agenda, usually political and colonial. The conspiracy generators often use social media to spread and perpetuate their disinformation, reflecting a masterful understanding of how falsehoods travel much more rapidly via social media than truth (Vosoughi et al., 2018). They are intentionally manipulating the conspiracy believers and driving wedges between people and groups of people.

Business entities may have taken advantage of the culture of conspiracy, finding profit in conspiracy generation and consumption. A high-profile employee whistleblower emerged during the fall of 2021 to allege that Facebook (and potentially other social media platforms) were profiting from the use of colonial splitting algorithms that encouraged conspiracy consumption based upon political leanings of platform users (Zubrow et al., 2021). In addition, certain social influencers (a.k.a., conspiracy generators) were *whitelisted* by the platform algorithm in ways that kept those influencers free from scrutiny of checks that detected and thwarted potential, misinformation and hateful and divisive content. Whitelisted is a term of privilege to describe when certain users are granted permissions to do things that other users are not allowed—even the term "whitelisted" conveys a sense of the privilege involved. The whistleblower alleged that the divisive (colonial splitting) tactics were used to generate greater interest in the platform and therefore greater profits—a strategy that encouraged divisiveness as a profitable business decision for the company (Zubrow et al., 2021). If true, the allegations certainly suggest that self-business decisions may have had a hand in exacerbating social divisions and the spread of conspiracy behavior in ways that ultimately contributed to civil unrest. The methods are reminiscent of other colonial practices engaged upon by businesses that in effect place business self-interests above the collective interests of the whole (Blume, 2020; see also Chap. 7 this volume).

Contemporary conspiracies include old themes of the past that used -isms to divide and put down people. How sad it is that there are people so lost or miserable that they feel the need to create alternative realities and alternative facts in this beautiful world. How indicting of colonial societies that there is the need for alternatives realities and alternative facts because colonial promises for societies have not panned out. The cults of conspiracy theories exist as a place where alienated people feel they belong, where they have identity and a sense of authority and belongingness that they do not apparently experience in the "real" colonial society. Colonialism has alienated so many over time that its many victims try to find ways to escape from the inequitable realities—and conspiracy generators are more than willing to assist. Conspiracy generation is yet another expression of privilege over others, and the existence of conspiracy movements is a sign of the illness inherent in colonial social orders.

One of the prominent generators of conspiracies on social media was an anonymous entity known as "Q." Many of the conspiracies included horrific visions of human nature and wild tails of misbehavior by certain politicians and celebrities. Q's conspiracies were packed with colonial -isms meant to split people and groups, making Q an excellent example of a master manipulator of those vulnerable to conspiracy thinking. Q generated a significant following resulting in a cult-like group referred to as QAnon (The Soufran Center, 2021). The relational psychopathology associated with QAnon has been so damaging to the mental health of individuals and their families that a QAnon support group has emerged on Reddit to assist in the healing from the QAnon cult (Reddit, 2021). During the pandemic, the COVID-19 conspiracies were merged with the conspiracies of Q to create a much larger alliance of conspiracy generators, believers, and manipulators, including Trump supporters, white supremacists, and antivaxxers (Spring & Wendling, 2020). Later, these allies would exercise considerable defiance against suggested public health measures to control virus spread and were key participants in the first US insurrection on January 6, 2021. One of the leaders storming the US Capitol publicly identified himself as the "shaman" of QAnon, an insulting and laughable assertion from a white supremacist manipulating others during an insurrection. Later it was found that the "shaman" had opposed being vaccinated while in the military and had made threats against the US vice president (Sharp & Jewers, 2021).

White supremacy, fear, and conspiracies Q and QAnon generate conspiracies that suggested child abuse, murder, and satanic practices of minoritized groups and liberals, beliefs that most certainly generate fear, hate, and sometimes violence (The Soufran Center, 2021). The underlying theme of many conspiracy theories is a commonly held belief that outsiders threaten the moral superiority and way of life of adherents. Those perceived threats result in externalized fear and rage common to the colonial experience. Outsiders from the perspective of modern conspiracy groups are typically the outgroups of colonial societies, such as BLM supporters during the pandemic, demonstrating how conspiracies are often racialized.

Colonial conspiracies suggest outside threats to colonial ways of life, especially the colonial perceptions of white supremacy. One very old colonial conspiracy is that minoritized groups will replace and cancel Whites as the dominant culture in those nations, a theme that supports the importance of white nationalism and supremacy movements as a form of resistance to the threats to Whites. Today, that very old conspiracy theme has a modern expression referred to as white replacement, with some adherents believing that minoritized groups are engaging in a form of genocide towards Whites (Bridge Initiative Team, 2020). An excellent example of appealing to this age-old conspiracy theory was when former Trump official Stephen Miller not so subtly suggested that the relocation of Afghan allies to the US was intended to change the nation (Fox News, 2021), promoting a xenophobic position he had been advocating for at least 3 years (Alvarez & Warren, 2021). The racist conspiracies suggest old colonial themes such as divinely sanctioned white supremacy dividing society through racialized anger, blame, and fear and disinformation.

The themes of white supremacy in widely circulated conspiracy theories set the stage for racialized defiance and distrust that eventually boiled over in the context of the COVID-19 pandemic. Those who were targeted by conspiratorial blame varied widely, from minoritized members of society to health care professionals and government officials. Misinformation, anger, and fear in the context of privilege suggested that white supremacy justified any and all activities in defense of the colonial way of life, including violence against others.

Conspiracies and colonial insurrection As discussed in Chap. 8, the American election brought about considerable unrest driven by misinformation and white supremacy. The federal Kerner Commission (1968) warned that inequities and civil unrest were a function of White racism, the real threat to peace in American society, but that evidence had been essentially ignored for over 50 years. At first the unrest was focused on state governments that were deemed contrary to colonial and white supremacy goals. The state of Michigan was an excellent example of the targeted protests and intimidation. A senior health adviser to former President Donald Trump who had advocated for infection-acquired herd immunity encouraged the people of Michigan through a tweet to resist public health precautions for COVID-19 (LeBlanc & Diamond, 2020). Additionally, a plot was discovered where several anti-government militia members planned to storm the Michigan state capitol, possibly shoot law enforcement officials, and kidnap Governor Gretchen Whitmer with nefarious intent to hold a kangaroo court and possibly execute her (Flesher, 2020). The idea that someone holds beliefs that their vision of their country is so superior to others that they are entitled to take the law into their own hands and execute mob justice is certainly evidence of a privileged perspective. In Michigan, those beliefs of superiority emerged often in late 2020, when white supremacists and conspiracy supporters opposed the counting of votes in communities of color and threatened violence against state election officials, exercising colonial privilege to overturn election results (Censky, 2021). The white supremacy and conspiracy driven threats against US states would eventually morph into threats against the US federal government.

January 6, 2021 An organized rally on January 6, 2021, coincided with the congressional session called to certify the federal election as required by US law. The rally was prescheduled and highly advertised and planned by supporters of Former President Trump, who recruited attendees, in some instances providing means and resources for people to attend (Dilanian & Collins, 2021; Lardner & Smith, 2021; Tanfani et al., 2021; Valou, 2021). Additionally, white supremacist groups appeared to coordinate their plans before the rally (Lucas, 2021). The former president and other Trump family members, Congressman Mo Brooks from Alabama, Rudy Guiliani, and Roger Stone were speakers at the rally who spoke inflammatory words (Bennett, 2021; Valou, 2021). Congressman Brooks was later found to have worn body armor to the rally (Newell, 2021), suggesting he was ready for violence. The rally dissolved into a march to the US Capitol that turned into a storming of the building while congress was in session to coerce elected officials not to certify the presidential election. The resulting insurrection was violent with several people including law enforcement officers hurt and killed.

During the insurrection, rebels used many different types of weapons including stun weapons, mace and bear spray. and flags on poles used to beat the police, including thin blue line flags meant to honor law enforcement officials. The mob included ex-military, police, and firefighters who fought against other public servants. There was also a group that seemed intent on capturing key politicians and perhaps even lynching US Vice-President Mike Pence and others on make-shift gallows near the Capitol (Associated Press, 2021b; Axon et al., 2021; Helsel, 2021; Perez & Prokupecz, 2021). The leaders were avowed leaders of QAnon and known white supremacist groups–the insurrection represented the first flying of the Confederate Battle Flag in the US Capitol (McLaughlin, 2021), a relic of the US Civil War and symbol of white supremacy and support for slavery and rebellion. Rebels looted and soiled the Capitol building and intimidated members of congress who were sheltered in place in the building, while police defended congress and mislead the rebels away from congressional representatives (Mendoza & Linderman, 2021; Murphy & Polantz, 2021). Shortly after the insurrection, the Federal Bureau of Investigation arrested a man who was carrying a "white privilege" card and found with thousands of rounds of ammunition, 49 guns, and material to make bombs (Riotta, 2021).

White supremacy was clearly at the heart of the insurrection, with symbols of hate clearly visible and with white supremacy groups front and center of the effort. White supremacy also impacted public reaction after the insurrection, when many groups attempted to downplay the events of the day or attempted to whitewash the history of that day. One only has to examine the differences between public and political responses to the terrorist attacks of September 11, 2001, compared to the attack of January 6, 2021, to see the impact of racism at work. When white supremacists were involved, they seemed to get a pass compared to the treatment of Arab Americans after September 11. Twenty years later, little had changed with regard to racial privilege.

The preponderance of evidence suggests that the insurrection was orchestrated by colonial rebels of privilege who flaunted superiority over others and therefore felt entitled to special treatment. One insurrectionist was a Chief Executive Officer of a corporation (Egan, 2021). Another insurrectionist flew to the insurrection on a private jet (Burke, 2021). A Trump administration insurrectionist insisted that he receive a cell without cockroaches (Williams, 2021). One insurrectionist requested permission to be married in Peru after being charged (Cohen, 2021a), and another insurrectionist requested permission to go on a working vacation in Mexico after being charged and received that permission from a federal judge in Texas (Chappell, 2021). Several insurrectionists apparently did not have enough interest in the election to cast a ballot (Ellis & Hicken, 2021). The shaman of QAnon discussed earlier went on a hunger strike to get an organic food diet, which was granted by a federal judge and he was transferred to another jail to accommodate those needs (Balsamo, 2021). Later, a federal judge expressed concerns about light sentences and plea deals for some insurrectionists (Tillman, 2021). Evidence suggests that White Americans often benefit from the privilege of plea deals when minoritized citizens do not, (Berdejó, 2018).

Also apparent in the inherent privilege of the insurrection was the narcissism of its participants. Narcissistic orientations are psychologically damaging and self-defeating consequences the emerge from the insecurity of colonial radical individualism and self-orientation (Blume, 2020). The privilege and narcissistic orientations of insurrectionists was obvious in their posting of selfies and videos in the Capitol Building and during the insurrection. These activities not only demonstrated privilege in that there was no fear of retribution for posting, it also was self-defeating by making insurrectionists vulnerable to being fired from jobs or arrested and charged with crimes (Axon et al., 2021; Stone & Bartz, 2021). Privilege in colonial nations often provides a false sense of security amidst the vulnerability of an interdependent world (Blume, 2020). For example, colonial political power could not protect Mr. Trump from civil lawsuits by police victimized by insurrectionists (Diaz, 2021). He and some allies were banned from social media platforms (Soo, 2021), and pressure mounted to suspend the accounts of prominent antivaxxers as well (BBC, 2021d).

Many public health officials were concerned the insurrection would become a COVID-19 superspreader event as a result of unmasked insurrectionists as well as certain individuals in congress defiantly unmasked when sheltering in place (Mitropoulos, 2021). Over 30 Capitol police officers tested positive for COVID-19 after the insurrection, as did several members of congress (Kounang & Wild, 2021; Peltz, 2021).

The political consequences of the insurrection were widespread and likely will reverberate through the American social order for years to come. First, the insurrection highlighted the fragility of the American social order as well as the elevated privilege of those who want to defend white supremacy and other colonials values. Second, the US Republican party experienced its own consequences of colonial splitting between conspiracy theorists and white supremacists with those who voted to impeach Donald Trump for the insurrection or those who wish for a return to the colonial "normal" that pre-existed Mr. Trump (e.g., Anderson, 2021; Gruver, 2021). When the Pennsylvania Republican party censured Senator Pat Toomey for voting for impeachment of Mr. Trump, a leading party official said Mr. Toomey was not elected to "vote his conscience" or "do the right thing" (Santucci, 2021). The event highlighted the depth of colonial deception and privilege involved in efforts to overturn the election and to defend misinformation and conspiracies that contributed to the insurrection and devasting health consequences of COVID-19. Some former Trump officials publicly opposed the acts of deception triggering the insurrection (Mena, 2021), but others remained quiet or committed to conspiratorial untruths. Congressperson Marjorie Taylor Greene of Georgia and QAnon proposed a new racialized congressional caucus post-insurrection dedicated to protecting "Anglo-Saxon values," a proposal withdrawn under party pressure (Gordon, 2021). Sadly for all Americans, the Republican party includes many white nationalists and QAnon conspiracy generators and consumers, racializing the focus of the party (Fox, 2021; Warren, 2021).

The US government expects more acts of terrorism and rebellion from white supremacy and conspiracy groups emboldened by the January 6, 2021, insurrection (Office of the Director of National intelligence, 2021). Political instability in the US has compounded pandemic-related stress in ways that significantly and negatively impact health and mental health (APA, 2021). Conspiracies and mistrust will have significant negative consequences on the psychological well-being for many post-pandemic years to come.

Beyond Privilege: An Indigenous Interpretation

Privilege is self-defeating in how it lulls people into a false sense of security. Vaccine nationalism is an excellent example of the false sense of security to privileged nations, which still leaves an interdependent world order vulnerable. A study from Rand projected that vaccine nationalism could cost nations trillions of extra dollars due to continued viral spread and mutations among the global community (Hafner et al., 2021). Chapter 9 shares many different examples of privilege in action during the COVID-19 pandemic, yet with each story, those who expressed their privilege simultaneously generated significant negative consequences to themselves and others as a result. Part of the reason I think that occurs is because privilege blinds people to the realities of their situation, leaving them vulnerable to the real-world threat they do not see—their own poor judgment. Poor judgment was on full display during the pandemic and frequently resulted in destructiveness and death.

Self-oriented belief systems naturally leave people vulnerable because the "self" is a lonely entity. True strength arises from relationships, and self-interests tend to interfere with healthy relationships. Colonial psychological beliefs have elevated autonomy as symbolic of psychological well-being and health, and yet autonomy is a myth in an interdependent world (Blume, 2020). Seeking autonomy quite literally means rejecting reliance on others, placing self above relationships, which from an Indigenous perspective compounds the loneliness of a self-oriented existence. In a very real sense, practicing self and autonomous psychology tends to enhance distrust and division. As interpreted by an IAPP, autonomy is more likely to bring one psychological sickness rather than psychological wellness. Self-oriented living tends to dehumanize both self and other through interrupting our natural connectivity to one another.

Conspiracy movements are also very lonely propositions even though they feign the appearance of a collective viewpoint. The paranoia inherent in conspiracies tend to drive mistrust toward others, seeing others as threats, when in fact the conspiracy beliefs are the true threats to psychological health and well-being. Conspiracy generators manipulate others for self-gain, and conspiracy consumers allow themselves to be manipulated. It is difficult to have healthy, balanced, and harmonious relationships when one suspects that others are threats. Colonial conspiracies have their roots in colonial splitting tactics and racialized themes reflecting supremacy viewpoints. The toxicity of conspiracies as colonial splitting cannot be overstated. Nations who wield such tactics internally are also likely to be vulnerable to those same tactics being delivered by other colonial nations hoping to destabilize their rivals and enemies (Cohen, 2021b). The toxicity of those beliefs weighs heavily on colonial societies. During COVID-19, conspiracy beliefs were major drivers of viral spread and death.

Expressions of anti-intellectualism and anti-science have been carried out in acts of defiance, fueled by externalized anger and fear and distrust of others. Confirmation biases ensure that people will continue to trust their own conspiratorial perceptions of the world, filtering the real world through misinformed minds. The Dunning-Krueger Effect suggests that some will have false confidence in their perceptions of reality potentially to their own detriment. The truth is that privilege benefits from ignorance—as long as the people remain mired in self-confirmed ignorance, they will not see the reality of their own circumstances. The inequitable status quo will remain unchallenged as a result. Inequities will be blamed on others rather than on the inherent injustices in the colonial social system. Colonial societies would be healthier if citizens took informed leaps of faith toward scientific evidence rather than blind leaps of faith toward their misinformed perceptions of reality.

White supremacy is also born out of externalized fear and results in externalized rage toward others. From an IAPP point of view, strategies to address these deeply-seated externalized emotions would be helpful to prevent significant divisiveness during future pandemics. Beneath supremacist beliefs of strength is an extremely fragile existence built upon a lie of superiority. When the lie clashes with reality, it threatens believers of the lie such that way they want to strike out at the world. White supremacy and nationalism are colonial cultural perspectives; adherents are the true believers in colonial culture. As a result, the culture of white supremacy and nationalism must be challenged and transformed systemically.

A critical strategy to address future pandemic threats is to transform the systems that generate and foster the misperception of externalized threats. Hierarchical social systems that allow for supremacy of any group or individual will not engender collective trust. Self-oriented social systems do not contribute to a sense of unity of purpose or vision. In fact, self-orientation creates the self-versus-other beliefs that generate externalized perspectives of threat. Societies that believe that one individual holds more esteem than another will always be vulnerable to inequities that risk sickness. Social systems that emphasize personal liberties over social responsibility are unlikely to do well in addressing collective threats. A social order that believes that one individual is entitled to that which another is not cannot adequately prioritize the needs of the whole above the needs of the few. It is unlikely such a social order will exercise restraint when restraint is necessary or consider the needs of others as equally weighted as the needs of the self. When privilege is involved, inconsideration of others is often inherent.

SARS-CoV-2 has demonstrated that colonial privilege leaves societies in unstable positions for addressing collective threats–stuck in the mire of its inequities. The pandemic, as destructive and painful as it has been, reopened the possibility for collective opportunities to recreate a post-pandemic world. Chapter 10 will examine those possibilities through Indigenous eyes and offer suggestions for how we move toward a healthier world together.

References

American Academy of Pediatrics. (2021, September 13). *Children and COVID-19: State-level data report*. : Author. https://www.aap.org/en/pages/2019-novel-coronavirus-covid-19-infections/children-and-covid-19-state-level-data-report/

Anderson, B. (2021, February 15). *NC GOP votes to censure Sen. Burr after impeachment vote*. : Associated Press. https://apnews.com/article/capitol-siege-donald-trump-richard-burr-north-carolina-impeachments-7fa6661bf9b7a2a2471e9512ec671926

Alonso, M. (2021, September 14). *Conservative radio host who swore off Covid-19 vaccine dies after contracting virus, co-host says*. : CNN. https://www.cnn.com/2021/09/14/media/bob-enyart-death-covid/index.html

Alvarez, P., & Warren, M. (2021, September 3). *Trump adviser Stephen Miller warned of "Iraqs and 'Stans' in the US while slow-walking the entry of Afghan allies*. : CNN. https://www.cnn.com/2021/09/03/politics/trump-adviser-stephen-miller-afghan-allies-us-entry/index.html

APA. (2020). *Building vaccine confidence through community engagement*. Washington, D.C.: Author. https://www.apa.org/topics/covid-19/equity-resources/building-vaccine-confidence.pdf.

APA. (2021). APA: U.S. adults report highest stress level since early days of the COVID-19 pandemic. Washington, D.C.: Authors. https://www.apa.org/news/press/releases/2021/02/adults-stress-pandemic

APA Working Group on Health Disparities in Boys and Men. (2018). *Health disparities in racial/ethnic and sexual minority boys and men*. Retrieved from http://www.apa.org/pi/health-disparities/resources/race-sexuality-men.aspx

Ashton, J. (2021). COVID-19 and the anti-vaxxers. *Journal of the Royal Society of Medicine, 114*(1), 42–43. https://doi.org/10.1177/0141076820986065

Associated Press. (2021a, January 27). *Canadian couple condemned for allegedly jumping vaccine line*. New York: Associated Press. https://apnews.com/article/vancouver-british-columbia-canada-conronavirus-pandemic-yukon-25d99a7547e71e6b54aedbb65ee7e960

Associated Press. (2021b, February 10). *The latest: House managers wrap up 1st full day of arguments*. : Author. https://apnews.com/article/trump-impeachment-trial-live-2-10-2021-c5a2717b25d339ec1746d6d0836d837f

Axon, R., Pulver, D., Stassen-Berger, R., Fraser, J., Salman, J., Penzenstadler, N., Wedell, K., Hines, M., & Baratz, D. (2021, April 2). *Capitol riot arrests: See who's been charged across the U.S.* : USA Today. https://www.usatoday.com/storytelling/capitol-riot-mob-arrests/

Balsamo, M. (2021, February 4). *Man who wore horns in US Capitol riot moved to Virginia jail*. New York: Associated Press. https://apnews.com/article/jacob-chansley-moved-virginia-jail-9a28be7295c76947aaf5b223411c1ddd

BBC. (2020, October 28). *Coronavirus cases increasing in European countries in recent* weeks. London: Author. https://www.bbc.com/news/world-europe-54716993

BBC. (2021a, January 27). *'Wealth increase of 10 men during pandemic could buy vaccines for all.'* : Author. https://www.bbc.news/news/world-55793575

BBC. (2021b, January 31). *Covid vaccination: Los Angeles Dodger Stadium 'closed by protests.'* : Author. https://www.bbc.com/news/world-us-canada-55875263

BBC. (2021c, February 24). *Covid: WHO pleads with Tanzania to start reporting cases.* : BBC. https://www.bbc.com/news/world-africa-56145510

BBC. (2021d, 26 March). *Covid vaccine: Social media urged to remove the 'disinfo dozen.'* : BBC. https://www.bbc.com/news/technology-56536390

Bennett, K. (2020a, November 13). *Ivanka trump and Jared Kushner's children withdrawn from school after administrators raised concerns about adherence to Covid precautions.* : CNN. https://www.cnn.com/2020/11/13/politicis/jared-kushner-ivanka-trump-children-school-covid/index.html

Bennett, K. (2020b, December 8). *Melania Trump cheers new White House tennis pavilion amid ongoing pandemic*. New York: CNN. https://www.cnn.com/2020/12/07/politics/melania-trumps-tennis-pavilion/index.html

Bennett, K. (2021, January 11). *Melania trump and adult trump children avoid the spotlight after one of nation's darkest days.* : CNN. https://www.cnn.com/2021/01/08/politics/melania-trump-white-house-capitol-riot/index.html

Berdejó, C. (2018). Criminalizing race: Racial disparities in plea-bargaining. *Boston College Law Review, 59*(4), article 2. http://lawdigitalcommons.bc.edu/bclr/vol59/vol59/iss4/2

Bernheim, B. D., Buchmann, N., Freitas-Groff, Z., & Otero, S. (2020). *The effects of large group meetings on the spread of COVID-19: The case of Trump Rallies.* : Stanford University Institute for Economic Policy Research. https://siepr.stanford.edu/sites/default/files/publications/20-043.pdf.

Blume, A. W. (2020). *A new psychology based on community, equality, and care of the earth: An indigenous American perspective*. ABC-CLIO/Praeger.

Bonds, A., & Inwood, J. (2015). Beyond white privilege: Geographics of white supremacy and settler colonialism. *Progress in Human Geography, 40*(6), 715–733. https://doi.org/10.1177/0309132515613166

Bradley, M., Ing, N., Mulligan, M., & Suliman, A. (2020, October 15). *France rolls out Covid curfews as Parisians lament new restrictions.* : NBC News. https://www.nbcnews.com/news/world/france-rolls-out-covid-curfews-parisians-lament-new-restrictions-n1243501

Bridge Initiative Team. (2020, February 3). *Factsheet: White genocide conspiracy theory.* : Georgetown University. https://bridge.georgetown.edu/research/factsheet-white-genocide-conspiracy-theory/

Brown, C. M., Vostok, J., Johnson, H., Burns, M., Gharpure, R., Sami, S., Sabo, R. T., Hall, N., Foreman, A., Schubert, P. L., Gallagher, G. R., Fink, T., Madoff, L. C., Gabriel, S. B., MacInnis, B., Park, D. J., Siddle, K. J., Harik, V., … Laney, A. S. (2021). Outbreak of SARS-CoV-2 infections, including COVID-19 vaccine breakthrough infections, associated with large public gatherings—Barnstable County, Massachusetts, July 2021. *MMWR*. https://doi.org/10.15585/mmwr.mm7031e2

Budryk, Z. (2021, January 27). *Inslee rebukes hospital over vaccine appointments for donors.* : The Hill. https://thehill.com/policy/healthcare/536130-inslee-rebukes-hospital-over-vaccine-appointments-for-donors

Burke, M. (2021, January 15). Texas realtor who took private jet is charged in Capitol riot. : NBC News. https://www.nbcnews.com/news/us-news/texas-real-estate-agent-who-took-private-jet-d-c-n1254453

Burnside, T. (2021, December 17). *Tennessee governor: 'One thing this vaccine will not solve or cure is selfishness.'* : CNN. https://www.cnn.com/2020/12/17/us/tn-bill-lee-coments-vaccines-covid-trnd/index.html

Bynum, R., Smith, M. R., & La Corte, R. (2021, January 30). *Playing favorites? Hospital boards, donors get COVID shots.* : Associated Press. https://apnews.com/article/technology-washington-coronavirus-pandemic-russ-seattle-c453fc84e9378ba4259715d3e0ad50d9

CDC. (2020, November 10). *Scientific brief: Community use of cloth masks to control the spread of SARS-CoV-2.* : Author. https://www.cdc.gov/coronavirus/2019-ncov/more/masking-science-sars-cov2.html

CDC. (2021, May 13). *Interim public health recommendations for fully vaccinated people.* : Author. https://www.cdc.gov/coronavirus/2019-ncov/vaccines/fully-vaccinated-guidance.html

Censky, A. (2021, January 1). *How misinformation lit the fire under a year of political chaos in Michigan.* Washington, D.C.: National Public Radio. https://www.npr.org/2021/01/01/952528193/how-misinformation-lit-the-fire-under-a-year-of-political-chaos-in-michigan

Chappell, B. (2021, February 6). *U.S. judge grants accused rioter's request to vacation in Mexico.* Washington, D.C.: National Public Radio. https://www.npr.org/sections/insurrection-at-the-capitol

Cilizza, C. (2020, November 17). *This republican governor is playing politics while Covid-19 burns through her state.* New York: CNN. https://www.cnn.com/2020/11/16/politics/kristi-noem-south-dakota-covid-19/index.html

CNN. (2021a, August 2). *Man's last text: 'I should have gotten the damn vaccine.'* : Author. https://www.cnn.com/videos/health/2021/08/02/jessica-dupreez-coronavirus-covid-19-last-text-vaccine-hesitant-newday-vpx.cnn

CNN. (2021b, September 9). *'I mean, come on': GOP governor rails against vaccine conspiracy theories.* New York: CNN. https://amp.cnn.com/cnn/videos/politics/2021/09/09/governor-jim-justice-vaccine-conspiracies-dons-take-dlt-vpx.cnn

Cohen, M. (2021a, February 9). *Alleged Capitol rioter asks judge to let him visit Peru to get married.* New York: CNN. https://www.cnn.com/2021/02/09/politics/capitol-rioter-peru-married/index.html

Cohen, Z. (2021b, April 19). *China and Russia 'weaponized' QAnon conspiracy around time of US Capitol attack, report says.* : CNN. https://www.cnn.com/2021/04/19/politics/qanon-russia-china-amplification/index.html

Collins, B. (2021, September 24). *'Vigilante treatments': Anti-vaccine groups push people to leave ICUs.* New York: NBC News. https://www.nbcnews.com/tech/tech-news/vigilante-treatments-anti-vaccine-groups-push-people-leave-icus-rcna2233

Collins, K., & Acosta, J. (2021), February 11. *Trump's Covid-19 condition was so concerning that doctors considered putting him on a ventilator, source confirms.* New York: CNN. https://www.cnn.com/2021/02/11/politics/donald-trump-covid-ventilator/index.html

Collins, K., Diamond, J., Acosta, J., Diaz, D., Liptak, K., & Klein, B. (2020, October 25). *At least 5 of Vice President Pence's aides test positive for coronavirus.* : CNN. https://www.cnn.com/2020/10/24/politics/mac-short-coronavirus-positive-test/index.html

Desmon, S. (2021, 21 January). *How to convince the COVID-19 vaccine hesitant.* Baltimore: Johns Hopkins Center for Communication Programs. https://ccp.jhu.edu/2021/01/21/covid-19-vaccine-hesitant/

Devi, S. (2020). COVID-19 exacerbates violence against health workers. *Lancet, 396*, 658. https://doi.org/10.1016/S0140-6736(20)31858-4

Diaz, J. (2021, March 31). *2 Capitol police officers sue trump for injuries sustained during the Jan. 6 riot.* Washington, D.C.: National Public Radio. https://www.npr.org/2021/03/31/982928605/2-capitol-police-officers-sue-trump-for-injuries-sustained-during-jan-6-riot

Dilanian, K., & Collins, B. (2021. April 20). *There are hundreds of posts about plans to attack the capitol. Why hasn't this evidence been used in court?* : NBC News. https://www.nbcnews.com/politics/justice-department/we-found-hundreds-posts-about-plans-attack-capitol-why-aren-n1264291

Egan, M. (2021, January 10). *CEO arrested for breaching the US capitol during trump-fueled insurrection.* : CNN. https://www.cnn.com/2021/01/09/business/capitol-hill-ceo-arrested-trump/index.html

Elliot, J. K. (2020, November 17). *Many COVID-19 patients insist 'it's not real' until they die, nurse says.* Vancouver: Global News. https://globalnews.ca/news/7467283/coronavirus-denier-deaths-nurse-hoax/amp/

Ellis, B., & Hicken, M. (2021, February 1). *They stormed the Capitol to overturn the results of an election they didn't vote in.* New York: CNN. https://www.cnn.com/2021/02/01/us/capitol-rioters-non-voters-invs/index.html

Erdman, S. L., Hoffman, J., & LeBlanc, P. (2020, November 17). *Stanford distances itself from Dr. Scott Atlas after he urges resistance to public health measures.* New York: CNN. https://www.cnn.com/2020/11/16/politcis/atlas-stanford-coronavirus-michigan/index.html

Flaherty, D. K. (2011). *The vaccine-autism connection: A public health crisis caused by unethical medical practices and fraudulent science.* The Annals of Pharmacotherapy, 45, 1302-1304. 10.13451aph.10318.

Flesher, J. (2020, December 17). : Associated Press. https://apnews.com/article/gretchen-whitmer-michigan-indictments-coronavirus-pandemic-traverse-city-10f7e02c57004da9843f89650edd4510.

Foran, C., & Wilson, K. (2021, February 8). *GOP Rep. Ron Wright dies following Covid diagnosis.* : CNN. https://www.cnn.com/2021/02/08/politics/ron-wright-congressman-dies/index.html

Fox, L. (2021, March 5). *Democratic Rep. Zoe Lofgren quietly releases massive social media report on GOP colleagues who voted to overturn the election.* : CNN. https://www.cnn.com/2021/03/05/politics/lofgren-social-media-report-gop-lawmakers/index.html

Fox, L., & LeBlanc, P. (2021, August 12). *Rand Paul reveals in late financial disclosure that his wife bought stock in company behind remdesivir in February 2021.* : CNN. https://www.cnn.com/2021/08/11/politics/rand-paul-wife-stock-gilead-sciences/index/html

Fox News. (2021, August 18). Stephen Miller: Afghanistan resettlements driven by politics, not humanitarian concerns. New York: Author. https://www.foxnews.com/media/stephen-miller-afghanistan-refugees-resettlement-politics-humanitarian

Gauchat, G. W. (2008). A test of three theories of anti-science attitudes. *Sociological Focus, 41*(4), 337–357. https://doi.org/10.1080/00380237.2008.10571338

Gauk-Roger, T., & Martin, J. (2020, November 7). *Days after winning the World Series, the Dodgers have five positive Covid-19 cases.* New York: CNN. https://www.cnn.com/2020/11/07/us/dodgers-covid-cases-world-series-spt/index.html

Gillies, R. (2021, August 13). *Canada to require air travelers to be vaccinated.* : Associated Press. https://apnews.com/article/lifestyle-business-canada-travel-coronavirus-pandemic-f504cb07e496c8569529bd5b8f5b2cf5

Goldhill, O. (2021a, February 11). *Covid-19 vaccination rates follow the money in states with the largest wealth gaps, analysis shows.* Boston: STAT News. https://www.statnews.com/2021/02/11/covid-19-vaccination-rates-follow-the-money-in-states-with-biggest-wealth-gaps/

Goldhill, O. (2021b, March 4). *In Palm Beach, Covid-19 vaccines intended for rural Black communities are instead going to wealthy white Floridians.* Boston: STAT News. https://www.statnews.com/2021/03/04/covid19-vaccines-for-rural-black-communities-going-to-wealthy-white-floridians/

Gordon, J. (2021, 18 April). *Marjorie Taylor Greene cans controversial America First caucus that wanted to promote 'Anglo Saxon traditions' after blowback from Kevin McCarthy.* : Daily Mail. https://www.dailymail.co.uk/news/article-9483437/amp/Marjorie-Taylor-Greene-cans-controversial-America-caucus-promoting-Anglo-Saxon-traditions.html

Government of Canada. (2021, October 6). Mandatory COVID-19 vaccination requirements for federally regulated transportation employees and travellers. Ottawa: Author. https://www.canada.ca/en/transport-canada/news/2021/10/mandatory-covid-19-vaccination-requirements-for-federally-regulated-transportation-employees-and-travellers.html

Griffith, J. (2020a, March 18). *Coronavirus: Trump says it may be 'the story of life' that well-connected get testing first.* : NBC News. https://www.nbcnews.com/news/us-news/coronavirus-nyc-mayor-slams-nets-over-testing-trump-weighs-n1162971

Griffith, J. (2020b, December 2). *Couple who tested positive for Covid are arrested after boarding flight.* New York: NBC News. https://www.nbcnews.com/news/us-news/couple-who-tested-positive-covid-arrested-after-boarding-flight-n1249753

Gruver, M. (2021, February 6). *Wyoming GOP censures Rep. Liz Cheney over impeachment vote.* New York: Associated Press. https://apnews.com/article/donald-trump-capitol-siege-censures-rawlins-wyoming-3d2a5ad3377bb748c22f632642ba23f1

Gupta, A. H. (2020a, October 22). *How an aversion to masks stems from 'toxic masculinity.'* : New York Times. https://www.newyorktimes.com/2020/10/22/us/masks-toxic-masculinity-covid-men-gender.html

Gupta, S. (2020b, December 6). *If the United States were my patient: Science cannot rescue us from ourselves.* New York: CNN. https://www.cnn.com/2020/12/06/health/coronavirus-us-patient-vaccine-rescue-gupta/index.html

Hafner, M., Yerushalmi, E., Fays, C., Dufresne, E., & Van Stolk, C. (2021). *The global economic cost of COVID-19 vaccine nationalism.* Santa Monica: Rand. https://www.rand.org/pubs/research_briefs/RBA769-1.html

Hamel, L., Lopes, L., Kearney, A., Kirzinger, A., Sparkes, G., Stokes, M., & Brodie, M. (2021, August 11). *KYY COVID-19 vaccine monitor: Parents and the pandemic.* : Kaiser Family Foundation. https://www.kff.org/coronavirus-covid-19/poll-finding/kff-covid-19-vaccine-monitor-parents-and-the-pandemic/

Helsel, P. (2021, April 1). *California man charged with attacking officer with stun weapon in Capitol riot.* New York: NBC News. https://www.nbcnews.com/news/us-news/california-man-charged-attacking-officer-stun-weapon-capitol-riot-n1262848

Holcombe, M., & Kaye, R. (2021, July 28). *Staff at a Florida hospital say they are hearing panic, fear and regret from unvaccinated patients.* New York: CNN. https://www.cnn.com/2021/07/26/us/florida-coronavirus-hospital-surge/index.html

Hollingsworth, H., & Salter, J. (2021, July 26). *Missouri AG sues over St. Louis area mask mandate.* New York: Associated Press. https://apnews.com/article/health-coronavirus-pandemic-michael-brown-st-louis-23f9b3da8c866cfffc617699b28caacb

Hotez, P. J. (2020). Anti-science extremism in America: Escalating and globalizing. *Microbes and Infection, 22*, 505–507. https://doi.org/10.1016/j.micinf.2020.09.005

Hotez, P. J. (2021a). America's deadly flirtation with anti-science and the medical freedom movement. *Journal of Clinical Investigation.* https://doi.org/10.1172/JCI149072

Hotez, P. J. (2021b). Anti-science kills: From Soviet embrace of pseudoscience to accelerated attacks on US biomedicine. *PLOS Biology.* https://doi.org/10.1371/journal.pbio.3001068

Islam, M. S., Sarkar, T., Khan, S. H., Kamal, A.-H. M., Hasan, S. M. M., Kabir, A., Yeasmin, D., Islam, M. A., Chowdhury, K. I. A., Anwar, K. S., Chughtai, A. A., & Seale, H. (2020). COVID-19-related infodemic and its impact on public health: A global social media analysis. *American Journal of Tropical Medicine and Hygiene, 103*(4), 1621–1629. https://doi.org/10.4269/ajtmh.20-0812

Johnson, C. K., Fingerhut, H., & Deshpande, P. (2020, November 6). *Counties with worst virus surges overwhelmingly voted Trump.* : Associated press. https://apnews.com/article/counties-worst-virus-surges-voted-trump-d671a483534024b5486715da6edb6ebf

Jolley, D., & Douglas, K. M. (2017). Prevention is better than cure: Addressing anti-vaccine conspiracy theories. *Journal of Applied Social Psychology, 47*, 459–469. https://doi.org/10.1111/jasp.12453

Joseph, A. (2021, July 27). *CDC recommends masks indoors even for some vaccinated against Covid-19.* Boston: STAT News. https://www.statnews.com/2021/07/27/cdc-recommends-masks-indoors-even-for-those-vaccinated-against-covid-19/

Kaiser Health News. (2020, October 9). *Fetal tissue research Trump opposes used to develop antibody therapy he praises as 'cure.'* : Author. https://khn.org/morning-breakout/fetal-tissue-research%2D%2Dtrump-opposes-used-to-develop-antibody-therapy-he-praises-as-cure/

Kaplan, A. (2020, November 14). *As Covid cases soar, GOP state lawmakers keep fighting to limit governors power to respond.* New York: NBC News. https://www.nbcnews.com/politics/politics-news/covid-cases-soar-gop-state-lawmakers-keep-fighting-limit-governors-n1247801

Kelleher, S. R. (2020, November 14). *Covid-19 alert: The 10 riskiest states to visit right now, ranked.* https://www.forbes.com/sites/suzannerowankelleher/2020/11/14/covid-19-alrt-the-10-riskiest-states-to-visit-right-now-ranked/

Kerner Commission. (1968). *Report of the National Advisory Commission on Civil Disorders.* Washington, D.C.: Government Printing Office. https://www.ojp.gov/ncjrs/virtual-library/abstracts/national-advisory-commission-civil-disorders-report

Kesslen, B., & Murphy, J. (2021, August 25). *South Dakota Covid cases quintuple after Sturgis motorcycle rally.* : NBC News. https://www.nbcnews.com/news/us-news/south-dakota-covid-cases-quintuple-after-sturgis-motorcycle-rally-n1277567

Kirzinger, A., Sparks, G., & Brodie, M. (2021). *KFF COVID-19 vaccine monitor: In their own words, six months later.* San Francisco: Kaiser Family Foundation. https://www.kff.org/coronavirus-covid-19/poll-finding/kff-covid-19-vaccine-monitor-in-their-yown-words-six-months-later/

King, A. (2020, November 25). *Embattled public health workers leaving at 'steady and alarming' rate.* Washington, D.C.: National Public Radio. https://www.npr.org/2020/11/25/938873547/embattled-public-health-workers-leaving-at-steady-and-alarming-rate

Klein, B. (2020, December 15). *Melania Trump breaks children's hospital rules by taking her mask off to read to patients.* New York: CNN. https://www.cnn.com/2020/12/15/politics/melania-trump-childrens-national-mask/index.html

Koenig, D. (2021, August 25). *Delta will charge unvaccinated employees $200 per month.* New York: Associated Press. https://apnews.com/article/lifestyle-business-health-coronavirus-pandemic-06f736ac985d59c38c2ae8201f717d91

Kounang, N. (2020, October 29). *Many counties that hosted Trump rallies had a significant increase in Covid-19 cases.* CNN. https://www.cnn.com/2020/10/29/health/covid-trump-rallies-counties-cases/index.html

Kounang, N., & Wild, W. (2021, January 24). *38 Capitol Police officers test positive for Covid-19 after capitol riot.* : CNN. https://www.cnn.com/2021/01/24/politics/capitol-police-riot-coronavirus/index.html

Kramer, J. (2021, January 8). *Why people latch on to conspiracy theories, according to science.* Washington, D.C.: National Geographic. https://www.nationalgeographic.com/science/2021/01/why-people-latch-on-to-conspiracy-theories-according-to-science/

Krueger, J., & Dunning, D. (1999). Unskilled and unaware of it: How difficulties in recognizing one's own incompetence lead to inflated self-assessments. *Journal of Personality and Social Psychology, 77*(6), 1121–1134. https://doi.org/10.1037/0022-3514.77.6.1121

Kupferschmidt, K. (2021, February 17). *Unprotected African health workers dies as rich countries buy up COVID-19 vaccines.* Washington, D.C.: Science. https://www.sciencemag.com/news/2021/02/unprotected-african-health-workers-die-rich-countries-buy-covid-vaccines

Kurtzleben, D. (2020, October 28). *Trump has weaponized masculinity as president. Here's why it matters.* Washington, D.C.: National Public Radio. https://www.npr.org/2020/10/28/928336749/trump-has-weaponized-masculinity-as-president-heres-why-it-maters

La Monica, P. R. (2020, October 5). *Trump has ties to drugmaker Regeneron—And now its stockis surging.* New York: CNN. https://www.cnn.com/2020/10/05/investing/trump-regeneron/index.html

Lamoureux, M. (2021, May 11). *Anti-maskers ready to start masking—To protect themselves from the vaccinated.* New York: Vice Media. https://www.vice.com/en/article/88nnwg/anti-maskers-ready-to-start-maskingto-protect-themselves-from-the-vaccinated

Lardner, R., & Smith, M. R. (2021, January 17). *Records: Trump allies behind rally that ignited Capitol riot*. New York: Associated Press. https://apnews.com/article/epection-2020-donald-trump-capitol-siege-campaigns-elections-d14c78d53b3a212658223252fec87e99

Lawless, J., Kirka, D., & Madhani, A. (2021, June 11). *G-7 pledge to share, but jostle for ground in the sandbox*. New York: Associated Press. https://apnews.com/article/government-and-politics-joe-biden-europe-g-7-summit-coronavirus-vaccine-f17540d6b68bd80561bea30d66059b60

LeBlanc, P. (2021, August 4). *Arkansas GOP governor says he regrets ban on mask mandates as Covid-19 cases surge*. New York: CNN. https://www.cnn.com/2021/08/04/politics/asa-hutchinson-arkansas-mask-mandate/index.html

LeBlanc, P. & Diamond, J. (2020, November 15). *Trump coronavirus adviser Scott Atlas urges Michigan to 'rise up' against new Covid-19 measures.* : CNN. https://www.cnn.com/2020/11/15/politics/scott-atlas-coronavirus-michigan/index.html

Lee, B. Y. (2021, August 9). *Anti-vaxxers using "I am legend" movie against COVID-19 vaccines*. New York: Forbes. https://www.forbes.com/sites/brucelee/2021/08/09/anti-vaxxers-using-i-am-legend-movie-against-covid-19-vaccines/?sh=7b2ba3101473

Levenson, E. (2020, November 17). *These GOP governors long resisted masks and coronavirus rules. Now their states are in crisis*. New York: CNN. https://www.cnn.com/2020/11/17/us/coronavirus-midwest-northern-governors/index.html

Lithwick, D. (2020, May 14). *Refusing to wear a mask is a uniquely American pathology*. New York: Slate. https://slate.com/news-and-politics/2020/05/masks-coronavirus-america.html

Lucas, R. (2021, March 24). *New evidence points to coordination among extremist groups ahead of Capitol riot*. https://www.npr.org/2021/03/24/980754255/new-evidence-points-to-coordination-among-extremist-groups-ahead-of-capitol-riot

Madani, D. (2021, February 2). *Missouri lawmaker indicted for allegedly selling fake stem cell treatments for Covid-19*. : NBC News. https://www.nbcnews.com/news/us-news/missouri-lawmaker-indicted-allegedly-selling-fake-stem-cell-treatments-covid-n1256551

Maxouris, C., & Levenson, E. (2020, November 11). *North Dakota allows infected health care workers to continue working as hospitals hit capacity*. : CNN. https://www.cnn.com/2020/11/11/health/us-coronavirus-wednesday/index.html

McCausland, P. (2020, December 13). *Rural doctors face vaccine distrust and conspiracies*. They have a plan. New York NBC News. https://www.nbcnews.com/news/us-news/rural-doctors-face-vaccine-distrust-conspiracies-they-have-a-plan-n1250953

McIntosh, P. (1989). *White privilege: Unpacking the invisible knapsack*. Peace and Freedom, July/August, 10–12.

McLaughlin, E. C. (2021, January 7). *Before Wednesday, insurgents waving confederate flags hadn't been within 6 miles of the US Capitol*. : CNN. https://www.cnn.com/2021/01/07/us/capitol-confederate-flag-fort-stevens/index.html

Meade, A. (2021, 1 August). *Sky News Australia banned from YouTube for seven days over Covid misinformation*. : The Guardian. https://amp.theguardian.com/media/2021/aug/01/sky-news-australia-banned-from-youtube-for-seven-days-over-covid-misinformation

Meitzner, M. (2020). Populist anti-scientism, religious polarization, and institutionalized corruption: How Indonesia's democratic decline shaped its COVID-19 response. *Journal of Current Southeast Asian Affairs, 39*(2), 227–249. https://doi.org/10.1177/1868103420935561

Mena, K. (2021, March 27). *Former Trump chief of staff calls ex-president's Capitol riot claims 'manifestly false.'* : CNN. https://www.cnn.com/2021/03/27/politics/mick-mulvaney-trump-january-6-riot/index.html

Mendoza, M. & Linderman, J. (2021, March 5). *Officers maced, trampled: Docs expose depth of Jan. 6 chaos*. : Associated Press. https://apnews.com/article/docs-expose-depth-january-6-capitol-siege-chaos-fd3204574c11e453be8fb4e3c81258c3

Miller, S., & Culver, J. (2021, July 4). *More than 99% of recent COVID deaths in US involve unvaccinated people, a 'sad and tragic' situation, Fauci says: Today's live updates*.

Washington, D.C.: USA Today. https://www.usatoday.com/story/news/health/2021/07/04/more-than-99-us-covid-deaths-involve-unvaccinated-people/7856564002/
Mitropoulos, A. (2021, January 9). *Capitol Hill riot could prove to be COVID-19 super-spreader event, experts say*. https://abcnews.com/Health/capitol-hill-riot-prove-covid-19-superspreader-event/story
Mueller, B. (2021, May 5). As Covid ravages poorer countries, rich nations spring back to life. New York: New York Times. https://www.nytimes.com/2021/05/05/world/europe/coronavirus-covax-vaccination.html
Murphy, P. P., Flores, R., Toropin, K., & Weisfeldt, S. (2021, February 18). *Florida county commissioner limited vaccine drive to the two richest zip codes and then created a 'VIP list.'* : CNN. https://www.cnn.com/2021/02/18/politics/manatee-county-vaccine/index.html
Murphy, P. P., & Polantz, K. (2021, January 10). *Man seen chasing Black Capitol police officer in video faces charges*. New York: CNN. https://www.cnn.com/2021/0/10/politics/doug-jensen-capitol-hill-police-officer/index.html
Newell, J. (2021, July 28). *Turns out Mo Brooks was wearing body armor to Trump's very peaceful Jan. 6 rally*. New York: Slate. https://slate.com/news-and-politics/2021/07/mo-brooks-body-aror-jan-6-rally.amp
Niebuhr, R. (1960). Moral man in immoral society. New York: Scribner.
O'donnell, C., & Aboulenein, A. (2021, August 18). *U.S. to begin offering COVID-19 vaccine booster shots in September*. London: Reuters. https://www.reuters.com/world/us/us-start-offering-covid-19-vaccine-booster-doses-september-2021-08-18/
Odula, T., & Muhumuza, R. (2021, March 17). *Tanzania's populist President John Magufuli has died at age 61*. New York: Associated Press. https://apnews.com/article/john-magufuli-dead-tanzania-president-1368d5d852ca2b8b35fe108c3abbc0a0
Office of the Director of National Intelligence. (2021, March 1). *(U) Domestic violent extremism poses heightened threat in 2021*. Washington, D.C.: Author. https://www.dni.gov/files/ODNI/documents/assessments/UnclassSummaryofDVEAssessment-17MAR21.pdf
Office of the Texas Governor. (2021, August 17). *Office of the governor statement concerning Governor Abbott*. Austin, TX: Author. https://gov.texas.gov/news/post/office-of-the-governor-statement-concerning-governor-abbott
Ogrysko, N. (2021, September 9). *Biden will now require vaccines for all federal employees via new executive order*. Washington, D.C.: Federal News Network. https://federalnewsnetwork.com/workforce/2021/09/biden-will-now-require-vaccines-for-all-federal-employees-via-new-executive-order/
Parker, L. (2017, April 21). *Why a 'war on science' puts us all at risk*. Washington, D.C.: National Geographic Society. https://www.nationalgeographic.com/science/article/david-titley-science-climate-change-sea-level-rise
Parramore, L. S. (2021, January 12). *Like QAnon's Capitol rioters, the Nashville bomber's lizard people theory is deadly serious*. New York: NBC News. https://www.nbcnews.com/think/opinion/qanon-s-capitol-rioters-nashville-bomber-s-lizard-people-theory-ncna1253819
Patra, K. (2021, July 22). *NFL informs clubs that COVID-19 outbreaks among unvaccinated players could lead to forfeited games*. New York: National Football League. https://www.nfl.com/news/nfl-covid-19-outbreaks-unvaccinated-players-forfeit-cancelled-games
Payne, D. (2020, October 13). *As public opposition to lockdowns grows, WHO seeks other methods to control virus*. Washington, D.C.: Just the News. https://justthnews.com/politics-policy/coronavirus/public-oppoition-lockdowns-grows-who-shifts-tone-calls-other-methods
Peltz, J. (2021, January 14). *NY congressman tests positive for virus, latest since breach*. New York: Associated Press. https://apnews.com/article/donald-trump-new-york-adriano-espaillat-coronavirus-pandemic-manhattan-f005987e15be6d422Ce3bc6acfb129dc
Perez, E., & Prokupecz, S. (2021, January 10). *Two men carrying plastic restraints during the Capitol riot charged by feds*. https://www.cnn.com/2021/01/10/politics/eric-munchel-larry-rendell-brock-capitol-riot/index.html

Perrett, C. (2021, January 24). *As he faced death threats, Fauci said he once opened an envelope that contained a 'puff of powder' he feared was anthrax or ricin*. New York: Business Insider. https://www.businessinsider.com/fauci-opened-envelope-containing-mystery-powder-during-trump-admin-2021-1

Ramos, E. (2021, August 20). *Child COVID-19 hospitalizations soar, filling pediatric wings, data show*. : NBC News. https://www.nbcnews.com/news/us-news/child-covid-19-hospitalizations-new-high-august-2021-n1277119

Reddit. (2021, February 14). *QAnon Casualties*. San Francisco: Author. https://www.reddit.com/r/QAnonCasualties/

Reny, T. T. (2020). Masculine norms and infectious disease: The case of COVID-19. *Politics and Gender, 16*(4), 1028–1035. https://doi.org/10.1017/S1743923X20000380

Reuters. (2021, September 23). *Delta Air says employee vaccination rate against COVID-19 rises to 82%*. London: Author. https://www.reuters.com/business/delta-air-says-employee-vaccination-rate-against-covid-19-rises-82-2021-09-23/

Richmond, T. (2021, February 17). *33-year-old Bucks exec Alex Lasry gets COVID vaccine early*. https://apnews.com/article/nba-milwaukee-wisconsin-milwaukee-bucks-coronavirus-pandemic-2a915698164e42ca4c31fb3f65916036

Riotta, C. (2021, January 28). *FBI charges man carrying 'white privilege' card who built bombs with alleged 'intent to attack Democrats.'* : Independent. https://www.independent.co.uk/news/world/americas/us-politics/fbi-trump-arrests-riots-ian-rogers-attack-democrats-b1794317.html

Romer, D., & Jamieson, K. H. (2020). Conspiracy theories as barriers to controlling the spread of COVID-19 in the U.S. *Social Science & Medicine, 263*, 113356. https://doi.org/10.1016/j.socscimed.2020.113356

Roozenbeek, J., Schneider, C. R., Dryhurst, S., Kerr, J., Freeman, A. L. J., Recchia, G., van der Bles, A. M., & van der Linden, S. (2020). Susceptibility to misinformation about COVID-19 around the world. *Royal Society Open Science, 7*, 201199. https://doi.org/10.1098/rsos201199

Satariano, A., & Alba, D. (2020, April 10). *Burning cell towers, out of baseless fear they spread the virus*. New York: New York Time. https://www.nytimes.com/2020/04/10/technology/coronavirus-5g-uk.html

Santucci, J. (2021, February 16). *Sen. Pat Toomey faces censure over impeachment vote: 'We did not send him there to do the right thing.'* : USA Today. https://www.usatoday.com/story/news/politics/2021/02/16/pat-toomey-faces-censure-over-impeachment-vote-republican-party/6759842002/

Savarese, M. (2021, February 8). *Brazil's wealthy cause a stir trying to score quick vaccines*. : Associated Press. https://apnews.com/article/brazil-wealthy-coronavirus-vaccine-c1e157ac56985dcb6f3931f31a1c3ff6

Schaper, D. (2021, September 28). *United Airlines says almost all its workers are vaccinated; some others may be fired*. : National Public Radio. https://www.npr.org/2021/09/28/1041360095/united-airlines-workers-vaccinated

Sergent, K., & Stajkovic, A. D. (2020). Women's leadership is associated with fewer deaths during the COVID-19 crisis: Quantitative and qualitative analyses of United States governors. *Journal of Applied Psychology, 105*(8), 771–783. https://doi.org/10.1037/apl0000577

Sharp, R., & Jewers, C. (2021, January 16). *QAnon shaman dehorned: MAGA Capitol invader's mom sees him denied bail in court where prosecutors claim he called Pence a 'child-trafficking traitor' and left a note for the VP saying 'it's only a matter of time, justice is coming.'* : Daily Mail. https://www.dailymail.co.uk/news/article-9150231/U-S-says-Capitol-rioters-meant-capture-assassinate-officials-filing.html

Sherman, C. (2021, January 24). *Mexico's president says he's tested positive for COVID-19*. New York: Associated Press. https://apnews.com/article/pandemics-marcelo-ebrard-mexico-coronavirus-pandemic-vladamir-putin-7c4ffeae9e363d519d5c336202be0ae6

Siemaszko, C. (2021, January 25). *Vaccine tourism on the rise as wealthy international tourists eye an opportunity in the US.* : NBC News. https://www.nbcnews.com/news/us-news/vaccine-tourism-rise-wealthy-international-tourists-eye-opportunity-u-s-n1255531

Smith, A. (2020, October 25). *'We're not going to control the pandemic,' Trump chief of staff Mark Meadows says in a heated interview.* : NBC News. https://www.nbcnews.com/politics/donald-trump/meadows-says-we-re-not-going-to-control-pandemic-heated-interview-n1244681

Smith, M. R., Weber, L., & Barry-Jester, A. M. (2020, June 12). *Public health workers fighting virus face growing threats.* New York: Associated Press. https://apnews.com/article/8839ed5e94eea718304820218919738e

Smith, P., & Chirbas, K. (2021, September 17). *Carmine's hostess attacked after asking diners for proof of vaccination.* New York: NBC News. https://www.nbcnews.com/news/us-news/carmine-s-hostess-attacked-after-asking-diners-proof-vaccine-n1279410

Soo, Z. (2021, January 26). *Twitter permanently bans My Pillow CEO.* : Associated Press. https://apnews.com/article/joe-biden-trump-media-elections-presidential-elections-ac34de7cb5844d96589a10ea6e653d50

Specia, M. (2020, September 28). *As Europe's coronavirus cases rise, sodo voices crying hoax.* : New York Times. https://www.nytimes.com/2020/09/28/world/europe/europe-coronavirus-protests.html

Spokane Public Radio (2019, July 18, 7:45 am). *Mayoral candidate interviews.* : Author.

Spring, M., & Wendling, M. (2020, September 2). *How Covid-19 myths are merging with the QAnon conspiracy theory.* : BBC. https://www.bbc.com/news/blogs-trending-53997203

Sprunt, B. (2020, October 4). *Despite risks to others, Trump leaves hospital suite to greet supporters.* : National Public Radio. https://www.npr.org/sections/latest-updates-trump-covid-19-results/2020/10/04/920181116/in-brief-drive-by-trump-waves-to-supporters-outside-of-walter-reed

Stafford, M. (2021, March 26). *Prosecutors add 3 fraud charges against Missouri lawmaker.* New York: Associated Press. https://apnews.com/article/indictments-missouri%2D%2Dtigers-mens-basketball-coronavirus-pandemic-2be640dc7681d31d498f50cd6389c64e

Stargardter, G. (2021, January 24). *'Get out Bolsonaro!' Say ex-supporters in Brazil as COVID-19, vaccines weigh.* London: Reuters. https://www.reuters.com/article/us-brazil-politics-idUSKBN29T0QZ

Stargardter, G., & Paraguassu, L. (2020, July 8). *Special report: Bolsonaro bets 'miraculous cure' for COVID-19 can save Brazil—And his life.* : Reuters. https://www.reuters.com/article/us-health-coronavirus-brazil-hydroxychlo/special-report-bolsonaro-bets-miraculous-cure-for-covid-19-can-save-brazil-and-his-life

Stone, M., & Bartz, D. (2021, January 7). *Some U.S. Capitol rioters fired after internet detectives identify them.* London: Reuters. https://www.reuters.com/article/us-usa-election-protests-fallout/some-u-s-capitol-rioters-fired-after-internet-detectives-identify-them-idUSKBN29C36M

Tanfani, J. Berens, M., & Parker, N. (2021). *How trump's pied pipers rallied a faithful mob to the capitol.* London: Reuters. https://www.reuters.com/article/us-usa-trump-protest-organizers-insight/how-trump-pied-pipers-rallied-a-faithful-mob-to-the-capitol-idUSKBN29G2UP

Taylor, S. (2019). The psychology of pandemics: Preparing for the next global outbreak of infectious disease. Cambridge, UK: Cambridge Scholars Publishing.

The Soufran Center. (2021). *Quantifying the Q conspiracy: A data-driven approach to understanding the threat posed by QAnon.* New York: Author. https://thesoufancenter.org/research/quantifying-the-q-conspiracy-a-data-driven-approach-to-understanding-the-threat-posed-by-qanon/.

Tillman, Z. (2021, July 29). *A judge questioned if Capitol rioters are getting off too easy for "terrorizing members of Congress".* New York: Buzzfeed. https://www.buzzfeednews. com/amphtml/zoetillman/capitol-riot-jan-6-defendants-plea-deals-too-lenient

Toropin, K. (2021, February 17). *DeSantis defends controversial vaccine deal with developer—And threatens to pull vaccines if officials don't like it*. New York: CNN. https://www.cnn.com/2021/02/17/politics/ron-desantis-vaccines/index.html

Treisman, R. (2020, November 1). *WH adviser Scott Atlas apologizes for interview with Kremlin-backed news outlet*. Washington, D.C.: National Public Radio. https://www.npr.org/2020/11/01/930149143/wh-adviser-scott-atlas-apologizes-for-interview-with-kremlin-backed-news-outlet

Valou, K. (2021, January 4). *Here's everything you need to know about the 'March for Trump' rally*. Washington, D.C.: WGRZ. https://www.wgrz.com/article/news/local/protests/march-for-trump-rally-dc-january-6-protest-pro-trump-demonstrators-event-details/65-2e019324-7861-48fa-8d78-d99b9617558b

Vargas, E. D., & Sanchez, G. R. (2020, August 31). *American individualism is an obstacle to wider mask wearing in the US*. Washington, DC: Brookings Institute. https://www.brookings.edu/blog/up-front/2020/08/31/american-individualism-is-an-obstacle-to-wider-mask-wearing-in-the-us/

Vosoughi, S., Roy, D., & Aral, S. (2018). The spread of true and false news online. *Science, 359*, 1146–1151. https://doi.org/10.1162/science.aap9559

Warren, M. (2021, January 16). *As Trump leaves the stage, republicans grapple with new conspiracy caucus*. New York: CNN. https://www.cnn.com/2021/01/16/politics/qanon-gop-trump-congress-future/index.html

Westcott, B., McKeehan, B., Renton, A., Woodyatt, A., Alfonso, F., Macaya, M., & Hayes, M. (2020, October 5). *October 4 Trump Covid-19 news*. New York: CNN. https://www.cnn.com/politics/live-news/trump-covid-19-updates-sunday/index.html

Wexler, M. N. (1995). Expanding the groupthink explanation to the study of contemporary cults. *Cultic Studies Journal, 12*(1), 49–71.

WHO. (2021, October 4). *Interim statement on booster doses for COVID-19 vaccination*. Geneva: Author. https://www.who.int/news/item/04-10-2021-interim-statement-on-booster-doses-for-covid-19-vaccination

WHO. (2020). *SARS-CoV-2 variants*. Geneva: Author. https://www.who.int/csr/don/31-december-2020-sars-cov2-variants/en/

WHO. (2020b). *How to report misinformation online*. Geneva: Author. https://www.who.int/campaigns/connecting-the-world-to-combat-coronavirus/how-to-report-misinformation-online

WHO, UN, UNICEF, UNDP, UNESCO, UNAIDS, ITU, UN Global Pulse, & IFRC. (2020, September 23). *Managing the COVID-19 infodemic: Promoting healthy behaviours and mitigating the harm from misinformation and disinformation*. Geneva: WHO. https://www.who.int/news/item/23-09-2020-managing-the-covid-19-infodemic-promoting-healthy-behaviours-and-mitigating-the-harm-from-misinformation-and-disinformation

Williams, P. (2021, March 5). *Federico Klein, former trump appointee charged in capitol riot, wants jail cell without cockroaches*. New York: NBC News. https://www.nbcnews.com/politics/justice-department/federico-klein-former-trump-appointee-charged-capitol-riot-requests-jail-n1259767

Zubrow, K., Gavrilovic, M., & Ortize, A. (2021, October 4). *Whistleblower's SEC complaint: Facebook knew platform was used to "promote human trafficking and domestic servitude."* New York: CBS News. https://www.cbsnews.com/news/facebook-whistleblower-sec-complaint-60-minutes-2021-10-04/

Chapter 10
Opportunities Created by COVID-19

Abstract Global crises such as COVID-19 simultaneously open doors to challenges and opportunities from an Indigenous perspective. Colonial backlashes have become more frequent, carried out in anger and fear when confronted with the failures and weaknesses of the colonial social orders have become more obvious. Colonial failures to promote social equity and humanitarian justice, and to promote sustainable planetary welfare for present and future generations, could not be ignored in the context of COVID-19. Colonial social orders not only failed to protect millions of people but also significantly exacerbated pandemic vulnerability. Self-orientations have left us vulnerable and resulted in conflict and retribution with one another and with the natural world. Awareness of colonial failures provide opportunities to decolonize and re-create societies with assumptions that better align with scientific evidence. The pandemic has provided the opportunity to retire artificial hierarchies and rebuild with egalitarian assumptions that engender trust and peace. Pursuit of intergenerational sustainability well-being for the whole of the planet, including human creatures, is possible. A restitutional approach to justice will enhance progress toward an equitable existence. Indigenous psychology provides perspective on how to seek reconciliation in relationships to enhance health and psychological well-being to build a more resilient planet.

Global problems represent both challenges and opportunities from an Indigenous perspective (Blume, 2020), so the psychological dilemma is how to address the problems and seize the opportunities simultaneously. The challenges associated with COVID-19 have been exposed to be the consequences of colonialism, therefore addressing the challenges means decolonizing societies so that global challenges such as pandemics become less of a threat to the collective whole. The opportunities associated with the COVID-19 pandemic are the result of exposing colonialism for what it has always been—an inequitable social system based upon a worldview with inherent myths and thinking errors that contribute to inherent vulnerabilities to all who reside in those societies. The opportunity before us is a choice to replace colonialism with a new prosocial worldview that will strengthen preparation for the next global crisis.

A. W. Blume, *Colonialism and the COVID-19 Pandemic*, International and Cultural Psychology, https://doi.org/10.1007/978-3-030-92825-4_10

Much of this book has chronicled the tragedies associated with colonialism. Colonialism has harmed and killed innumerable people over the last several centuries and has worked to dehumanize and discount the lives of hundreds of millions of people who were conquered, enslaved, oppressed, neglected, and sickened. As discussed in Chaps. 8 and 9, colonial cultures are finally becoming the subject of public debate, sometimes through peaceful discourse and sometimes with violent intent. Proponents of the colonial way of life have been fighting tooth and nail to conserve the colonial way of life out of fears of changing demographics that favor growth of minoritized populations. Those demographic changes elevate racialized colonial fears, contributing to significant acts of colonial backlash and other examples of fragility by colonial proponents—mainstream psychologists might refer to these processes as a colonial extinction burst. Another example of a colonial backlash and the fragility of privilege occurred when those who opposed masking and vaccine mandates became increasing menacing and hostile towards school and other public officials during the highly transmissible delta variant surge (Kelleher et al., 2021). However, despite the colonial backlashes or extinction bursts, for the first time in centuries people are openly debating the value of colonial culture in a world seeking health and equity.

Colonialism has contributed to what can only be referred to as a vast global wasteland—a wasteland fully exposed by the COVID-19 pandemic. Global climate change threatens the health of the entire planet. Environmental degradation is contributing to unbelievable global losses of species and long-term threats to human health. Economic, education, and health inequities are growing by leaps and bounds, compounded by colonial -isms. Within the human community, it is hard to imagine in a so-called civilized world that creatures, including humans, are discarded so easily. The intergenerational nature of poverty and hunger is indefensible from an IAPP perspective as a chronic source of psychological victimization. The colonial wasteland has been dehumanizing and destructive. It has left us vulnerable and brought us to a place of intergenerational grief. Action is required to retire the collective threat of colonialism.

Exposing the Challenges and Opportunities of Colonialism

The response to COVID-19 in many colonial nations, especially those with populist-nationalistic governments aligned with traditional colonial values, has been interpreted by many professionals to have been disastrous. Although there were many scientific breakthroughs as a result of the pandemic (STAT News, 2020), those breakthroughs in many instances were squandered or threatened by the activities of those more interested in exercising self-interests and liberties. Selfishness and its resulting political divisiveness were viewed with great concern, especially in the US (Altman, 2020; Brooks, 2021).

The many challenges that have emerged during the COVID-19 pandemic have contributed to excellent opportunities to transform colonial societies into compassionate nations better ready to address future pandemics (see Table 10.1). One

Table 10.1 Colonial challenges exposed by COVID-19 that represent opportunities

Challenges of colonialism	Opportunities presented during the pandemic
Superiority and hierarch-cracy	Challenge and retire artificial social hierarchies
Exceptionalism	Rebuild with egalitarian assumptions
white supremacy	Challenge artificial hierarchies; to challenge -isms
Self-orientation	Embrace collective interests over self
Impatience and immediacy	Embrace intergenerational connectivity in the flow of time and the process of becoming
Borders and boundaries	Challenge the efficacy of reductionism and radical autonomy in an interdependent world
Hierarchical relations	Decolonize relationships from hierarchical to sacred and respectful
Necessity, privilege, and exploitation	Honor collective necessity by prioritizing holistic values
Control, deceit, and manipulation	Instill values of consensus, honesty, and transparency into social structures and relationships
Values prioritizing the empowered	Prioritize the needs of the vulnerable to improve collective wellness
Emphasis on material well-being	Pursue policies that ensure collective well-being and intergenerational sustainability
Emphasis on competition and conflict	Embrace restitution rather than retribution as a way of restoring relationships; seek harmony and balance rather than advantage

primary opportunity that has arisen is to address the environmental degradation and climate change that has challenged health and exposed humans to novel viruses. Appropriate responses to prevent future pandemics begin with reduction of human consumption of natural resources. Human beings will have to learn to live within natural sustainable limits, which can occur through a reduction of colonial materialism. Human creatures have greatly exceeded fair shares of global natural resources, continuing to crowd out nature by slashing, burning, and urbanizing previously pristine or nearly pristine areas. The pandemic has awakened us more to the threats of climate change and environmental exploitation, therefore presenting a golden opportunity to articulate and motivate people to change wasteful and harmful overconsumption.

An Opportunity to Retire Colonial Superiority The foundation of colonialism was constructed on an inherent belief in hierarch-cracy--societies organized according to the basic tenets of a divinely sanctioned and ordained conquest that exploited and subjugated others. Beliefs in colonial superiority and white supremacy resulted from those basic tenets. From the very beginning, these societies were inherently disunified and stratified. The social orders and their social systems and institutions were infused with the implicit colonial biases that reflected the basic tenets of superiority-inferiority of certain peoples and cultures, contributing to superior-inferior outcomes over time. Inequitable experiences for people in colonial cultures resulted. Those inequitable circumstances were easy to ignore as long as the privileged in society were not confronted with risks to themselves as a result of the inequities. However, the COVID-19 pandemic unsettled even those who had benefitted directly or indirectly from colonialism over time. Exposing them to the risks of a disunified and inequitable society. The pandemic has been a wake-up call to the challenges of colonialism to all.

Colonial superiority, rather than elevating nations, resulted in significantly weakened nations. The perspective of superiority was confined only to a few within those societies, therefore when evaluated in a holistic way, superiority societies contributed to their own vulnerabilities. Superiority was achieved artificially, a myth that was built on the backs of others, resulting in a ridiculous notion that certain people were inherently different, better, and entitled, despite the overwhelming evidence of shared vulnerability within the natural world. The myth of superiority contributed to inherent white supremacy in colonial societies today.

Exceptionalism views one demographic group as divinely blessed, and therefore destined to dominate others. Colonial exceptionalism is rooted in the belief of white supremacy and assumes white privilege as a result of exceptional beliefs. The SARS-CoV-2 virus exposed the myth of exceptionalism in that colonial nations were often arrogantly and pathetically unprepared for a pandemic or any other global crisis. Using the US as an example, the response to the pandemic was anything but exceptional and clearly did not match the narrative of a mighty and invulnerable nation. The pandemic also exposed the myth of colonial superiority as well, illustrating how truly fragile these societies are since they have been built on the backs of others. Artificial superiority only exists in those nations because of an exceptional myth that some had the right to take equity away from others. The mythic stories of superiority and exceptionalism perpetuate beliefs about false hierarchies in society that harm people (Lemon, 2021). Superiority and exceptionalism made a unified response difficult to impossible.

The myth of white supremacy accounted for innumerable pandemic missteps, making it easy for some to believe in the lies spun by Whites yet difficult to accept the truth from minoritized people. Some weaponized fear, externalized toward outgroups deemed inferior to Whites. Some believed that as entitled people they were invulnerable to the pandemic and therefore acted without consideration for others. Some saw the pandemic as an opportunity to bully others or even seize power. None of these acts of superiority helped the pandemic response.

The myth of colonial white supremacy created the -isms in societies that have facilitated oppression and discrimination. This myth has created divided societies ill prepared for unified responses to any crisis facing the whole and contributed to perpetual acts of divisiveness and blame. Colonial splitting has been used by proponents of colonialism to manipulate and weaken others. Many have blamed immigrants for problems created by colonialism, such as the inequities in society that have left many Whites in society just as impoverished as minoritized communities. Some impoverished White Americans will embrace the myth of the American Dream despite their own circumstances, blaming minoritized groups instead of the privileged in society for not living the dream. As another example, many have blamed Asians and Asian Americans for the SARS-CoV-2 virus, a virus from the wild that likely would still be in the wild without colonial exploitation of the global environment. Many adherents to the myths of colonialism cannot accept the truth that acts of white supremacy have contributed to the misery of many, including a sizeable number of White citizens in colonials societies. Beliefs in white supremacy represent major barriers to collaborative approaches toward addressing the next pandemic. An IAPP perspective would suggest that the psychological well-being and health will rely upon challenging the colonial myths of exceptionalism, superiority, white supremacy, and privilege and its implied immunity from collective problems that impact all.

An Opportunity to Be Less Self-Oriented Another major area of concern for addressing the next pandemic is the colonial emphasis of self as the pre-eminent unit for understanding human existence. Autonomous activity was not functionally healthy or helpful for pandemic response when people did as they pleased under the guise of personal freedom and liberties. Individual expressions of personal liberty contributed to community spread, divisive behavior, and violence during the COVID-19 pandemic. Expressions of autonomy also reflected the colonial perspective that one was entitled to act a certain way with the perception of personal immunity (invulnerability) to the consequences of such self-oriented behavior.

The difficulties the US experienced with vaccine resistance interfering with vaccine-acquired herd immunity is a valuable lesson about how colonial individualism hinders addressing collective global crises like pandemics. In a previous book on Indigenous psychology (Blume, 2020), I discussed how a colonial self-orientation siloes perspectives. A single person may not see the collective threat of a particular situation. Even though many view portions of the whole picture, they are not interpreting those pieces collectively, missing the whole picture. This is what has happened with environmental degradation of the planet—a view of one person at one point of time saw no problem with exploitation—it is only when the consequences are viewed collectively across time that the true threat is revealed. The result is a perspective that is narrowly focused and near-sighted, missing a holistic view of what may be happening.

One person may view the choice to abstain from a vaccine as one's personal choice and a way to exercise one's liberty. Perhaps an individual cannot see the collective risks of many individuals abstaining from vaccines overtime because they are viewing the world as an individual entity rather than as a collective member of the whole of Creation. One may naturally resist the idea that one's personal choices are harming others, but the self alone is unable to anticipate holistic consequences. Colonial tunnel vision and myopia seriously threaten collective well-being (Blume, 2020). A colonial autonomous perspective on life compounds the collective wounding when personal willfulness dictates stubbornly standing one's ground despite the evidence of harm towards others and self. Viral surges among the fearfully or stubbornly unvaccinated resulted, providing the opportunity for SARS-CoV-2 to mutate into variants that threatened immunity to even those who had chosen to vaccinate. The unvaccinated would become at even greater risk if the vaccinated were to end up surviving a more virulent variant and then passing it along to those without any protection (Mackenzie, 2020). One person has limited view of the scope of their potential impact in an interdependent world. Addressing the pandemic through the eyes of one risked harm to everyone whether one intended it or not. The virus demonstrated the weaknesses of a self-orientation again and again despite individual resistance, and hostile variants thrived under libertarian pandemic responses.

Interestingly, scientists rarely consider an individual (n = 1) as sufficient for understanding anything scientifically meaningful. Scientists often desire population level data to understand the nature and activities of species, including humans. Using n=1 data leaves the observer-interpreter open to a wide variety of biases that can lead the individual to confident ignorance in one's personal reality of the world (remembering the Dunning-Krueger effect). How colonialism settled on an n=1 worldview was a philosophical proposition rather than a scientifically informed decision (Descartes, 1637). Yet, even in a scientifically advanced world, people in colonial nations often continue to think of the world through the lenses of me (n = 1).

The conceptualization of "self" is nothing but a myth (Blume, 2014; 2020). Human beings are really a collection of life entities cohabitating a body encircled by a permeable boundary referred to as skin. Skin is not a defining barrier between humans and the rest of the world. No one could exist in a healthy state without the colony of other entities accompanying us through life. Ironically, viruses have played an important role in our evolutionary development and are associated with 8% of human DNA (Quammen, 2021). Humans are never the same from moment to moment, due to the exchange of molecules through consumption, excretion, perspiration, and respiration. Entities are in reality colonies, perceived boundaries between the self and others are in reality permeable, and the self in reality changes moment by moment.

The self exists as an interdependent colony of entities within the larger web of the natural world. Autonomy is out of the question because there is no way a symbiotic colony-entity could be self-reliant. Survival is only possible in the context of the whole of the natural world. True independence and autonomy are myths as well, informed by the colonial myth of self. From the perspective of IAPP (Blume, 2020), to act as if one is independent and capable of real autonomy is to live a lie. Such behavior creates problems for the self rather than enhancing the viability of the self, since independent and autonomous behavior often reflect self-interests rather than interests in the collective well-being of an interdependent natural order.

Selfism must also be challenged since it defies the reality of an interdependent world. Societies cannot address global crises if radical autonomy and individualism are suggested as aspirational expressions for psychological wellness. Self-orientation presents barriers to holistic responses to address global challenges such as pandemics. Psychology has a prominent role in transforming the understanding that psychological health is a collective activity of the whole rather than an individual pursuit. A transformative role of psychology is especially important since it has perpetuated a colonial worldview with self-oriented myths since its inception.

Frankly, little if any evidence from modern life sciences has suggested that the individual should be the pre-eminent unit of existence. Life systems function better with cooperation and collaboration, when systems are harmonious and balanced.

Indigenous people as great observers of the natural world knew these things well before the birth of modern natural sciences. Indigenous ancestors knew that when they co-existed as equals with the natural world, human life was more settled—balanced and harmonious. They also knew when they overstepped by encroaching too much on the natural world and resource consumption overshoot occurred locally, the consequences were human suffering. Indigenous people did not arrive at the conclusion that seeking harmony and balances in relationships with others, human or otherwise, was a wise choice for experiencing peace and prosperity by accident.

They also knew that self-orientation overemphasized seeking self-interests at the expense of social responsibility. An inordinate focus on self-interests inevitably contributes to a narcissistic orientation toward others by assuming the pursuit and defense of self-interests justifies consequential harm that may result to others as a result (Blume, 2020). The pandemic exposed the narcissistic orientation inherent in wealth building by individuals and corporations at the expense of others already victimized by colonial inequities. A narcissistic orientation eventually impacts the entire system, rippling harm throughout an interdependent natural order, resulting in systemic illness. The pandemic response would have been greatly improved if social responsibility had superseded the pursuit and defense of self-interests.

Collective cultural approaches were effective during COVID-19. Puerto Rico, as an example, offered free COVID-19 testing at highway toll booths, bringing the tests to the people rather than the more passive approach toward testing seen on the mainland (Associated Press, 2020), and enforced strict mitigation measures that prevented spread and death (Acevedo, 2021), demonstrating concern for the collective whole rather than self-oriented libertarianism. It worked. Collectivism also worked for Indigenous Americans who took seriously the importance of strict mitigation efforts to protect reservations (Hardy et al., 2020). Other acts of collectivism demonstrated concern for the whole, such as the Blackfeet Nation donating vaccines to their Canadian neighbors (Samuels, 2021).

Accepting an interdependent life is the only rational choice in an interdependent world. Psychologically speaking, Indigenous people found that self-oriented living contributed to big trouble in societies, disrupting balance, harmony, and peace. Seeking self-interests meant unhealthy competition and divisiveness—it encouraged hoarding and greed rather than providing for and sharing with others. Emphasizing a self-made identity makes it tempting to rank order the world compared to me, resulting in the possibility of hierarchy and superiority. Emphasizing the self-made identity made it easy to forget about social responsibilities to others, including future generations. Emphasizing the self-made identity made it easy to forget the needs of the community. Forgetting about the community made it easy to slip into arrogance and privilege, tarnishing the sacredness of Creation. In reality, accepting the reality of an egalitarian and interdependent natural order. and what that reality suggests about relationships with others, is the only rational choice for any creature in Creation. If there was an original sin in colonialism, it was likely the foundational belief in the pre-eminence of the self.

An Opportunity to Increase Patience A worldview oriented around the self in the context of colonial perspective for time can create a sense of urgency and immediacy in self-oriented goals and gratifications. Increased exposure to novel viruses is due to the sense of urgency and immediacy for satisfying the material needs for the privileged few of the current generation. Self-orientation has lost perspective on how to provide for a sustainable existence in which humans tread lightly in the environment to benefit the whole of the natural world. A world where global overshoot of resource consumption and global climate change rapidly threatens life suggests the colonialism is impatiently unable to delay immediate gratification for its current generation, and therefore the natural world sickens intergenerationally.

Colonial citizens are not only impatient with satisfying self and national interests, they exhibited impatience with the process of addressing a global crisis. Many people experienced increasing difficulty adhering to safe practices with the passage of time, impatiently insisting that societies re-open and everything go back to "normal." Impatience cost lives during the COVID-19. One example was how impatience left the US vulnerable to the delta variant surge during the summer of 2021. The reversal of CDC masking policy was exposed to be premature and ill-conceived as delta surged. President Biden may the mistake of suggesting in a speech on July 4 that the country was heading toward independence from SARS-CoV-2 only to walk back the claim of independence through reinstatement of mitigation measures before autumn (CDC, 2021; Todd et al., 2021). Impatience generated carelessness in the face of a powerful virus. The lesson was a valuable lesson to approach relationships with viruses with humility. Colonial impatience is a serious barrier to sustainable change, especially problematic when many global problems will likely require intergenerational efforts toward change.

A more broad and distal vision of time would be helpful to maintaining patience with mitigation methods and with the ebb and flow of viral surges. In addition, the broad and distal view provides an opportunity to see the global picture and how the local presentation fits into the larger presentation of the virus. The broad and distal view reminds of the importance of considering interconnectivity and broad impact in public health initiatives, impacts that may be intergenerational in scope. The broad and distal view also permits delayed gratification that better matches the duration of pandemic threats. An IAPP perspective illustrates one model for instilling a broader and more distal vision of addressing global crises including pandemics.

An Opportunity to Remove Artificial Barriers Indigenous perspectives would also suggest the importance of breaking down divisive artificial barriers. Mentioned earlier was the artificial barrier of the body being a barrier between self and world. As discussed in Chap. 1, barriers, boundaries, and even fences and walls are colonial artifacts constructed as artificial barriers to protect self-interests and defend against externalized fears. Personal boundaries did not protect the self from the consequences of SARS-CoV-2. National boundaries were also insufficient to protect from virus spread. A critical lesson of the COVID-19 pandemic was that artificial boundaries provided an artificial sense of security. From an Indigenous perspective, the source of threat in colonial societies has been misdirected toward others rather than self. Misguided expressions of individual liberties within nations appeared to be the greatest threat during the COVID-19 pandemic rather than the external racialized and xenophobic threats that borders and boundaries are intended to defend. In reality, the shared vulnerability that all creatures experience in the interdependent natural order demands that real security comes from engaging in right relationships with the whole. If colonial nations treated others with equal respect, there would be little left to fear. Colonial nations have generated their own threats and fears from the consequences of unethical behavior towards others.

Decolonizing relationships would go a long way towards creating a secure world. Accepting personal responsibility for anger and fear would be much more psychologically healthy than blame and victimization. Retiring colonial exploitation of others (including nature) and hierarchical social systems would reduce the threat of colonial wounding to all in the natural world. Retiring acts of divisiveness such as colonial splitting and backlashes, as well as oppression, manipulation, and inequities would reduce the likelihood of blaming, bullying, and other conflict. Externalizing anger, anxiety, and fear would no longer be appealing since colonial divisiveness and threats would be mitigated. An IAPP can be one helpful way in preparing psychology to help others to find new, healthy ways to relating to others (Blume, 2020).

Preparing for the Next Pandemic: An Opportunity to Transform Colonial Values

The lessons of COVID-19 suggest that two broad areas of change must occur in colonial social orders to reduce pandemic threat. First, the natural world must be better protected and less exploited. Pandemic threat is positively associated with environmental degradation. Respecting nature and protecting wilderness would reduce novel virus contact. Indigenous perspectives related to wasting nothing should be incorporated into sustainable policies to avoid unnecessary encroachment. Second, the vulnerable in society need to be made less vulnerable to health risks. Inequities must be eliminated to reduce the threats, requiring a significant change of values from colonial to humane. It will require social transformations to economics, education, and health care, and the elimination of -isms due to social hierarchies.

Details concerning how to address these two broad areas of social change begin with processes to retire the colonial worldview and its institutions and systems that perpetuate environmental injustice and social inequities. These changes will require transformative and intentionally persistent and patient intergenerational interventions to be effective.

An Opportunity to Prioritize Collective Necessity The COVID-19 pandemic taught those who were paying attention life lessons about priorities. For example, early in the pandemic, before events were heavily politicized, it was clear that the necessary workers of society were not the same as those who were considered prestigious and important in the hierarchies of colonial social orders. Many participants of the necessary workforce were the working poor, conducting work that the privileged would turn their noses up at doing themselves. Certainly, many of those necessary workers should have been compensated more generously for their skills and services than the CEOs who engaged in wealth building activities at the expense of others during the same time period! Necessary health care workers were threatened so many times during the pandemic that some hospitals installed panic buttons on their name badges (Horner, 2021). Colonial societies seemed to have forgotten or never fully recognized what skills and tasks were truly indispensable, especially during a global crisis. Pandemic responses would have been much more effective and efficient if necessary workers had been fully protected by the societies that valued their services. Perhaps the profits of CEOs should have been used to fund such protections.

Here may be a controversial suggestion concerning value in society: Profiting from the activities of others is a non-essential activity outside of a colonial point of view. During a global pandemic we needed feet on the streets to keep society running rather than socially isolated profiteers. Those who built wealth were a burden rather than a benefit to the social order—their wealth building increased social inequities that in turn increased the likelihood of social divisiveness and conflict. The material orientation of colonial societies, including the US, has long perpetuated the belief that it was okay for a privileged few to materially profit from the services of others who labored at risk to themselves and their families. This level of exploitation does nothing to advance equity, justice, or peace in societies, but rather enhances social instability, increasing collective risk during any future global crisis, including a pandemic.

To adequately prepare for future pandemics, social priorities need to reflect the realities of collective necessity, which has never occurred in colonialism. The most necessary workers in colonialism have historically been the most exploited. Economic equity ensures that all in society are considered equally necessary to the efficient workings of the social order. Artificial hierarchies that reward the privileged are neither necessary nor efficient. Privilege only exists because leeching off others is sanctioned in colonial worldviews. Privilege has resulted from the violation of the human rights of necessary workers in society.

An Opportunity to Prioritize Consensus and Honesty The era of social media has made it easy to believe that opinions are facts. From an IAPP perspective, opinions are expressions of individual beliefs generated from the experience of a n = 1. Opinions take on greater value in cultures when self is held as the foundational unit for understanding healthy behavior. Colonial nations have a lengthy history of certain opinions and opinion-makers being counted and others being discounted. It comes as no surprise that opinions and opinion-makers are organized hierarchically by citizens in hierarchical societies, but the ranking like other artificial hierarchies do not have a basis in reality in an egalitarian world.

So-called "social influencers" have found the ability to wield their opinions with a great deal of power to persuade others to think and behave in certain ways. The problem with social influencers is that their opinions are often not supported by evidence, let alone facts, and their comments are not subject to the tests of peer review as one would see in scientific circles. During COVID-19, some social influencers were responsible for super-spreading misinformation and falsehoods that ultimately harmed pandemic response, with examples of that misinformation discussed in Chap. 9. Social influencers expressed their opinions under the liberties of freedom of speech, but those protected liberties suggest nothing about the veracity, quality, or healthiness of what is communicated. Freedom of speech does not simultaneously include assurances of social responsibility in what is said or written, therefore allowing for unhealthy circulation of conspiracy theories and misinformation as a result.

Indigenous people do not hierarchically rank order opinions or opinion-leaders. Indigenous people have opinions, of course, but value weighing consensus of the whole over the opinions of the one or the few. Seeking consensus is an excellent way for all to have their opinions heard or reviewed and operates to distill those opinions into a collective response. Consensus is a community-oriented method to peer review opinions to prevent one idea or one person from wielding hierarchical power or privilege over the views of the collective. Social influencers arise because colonial hierarchies allow a privileged few to manipulate others.

Another inherent weakness in colonialism exposed by the COVID-19 pandemic was the level of distrust created by dishonesty. Colonial government officials have abused the truth in order to manipulate and control minoritized others. Misinformation and abusing the truth have been very effective colonial weapons to dehumanize and disempower people. Many populist-nationalist leaders widely abused the truth during the COVID-19 pandemic in ways that contributed to palpable harm to their nations as a result. Rarely have the negative, self-inflicted consequences of colonial alternative facts, misinformation, fake news, and conspiracy theories been so readily apparent as they were during COVID-19. The result was palpable social tensions that interfered with coordinated and evidence-based responses to protecting health.

Dishonesty tends to be an exceedingly selfish behavior that destroys trust. When colonial leaders continue to use the same dishonest strategies that created the social inequities in the first place, they lose all credibility with those they seek to lead. Weaponizing dishonesty is an attempt to manipulate others into accepting fantasy as reality. Since the goals of dishonesty are to intentionally manipulate or deceive others, the practice leaves nations in tremendously disadvantageous positions to respond collectively to a common threat. It is difficult to respond effectively when the basis for those responses are founded in fantasy.

The problem is that colonial cultures assume that chronic dishonesty in service of privilege is acceptable. The acceptability of chronic dishonesty as normative is another reason why democracy is not well-matched to a colonial worldview. Dishonesty is not conducive to promoting a unified vision or to promoting an inclusive social covenant—chronic dishonesty is neither prosocial nor psychologically healthy. Preparing for a more effective pandemic response in the future will be better served by enhancing trust through complete transparency rather than through manipulation, obfuscation, and outright lies (e.g., Jonas, 2013).

Indigenous Americans have a long history of utilizing consensus to discern wisdom. Social consensus as a way to test the veracity of different viewpoints provides a check on manipulative disinformation campaigns and conspiratorial messaging meant to control others. Consensus draws conclusions from collective wisdom rather than one person. It would be a helpful process to prevent misinformation from derailing future pandemic responses.

An Opportunity to Prioritize the Vulnerable among us An Indigenous worldview helps to understand that we are only as strong as our most vulnerable members. Paradoxically, perhaps, it is in our best interests to prioritize care for our most vulnerable to overcome collective vulnerability. During the COVID-19 pandemic, many in the US were willing to sacrifice elders for the sake of economic opportunity. Children were an afterthought, and years of neglecting children left them at high risk for poverty and with limited resources to receive a quality education, pandemic or not. American educational inequity has negatively impacted children whereas American health inequities have negatively impacted children and elders.

Prioritizing care for elders and children is valued by Indigenous American people, unlike many colonial societies where both demographic groups are considered economic liabilities rather than valuable assets. Elevating the status of children and elders in society would be a very positive step toward reducing ageism in colonial societies. In addition, by addressing the needs of our most vulnerable age groups, the overall vulnerability of the population to pandemic health and education consequences would be circumvented. Questions concerning how to protect older adults and how to educate younger children under pandemic conditions will have already been considered and thoughtfully addressed.

Those with pre-existing health and mental conditions also constitute some of our most vulnerable. The COVID-19 pandemic compounded those vulnerabilities for decades to come. Elevating care in general and considering how to protect those with pre-existing conditions is a significant priority to address threats of future global illnesses. An equitable and healthy society does not stigmatize others. Neglecting health and mental health comorbidity contributed to expensive treatment when prevention would have been much more cost effective. More needs to be invested into a collective and equitable health care model that does not discriminate, rather than a hierarchical system that delivers unequal care and little in preventive methods.

The Opportunity to Pursue a Global and Timeless Perspective A unified "planetary" approach is needed to reduce the threats of global health emergencies (Jowell & Barry, 2020). Rather than each nation attempting to approach a pandemic as individuals with individual national interests, a collective vision is needed for a globally comprehensive plan to address the next pandemic. The lesson from COVID-19 has been clear--as long as nations respond variably, there will inevitably be lapses, gaps, and vulnerabilities that viruses will capitalize upon. Vaccine administration will need to be globally equitable, advanced health care services globally accessible, and health care resources globally available. The haves-versus-have-nots approach to pandemic control was an abysmal failure. The lesson from that failure is clear: A global pandemic response is only as effective as the response of its most vulnerable nation.

Artificial boundaries and borders are not respected by a virus (Jonas, 2013); therefore it makes sense to consider pandemic response and prevention as boundaryless. Pandemic responses must become global enterprises rather than national enterprises. Pandemic responses need to reflect the needs, interests, and priorities of the collective whole rather than the needs, interests, and priorities of the privileged few. Pandemic prevention efforts will also need to be carried out as global enterprises and reflect the needs, interests, and priorities of the global community rather than individual nations. With very few exceptions, nations failed to protect their people because they lacked the broad global vision needed to understand and anticipate interdependent vulnerability. Competition and conflict resulted as self-interests clashed. Vulnerable nations were not well-protected by privileged nations, leaving colonial powers vulnerable to global outbreaks with the possibility of dangerous mutations that existing vaccinations would not prevent. Pandemic prevention also requires an intergenerational vision and the development of a sustainable planetary intervention plan in perpetuity.

The Opportunity to Seek Collective Peace: An Indigenous Interpretation

The colonial world has never been one that promoted peace. Hierarchical beliefs that assume superiority and supremacy will never be conducive to the fundamental trust and fairness that is required for genuine peace. Splitting the world into us versus them inevitably contributes to conflict. The resulting -isms have left a divided people that have little incentive to seek the path of social responsibility rather than the path to defend self-interests. Exploiting, controlling, and manipulating others inevitably contributes to deep-seated toxic anger and fear that creates obvious barriers to peacemaking. Peace has always seemed like an unrealistic dream only because we were approaching the idea through the lenses of hierarchical colonial existences—of course it seems unrealistic under that perspective. However, a peaceful world would have enhanced pandemic response, so pursuit of peace is worthy of examination.

An Indigenous conceptualization of peace is one in which egalitarian creatures co-exist in balance and harmony for the good of the whole of Creation. Peace is not permanent--no utopian vision, but rather dependent upon the quality of relationships at any given moment. Peace is not a state of being, but rather an ongoing process to maintain and restore right relationships with others. A disturbance in the peace is a sign to work on relationships.

An Indigenous worldview allows for peace through restitution. Living realistically as an egalitarian being in an interdependent world generates the humility necessary to engage in restitution. Seeing the world as a collectively vulnerable community helps to diminish the unrealistic perceptions of externalized threats that drive retribution. Living spiritually in balance with the material existence provides checks on the imbalances of a material appetite. Treating others with the respect that sacred creatures warrant allows for sharing and collaboration to evolve and a vision for community to emerge. Living in cyclical time allows for multiple opportunities to correct similar and repeated mistakes over time—to improve in the process of becoming. The cyclical flow of time allows for patience over urgency and provides a broad view of how peace may methodically be made if we persevere together in our acts of reconciliation.

Peace is possible if one holds realistic assumptions that align with an interdependent and egalitarian existence. However, peace seems unlikely through colonial lenses that suggest the world is naturally hierarchical, inequitable, and unfair. How one believes is a choice and that choice determines what appears possible and what appears improbable. Ceasing hostilities with the planet is also an important part of the process of peacemaking (Blume, 2019). Humanity will not experience peace if it remains at war with the planet that nurtures and sustains all creatures. Warring with the planet has increased pandemic vulnerability. Peacemaking with the planet will reduce that vulnerability. It is much easier to make peace with our planet when prioritizing the needs of the whole. As long as humans insist on assigning value to self-interests, peacemaking will remain a difficult enterprise. To seek peace, proximal generations will be required to delay or postpone material gratification for the benefit of distal generations. Peace is possible if one wholeheartedly embraces the selfless preconditions for peace, stepping away from self-interests toward collective responsibility.

Optimism also emerges from living with peace toward others. It has been very difficult to imagine a colonial world at peace because self-orientations are inevitably conducted at cross-purposes with others. This is bound to happen when placing the utmost value on the individual liberties of billons to pursue their own self-interests without consideration for what might be valuable to the collective whole instead. Unfortunately, some find it more important to stand for liberties than to stand for life. Peacemaking is Creation-centric rather than anthropocentric, therefore eliminating the possibility of acting at cross-purposes with others. Peacemaking collectively restores relationships through acts of reconciliation, generating an optimistic view of what is possible when we unite in purpose rather than fall into divisiveness.

References

Acevedo, N. (2021, March 15). Puerto Rico enacted strict Covid measures. It paid off, and it's a lesson for the mainland. NBC News. https://www.nbcnews.com/news/lation/puerto-rico-enacted-strict-covid-measures-it-paid-s-n1260998

Altman, D. (2020). Understanding the US failure on coronavirus—An essay by Drew Altman. *BMJ, 370*, m3417. https://doi.org/10.1136/bmj.m3417

Associated Press. (2020, November 6). Puerto Rico to provide free virus testing at toll booths. Author. https://apnews.com/article/us-news-virus-outbreak-health-puerto-rico-c72d5739378f738f77c268ae9d3f30e0

Blume, A. W. (2014). Sharing the light of the sacred fire: A proposal for a paradigm shift in psychology. *Journal of Indigenous Research, 3*, Article 4.

Blume, A. W. (2019). Views from indigenous psychology: How people can make peace with the planet. *Psychology for a Better World: A Cross-cultural Journal on Emotional Intelligence, 7*, 45–58.

Blume, A. W. (2020). *A new psychology based on community, equality, and care of the earth: An indigenous American perspective*. ABC-CLIO/Praeger.

Brooks, D. (2021, May 6). Our pathetic herd immunity. New York Time. https://www.nytimes.com/2021/05/06/opinion/herd-immunity-us.html

CDC. (2021, August 26). Delta variant: What we know about the science. Author. https://www.cdc.gov/coronavirus/2019-ncov/variants/delta-variant.html

Descartes, R. (1637). *Discourse on the method. Translated in 1983 by V. R. Miller and R. P. Miller*. Springer.

Hardy, L., Saul, G., & Thompson, K. F. (2020, December 2). Tribes mount organized responses to COVID-19, In contrast to state and federal governments. Nation of Change. https://www.nationofchange.org/2020/12/02/tribes-mount-organized-responses-to-covid-19-in-contrast-to-state-and-federal-governments/

Horner, M. (2021, September 20). *Cox Medical Center Branson adding panic buttons to employee badges after reports of increased staff assaults*. KY3. https://www.ky3.com/2021/09/20/cox-medical-center-branson-adding-panic-buttons-employee-badges-after-reports-increased-staff-assaults/

Jonas, O. B. (2013). *Pandemic risk*. World Bank. https://www.worldbank.org/content/dam/Worldbank/document/HDN/Health/WDR14_bp_Pandemic_Risk_Jonas.pdf

Jowell, A., & Barry, M. (2020). COVID-19: A matter of planetary, not only national health. *American Journal of Tropical Medicine and Hygiene, 103*(1), 31–32. https://doi.org/10.4269/ajtmh.20.0419

Kelleher, J. S., Tang, T., & Rodriguez, O. R. (2021, August 22). Mask, vaccine conflicts descend into violence and harassment. Associated Press. https://apnews.com/article/health-coronavirus-pandemic-2eba81ebe3bd54b3bcde890b8cf11c70

Lemon, D. (2021). *This is the fire*. Little, Brown and Company.

Mackenzie, D. (2020). *COVID-19: The pandemic that never should have happened and how to stop the next one*. Hachette Books.

Stat News. (2020, December). How Covid-19 has fueled unprecedented advances in medicine. Author. https://www.statnews.com/wp-content/upload/2021/01/STAT_ebook_dec2020_covid19_final.pdf

Quammen, D. (2021). How viruses shape our world. *National Geographic, 239*(2), 41–67.

Samuels, (2021, May 5). US tribe shares vaccine with relatives, neighbors in Canada. Associated Press. https://apnews.com/article/montana-canada-coronavirus-pandemic-coronavirus-vaccine-government-and-politics-00e0f7a7ee6e75d7abdb67d03a067f82

Todd, C., Murray, M., & Kamisar, B. (2021, September 9). Biden resets after Delta frustrates his hope to declare Covid independence. NBC News. https://www.nbcnews.com/politics/meet-the-press/biden-resets-after-delta-frustrates-his-hope-declare-covid-independence-n1278793

Chapter 11
Indigenous Psychology and the Next Pandemic

Abstract Decolonizing hierarchical social orders is a necessary process to restore egalitarian and sacred relationships that align with the realities of dwelling together in an interdependent planetary system. Future pandemic preparation requires the reconciliation of a divided people and prioritizing movement toward education, economic, and health equities. Psychologists in particular have a social and planetary responsibility to help to eliminate the sources of psychological stress and sickness emanating from hierarchical societies—to address those root causes of psychological trauma and distress. Decolonizing attitudes, beliefs, and behavior is an essential part of the transformation, a role for which a decolonized psychology would be well-suited to address. Hierarchies in academic, health and mental health care, the legal system, science, and public policy represent threats to planetary equity and places where decolonized psychology can make a difference. Indigenous Psychology proposes a more egalitarian and holistically-focused perspective of health and wellness, enabling psychologists to work as agents for intergenerational behavior change in partnership with other disciplines to restore a sustainable world, to challenge and modify errant beliefs that contribute to inequitable consequences, and to advance justice and peace as a result of those interventions.

Facing the consequences of COVID-19 will be a defining feature of the post-pandemic world. Psychologists and other health and mental health care professionals will be asked to address the cognitive symptoms of COVID-19, the prolonged trauma of the disaster, and the compounded psychological scarring to already victimized and wounded people. Societies will face the psychological consequences of racism and xenophobia, of conspiracy theories, misinformation, and political divisiveness. Inequities worsened as a result of the pandemic, especially among minoritized people. In the colonial US, the January 6 insurrection and other subsequent efforts toward political oppression have generated additional layers of fear and distress that challenge the psychological well-being of the population. Human scarring is compounded by the scarring of nature through environmental degradation and global climate change. Each of the post-pandemic concerns mentioned above are the result of potentially modifiable human behaviors that may be addressed with psychological interventions.

A. W. Blume, *Colonialism and the COVID-19 Pandemic*, International and Cultural Psychology, https://doi.org/10.1007/978-3-030-92825-4_11

Colonialism has directly or indirectly perpetuated or worsened the psychological issues discussed above—it has also represented a barrier to addressing those problems with unity of purpose (Blume, 2020; Bump et al., 2021). Psychology as a discipline has the capability and responsibility to heal individuals who were psychological victimized during the pandemic, as well as address the human exploitation of the environment associated with pandemic risk. Psychology must help to decolonize hierarchical social structures and institutions that have contributed to environmental and human misery to prevent further psychological wounding.

Overcoming Colonial Hierarchies that Enhance Vulnerability

Hierarchical systems contribute to inequity and relational psychopathology, and thus consequentially to persistent psychological challenges for social orders. In order to reduce pandemic risk (see Table 11.1), hierarchical assumptions must be challenged as irrational and contrary to research concerning the egalitarian interdependence of the natural order. Hierarchy is an artificial human construct anthropomorphically superimposed onto the rest of the world by those who assumed their superiority in that hierarchy. Humans have long misunderstood their role in the social order as one of superiority and exceptionalism as a species. Colonial cultures

Table 11.1 How psychology can prepare for the next global crisis (pandemic or otherwise)

Action	Areas of Impact
Psychologists can help to retire hierarchical thinking, including ceilings and walls	Academic culture Classrooms Health care Mental health care Public policy Science
Psychologists can help to retire the *out-of-sight-out-of-mind* colonial mindset	Creating a global and intergenerational focus for psychological education, science, and practice Moving psychology from a proximal orientation to a more distal focus
Psychologists can help to decolonize what is considered functional and dysfunctional by: Challenging colonial self-oriented assumptions Challenging colonial anthropocentric assumptions Challenging colonial assumptions concerning materialism Helping to construct health care that addresses psychological victims AND systems that victimize Restore psychological Well-being through planetary health	Decolonizing psychology as a discipline Aligning psychology with the empirically derived assumptions of other life sciences concerning interdependence Redefining health and wellness holistically and collectively Treating those as we serve with the respect sacred entities deserve Restoring relationships with nature to improve psychological Well-being

have treated the natural world as hierarchically beneath the human world, and therefore disrespecting the natural world as a resource to be plundered (Deloria, 2003). In IAPP, humans are considered sacred entities, just as all entities of nature are sacred. Humans, however, are not more sacred or important than other species. In fact, the sacred role of humans is the same as all other creatures—to seek relations with others that enhances the whole of the sacred Creation. Thinking like an apex creature ignores the reality of an interdependent world. Egalitarianism encourages psychological wellness not apex thinking.

Hierarchical thinking errors, therefore, must be transformed into egalitarian reframes in order to reduce the risk of a next pandemic. In order to pursue this transformation, the first hierarchical thinking error in need of decolonization is the belief that some humans are superior creatures when compared to other creatures, making environmental exploitation a possibility due to that sense of superiority. Psychology can aid in this process by elevating the importance of the natural world to collective health and mental health. An IAPP perspective values the role of the natural world in healing and restoration, a perspective that would help colonial psychology to transition from a reductionistic to a global perspective. Psychological models would be enhanced by inclusion of the natural world in all considerations related to psychological health and wellness. An important disciplinary consideration becomes how to neutralize the environment impact of humans today so it will not psychological harm non-human and human life now and in perpetuity. The belief that some humans are superior creatures should be treated as a pathological thinking error to be challenged.

Part of decolonizing the humans are superior creatures thinking error is to consider the virus-human relationship. During the COVID-19 pandemic, the SARS-CoV-2 virus was dominant over humans despite its tiny size. Despite evidence of this domination, many people disrespected the virus' power. As a result, many people suffered and died needlessly. Others reacted with fear because they had felt the impact in their own lives, fear that could have been prevented if human relationships with viruses pre-pandemic had been more circumspect. Humans may have fared better by humbly respecting the virus and its environment pre-pandemic. Humans will need to become more respectful of viruses to avoid future pandemics.

The second hierarchical thinking error in need of decolonization is the belief that some demographic groups are naturally superior to other groups, contributing to false beliefs in the exceptionalism of a particular people, nation, and culture. This colonial thinking error has contributed to white supremacist views resulting in centuries of mistreatment of Black and Brown people, as well as artificial hierarchical constructions I have referred to as -isms in this book. Life sciences do not support the notion that certain people and their cultures are superior, and in fact, much of this book has exposed the inherent flaws in colonial culture as it relates to pandemic risk. The belief that some demographic groups are naturally superior to other groups needs to be treated by psychologists as the pathological thinking error it is.

Psychologists can help to retire colonial ceilings and walls There are also thinking errors related to artificial boundaries in need of decolonization. The first thinking error to decolonize is the belief that there are boundaries between material and spiritual existences that make the spiritual irrelevant for a material existence. Compartmentalizing the material from the spiritual in colonialism has contributed to a couple of dysfunctional outcomes from an IAPP perspective. First, the artificial distinction in colonial culture of the material world from spiritual world contributes to an emphasis on the observable world for this life, whereas the unobservable is viewed as irrelevant or disconnected from this reality. Second, the emphasis in colonialism on the observable world has contributed to colonial materialism as a visible sign of power and success, contributing to material exploitation of other humans and the rest of the natural world. Even psychology has fallen into the colonial trap of believing that the visible, observable world is the primary concern of psychological science. This has not been true for other sciences. Physics is an example of how science can respect the spiritual mysteries of the universe, which studies the impact of the invisible routinely. From an IAPP perspective, factors influencing human behavior are not always visible, but they are relevant to psychology.

A second boundary thinking error in need of decolonization is the belief that there are discrete boundaries between self and others (Blume, 2020). Human skin is not a wall from the world, and in fact, there are constant exchanges of molecules and microorganisms. Self is dynamic: What is considered the self today may become the other tomorrow. Humans are interconnected creatures rather than isolated entities from the natural world. Our skin does not prevent interdependence. A third and related boundary thinking error in need of decolonization is that community and national boundaries are impermeable. National boundaries do not stop the natural consequences of an interdependent world at the border. The air and water of one nation is the air and water of the world. If polluted by one, it is felt by all. National boundaries are artificial constructs that serve as barriers rather than assets to addressing global problems.

A fourth colonial boundary thinking error in need of decolonization is the belief there are boundaries between present, past, and future. Logically, the present is utterly reliant on the past, and the future reliant upon both past and future. In a single moment, past, present, and future co-exist when considering cyclical time (Blume, 2020). The activities of the present moment do not occur in a void—they have been informed by the past and impact the future simultaneously. Human activities have broad and lasting impact within the natural order in which they reside. A broad vision that does not wall off the present from past and future is important to creating sustainable healthy relationships with others. Happiness in the present is linked to healthy relationships with past and future. Challenging the thinking error boundary around the present moment will broaden the focus on the consequences of human behavior from proximal outcomes only to proximal and distal outcomes simultaneously.

Psychologists can help to retire the *out-of-sight-out-of-mind* colonial mindset The conceptualizations of artificial boundaries and proximal time makes it easy for people in colonial societies to forget the world beyond the self in this moment.

Another thinking error to challenge is the belief that if something is not visible or obvious, it is not real or relevant. Assuming the interconnectivity of all things in the natural world, consequences are neither place-bound nor time-limited. Our activities reverberate across time and space in ways where small activities can have large and long-term consequences to self and others. In order to decolonize human activity, the out-of-sight-out-of-mind thinking error must be challenged. Our activities must be reconsidered in light of their potential impact across both time and space. Treading lightly through life is responsible living and a step toward decolonizing the self.

Psychologists help to decolonize what is considered functional and dysfunctional Psychopathology should be viewed from the perspective of relationships rather than symptoms. White supremacy is a thinking error that interferes with egalitarian relationships in societies, therefore it is a precursor to relational psychopathology. White nationalism is a political belief developed from the thinking error of white supremacy, and therefore a political view that promotes psychopathology. These forms of relational psychopathology have been infinitely more toxic to colonial societies than the disorders often treated by psychologists today. Psychologists will need to refocus from only addressing individual presentations of clinical disorders to transformative acts of challenging colonial cultural thinking errors in public, in classrooms, and in clinical practice and research. Helping to decolonize thoughts and behavior psychologically strengthens societies in preparation for the next global threat.

A psychologically functional approach to address the next pandemic will involve a collective global movement toward egalitarian relationships to enhance collaboration, emphasize equity and transparency, and increase trust in the social structures and science. To prevent a pandemic, a broad holistic view of methods across space and time will be required, including intergenerational interventions on human behavior to simultaneously reduce environmental exploitation and degradation, to improve global physical and mental health, and to reduce risks related to inequities. Decolonizing societies is an important step in this process. Decolonizing society's social systems and institutions are an important part of decolonizing the society, including decolonizing psychology to enhance its capabilities to aid in global and intergenerational behavioral interventions. A nation cannot stand alone against a novel virus. Individual responses were found to be wholly ineffectual during COVID-19, but a collective response will be much more functional for a collective threat and generate inherent resilience.

Wellness of Society Requires Ending Colonial Divisiveness

Effective pandemic responses in the future will also depend upon challenging and ending colonial divisiveness. Colonial splitting and other divisive activities, such as blaming and bullying, serve no useful purpose for the whole and contribute to relational psychopathology that hinders crisis response. To prevent future pandemics, national leaders will need to align national interests with global interests. Pursuit of self-interests and the privilege that results from those pursuits will be challenged as psychologically dysfunctional. Exercising power or utilizing disinformation or untruth to control, manipulate, or coerce others increases pandemic risks. These colonial methods of individual leadership have no basis in reality within an interdependent world and should be called out as the delusional approaches they are.

Decolonizing colonial leadership will occur naturally if those who lead fully grasp the implications of dwelling equitably in a sacred and egalitarian natural order (Blume & Trimble, in preparation). Effective leaders during the next pandemic will need to be collective thinkers with collective visions for addressing collective threats–a broad and holistic view of the challenge and how to respond to the challenge. They will govern and lead by example and with transparency. The decolonized leader will place others first and themselves last, always, understanding that leadership is a transitory service rather than an entitlement or a career. Encouragement and optimism promote trust and confidence in leadership. Humility helps to convey the shared vulnerability that all have as equal entities in Creation.

Decolonizing divisive colonial societies and leadership will reduce conflict and enhance processes toward peace. Most colonial conflicts have been focused on national self-interests over material assets and resources. When colonialism is retired, competing self-interests would be replaced with collaborative global interests. Exploitation and predation will no longer be considered justified for the privileged few. Superiority of nations and peoples will be seen as irrational and privilege retired. Eliminating expensive colonial conflict will allow defense budgets to be redirected to education, health, and infrastructure that enhances personal security rather than conflicts that destabilize the whole.

Transforming colonial values Colonialism has long valued material acquisition in the here and now, reflecting the proximal self-orientation of the worldview. Proximal outcomes are helpful to consider, but distal outcomes provide a broad view of how human activities impact future generations. Colonial impatience has created a sense of urgency, mostly about non-urgent self-interests in the here and now. What demands urgency considering how colonial materialism negatively impacts the future of the planet by exploiting nature and other humans.

The colonial forces that have contributed to environmental degradation and climate change have been mindlessly at work for centuries. It will take some time to thoughtfully and patiently move toward goals of equity and sustainability that will restore human relationships with the rest of the planet (Blume, 2022). Humans will need to find their patience whether it is culturally comfortable or not. The imbalances and disharmony of colonial activities have caused intergenerational problems that will require patience to address. An Indigenous understanding of the cycling of time allows for multiple opportunities to get things right over time, providing patient optimism that our activities now will be sustainable over time and will eventually benefit the whole (Blume, 2020). Humans are in the process of becoming, with each generation aiding in that process. It will take time, time that we have if we are patient.

The importance of adequate ventilation was rediscovered during the pandemic. I have used the word "rediscovered," because we know that ventilation was used in Alghero against the plague in sixteenth century Europe (see Chap. 7). When businesses had better ventilation, they had less spread of SARS-CoV-2. Being outdoors was found to be much safer than being indoors in terms of ventilation. Indigenous people have long understood and appreciated the importance of the natural world for human healing. Being indoors is not a natural state of being for human creatures. Staying indoors tends to provide an artificial sense of security, but ironically, being outdoors was typically healthier. People also turned to the outdoors for recreation, which was psychologically helpful during a time when indoor recreational activities were risky. An essential lesson during COVID-19 was the importance of nature in healing.

Happiness from an IAPP perspective is a result of right relationships with other, including with others across time and space. Patience is required to restore those relationships with nature and future generations of non-human and human creatures. Our happiness is dependent upon patience in the collective processes of becoming and patience with our intergenerational interventions to retire colonialism and restore humans to sacredness as egalitarian creatures. Humility is also required, replacing human hierarchy and superiority with more equitable social systems. We will all be significantly more psychologically healthy and happy as result of these transformations, but the transformation will take time and patience.

Addressing inequities and poverty Global priorities will need to focus on the health and well-being of the whole to better prepare the planet to respond to global crises. Colonial belief systems that tolerate income and wealth inequities and allow persistent poverty are completely unethical and unsustainable. Global economic equity is far from a reality but represents an aspirational goal as we dismantle the economic disparities between colonists and colonized.

Capitalism as an economic system reflects the hierarchical structures of colonialism. During the COVID-19 pandemic, many exploited the capitalistic economic systemic to their advantage, including many health care businesses that shamefully gouged the people (Garber & Brownlee, 2021). Many assume that capitalism is the only rational approach to economics, but capitalism has not consistently demonstrated that it can prevent or reduce economic injustices in colonial societies. The COVID-19 pandemic exposed significant shortcomings in capitalistic economies, and as a result, some have suggested that capitalism needs to evolve or perhaps be replaced (King, 2021). Pre-pandemic scholarship demonstrated that the material economies of colonial nations are not globally sustainable due to resource overshoot habits or expectations for economic growth on the backs of others (Hickel, 2019). Strong arguments can be made that capitalism compounded COVID-19 health risks with its intergenerational inequities, wealth building at the expense of others, placing economic performance ahead of basic human need, and aversive environmental consequences risking novel virus exposure. Capitalism is profoundly wasteful and inefficient from an Indigenous perspective.

Some have suggested socialism as an alternative, but socialism is also a Eurocentric economic model that places material well-being as foundational, reflecting its colonial Eurocentric roots. Both capitalism and socialism are anthropocentric models for conceptualizing resource allocation and needs, prone to human abuse of nature. Socialist nations have contributed to environmental degradation in the same way that capitalist nations have from an Indigenous perspective—allocating resources according to human standards does nothing to protect from environmental exploitation. The world would greatly benefit from a model where Creation-centric needs of the planet drive resource use—to create an economic model that is consistent with healthy relationships for humans and non-human alike. What is needed is an economic model not driven by profit motives and self-interests, but, like Indigenous bartering economies (Chap. 3), focused on economic necessity for the well-being of the whole.

Economic policies will need to be evaluated with regard to how they create equity for the whole rather than how they create opportunity for a few. Any policy that creates inequity needs to be retired. As an example, in 2021 the US experienced perceived shortages in the workforce that annoyed businesses. Certain states cut unemployment benefits under the assumption that people were staying home because they earned more on unemployment benefits than at work (Luhby, 2021), but after those states dropped those benefits, there were only marginal improvements to the labor shortages were noted (Campbell, 2021). However, the reality was that lack of childcare and unjustly disparate salaries in those states were the real issues, and that cutting off unemployment benefits risked sending more children into poverty. In addition, frontline health care staffing issues emerged later in the pandemic as a result of burn-out, insufficient wages, and mistreatment by the public ib. both the US and UK (British Medical Association, 2021; Kirzinger et al., 2021). One example was the significant shortage of first responder Emergency Medical Technicians that threatened appropriate response times to medical emergencies in many regions of the country (McCausland, 2021).

Compensation and benefits to employees will need to be re-evaluated to align with the economic necessity of the work, including provisions for childcare and with a perspective that acknowledges the sacredness and the equity of the workforce. Tax laws need to be modified toward equity, retiring wealth building protections for the very few. Those nations, corporations, and individuals who have benefitted most from colonial economic systems should compensate those who have been victimized with a safety net compensatory income. Health benefits need to be equitable for all employees, period, to prevent inequitable access to quality health care.

An Indigenous conceptualization of justice would be a very helpful lens in which to formulate how to restore equity in colonial societies. Colonial justice tends to operate under principles of retribution. The goals of retribution tend to be more inclined toward punishing what is considered wrongdoing rather than restoring prosocial behavior—in the US, punishment is often used instead of rehabilitation as an example. The 2021 reversal of the masking policy by the CDC (see Chap. 9) is an excellent example of how retributional justice, operating implicitly in colonial societies, may be used unwittingly to punish and dehumanize people for being different or not behaving in a certain way—in this instance, used to punish the unvaccinated. The exasperation of one writer who had fully complied with mitigation measures and was fully vaccinated illustrates the point—she stopped masking-up along with most other people after the CDC reversal of the masking policy, justifying that any risks to the unvaccinated as a result were on them (Estrich, 2021). A lot of people in colonial nations acted similarly, understandably frustrated with vaccination, masking, and social distancing non-compliance. However, from an IAPP perspective, non-compliance with public health methods to addressing COVID-19 were acts of relational psychopathology for many, suggesting that anti-vaxxing attitudes were likely symptoms of psychological unwellness. Restitution for the consequences of that sickness would be a much more psychologically functional approach than punishment or vengeance because of its insistence on acknowledging the pathology and the harms it has caused, then committing to righting the wrongs through restorative justice.

Colonial societies have historically used retributional justice as a weapon to minoritize groups that the privileged perceive to be inferior. An Indigenous conceptualization of justice assumes that justice involve restitution rather than retribution—that wrongdoers be held accountable for fixing the injury that has occurred as a result of the wrongdoing (Becker, 1997). Restitution oriented justice emphasizes activities that restore relationships to balance and harmony. When considering colonial economic wrongdoing against others from an Indigenous perspective, economic restitution through providing compensatory resources and transforming the economic rules of the social system would be natural first steps toward equity.

Restitution as a strategy to end inequity should involve some form of reparations to colonial victims that would have the effect of levelling the playing field. Reparations in kind might involve educational and health care advantages designed to address the colonial wounds in society. With regard to Indigenous Americans, reparations also should be linked to the land that was lost. One idea might be for the US federal government to turn over control of the Bureau of Land Management and the land it administers to a tribal collective who would act with greater respect toward the land than colonial forces have ever shown. Restitutional justice is the reasonable approach to transforming historic retributional injustices.

Instilling economic equity means instilling educational equity. Obviously, not everyone will have the same goals for education, but it is incumbent upon a fair and just society to make educational opportunities equitable. Barriers to education should be identified and dismantled. Public schools should be provided similar resources regardless of which neighborhoods they serve, and they should not have to endure fewer resources than privileged private schools. Teachers who work with our sacred children should be able to access whatever is needed to advance the next generation. Technological parity needs to be provided to schools, students, and their families before the next pandemic. Rich nations will be expected to share educational resources with poorer nations as restitution for centuries of colonial exploitation.

Education and economic equity would go a long way toward addressing health inequity. The model of restitution is also helpful to effectively address health disparities. Educating the next generation of health care professionals from minoritized communities needs to be prioritized and resources provided. Sharing of health care expertise and resources should become routine, especially by wealthier nations to poorer nations. Restitution by colonial societies would make equitable health prevention programs more accessible, and provide equitable access to basic human needs such as clean water and nutritious food.

Frankly, economics have been overly emphasized as a value in colonial societies due to the materialistic perspective of colonialism Economic considerations have driven both education and health care policies for too long. In an egalitarian and interdependent world, education and health care are much more essential to the whole than material gain to the few. Decolonizing pandemic responses means that education and health care policy need to drive economic decisions rather than economics driving education and health care policy.

For those who balk at these suggestions, it is worth reflecting upon the economic, education, and health and mental health costs of victimization associated with the vast wasteland of colonialism. Investment to ensure economic, educational, and health equity of the whole makes much more sense over the long-term than protecting the few and risking the whole. The COVID-19 pandemic illustrated how ineffectual the protection of the few was. Seeking equity is also seeking inoculation from the risks of inequity. The only logical approach in an interdependent world is to seek equitable protections for all as an important step for reducing global threats. Equity is herd immunity: Global economic, educational, and health equity is our collective herd immunity to effectively thwart pandemics of the future.

Unifying health care The splintered health care system of the US was exposed as organizationally dysfunctional and unable to mount a unified plan and collaborative effort to address the COVID-19 pandemic. Individual health care entities obviously do not have the capacity to address holistic health care problems. Asking health care entities to compete with one another for lifesaving equipment was a tremendously wasteful mistake. Allowing municipalities, counties, and states to set their own unique policies based on science or politics was an exceedingly ineffectual response that ignored the risks to the whole. Not fully preparing years before the onset of the pandemic was another colossal mistake that cost thousands of lives, mistakes often driven by colonial economics rather than science and common sense.

The Biden administration announced an interesting space-race type of approach to proactive vaccination research to reduce time to production, to promote better medical equipment and testing to use during a pandemic, and to create better PPE to protect health care professionals (Facher, 2021). Each of these proposals is a step in the right direction to promote pandemic preparation. However, what is missing is decolonizing health care systems and their racialized biases and competitive and disunified approach to care.

Unifying health care will enhance future responses to pandemics. A unified national health care system would provide uniformity and make equity of care across neighborhoods and communities more likely. A comprehensive plan for addressing the next pandemic should be available to all citizens and provide a clear blueprint for pandemic response. Politics should not derail such a plan if it is available to all citizens. Prevention should be equally considered with treatment. Vaccination development should be an ongoing enterprise as novel viruses are discovered. Economics should not drive vaccination development. Stockpiles of PPE and other medical equipment enough for everyone should be prepared (Mackenzie, 2020). Psychologists can prepare resources to improve the mental health outcomes during a pandemic by addressing social isolation and stress. A new unified model of health care would anticipate and prepare holistic responses to address regional surges in hospitalizations.

Unifying health care also means unifying physical health and mental health services. Health should be conceptualized holistically and systemically rather than compartmentally. Too often health is conceptualized as medicine rather than as a holistic response with allied health care professionals. Unified health care means having mental health and physical health services collaboratively serving clients under one roof, making accessibility easier. Cross-disciplinary work should be encouraged rather than turf wars fueled by economics. Mental health services should have parity with physical health services. With a holistic view of wellness, mental and physical health should not be artificially siloed from one another. Health is not simply defined by a physical dimension—health is also reliant upon mental, emotional, and spiritual well-being.

Individual health is not necessarily wellness, which is focused on the collective whole and heavily influenced by environmental well-being. Wellness is a function of healthy relationships with others. People often forget the importance of healthy environmental relationships to wellness. From an IAPP perspective, wellness is a source of resilience due to healthy connectivity to the inherent strengths of the whole of Creation.

Finally, unifying health care must occur on a global scale to address global pandemics. In reality, the WHO as a global health care entity was an appropriate entity to coordinate a global pandemic response. If the WHO is not up to the task, then it is the collective responsibility of the UN member nations to recreate a global health organization that is up to the task before the next pandemic. A world health-like organization should have the ability to distribute equitable health care globally. It should have the responsibility for developing an equitable plan to address the next pandemic on a global scale. It should have the ability to interpret global health care need and the power to address that need as it arises, including decisions about who should be first on the vaccine lists. Rather than blaming the organization or circumventing its sphere of influence, nations should be working to strengthen this important organization. It was unequivocally clear that national responses were ineffectual to a global health threat. It makes absolute sense to strengthen the one global health authority that exists to improve global pandemic responses. Nations will need to decolonize their own health policies to create the space necessary for a unified global response that is liberated from the nationalistic barriers.

Lessons from storytelling cultures One important life lesson would be to remember the history of this and other pandemics in such a way to honor collective sacrifices and grief. Millions of our ancestors have died so that we may learn the lessons from viruses—we disrespect them by forgetting these lessons. We also disrespect our progeny by not passing along the stories so that they, too, may learn the lessons. Indigenous cultures have preserved those stories and have been able to share the lessons, which is one important reason they took the pandemic seriously before many others. In fact, some people never took it seriously. Families can communicate the stories intergenerationally to improve pandemic preparation. Indigenous people may be looked to as a model for infusing the importance of storytelling into cultural values. The stories at their essence appear to have decolonizing benefits in that people will likely be less vulnerable to the toxicity and callousness of colonial amnesia.

Circling Back to Wellness: An Indigenous Interpretation

The story of COVID-19 is likely not over, despite the desire of human beings that it be finished. The development of Merck's antiviral medication molnupiravir to address COVID-19 showed preliminary promise to effectively reduce hospitalizations and mortality (Herper, 2021), but there were also concerns that its appearance might hinder vaccine seeking by those already disinclined to do so. Vaccines were found to be less efficacious with preventing infection and transmissibility of the delta variant, although still providing strong protections against severe illness (Fowlkes et al., 2021). There is the constant threat of variants that may have the capacity to evade known vaccinations. Without a vaccinated global population, there is the possibility of more variants as long as there are available hosts. Libertarian responses in defiance of seeking vaccinations or other forms of mitigation only make that possibility more probable. The UK modeling projections have suggested four possible future tracks for SARS-CoV-2, ranging from becoming less threatening to becoming more threatening before becoming less threatening or even morphing into another virus with the help of a zoonotic exchange from human to animal to human (Scientific Advisory Group for Emergencies, 2021). Even if COVID's story is drawing to a close, the story of viruses and humans will likely be repeated until we have learned the lessons we are supposed to learn.

Indigenous people look lessons in each life experience, hoping those lessons make us more fully human beings in the process of becoming. A lesson that is before us is how can we take a tragic event such as the COVID-19 pandemic and transform tragedy into resilience--convert personal crises into opportunities to improve us. Colonialism has created resilient people out of necessity. Indigenous Americans have defied the odds in surviving systematic efforts to erase both people and cultures, and have emerged wounded yet collectively stronger.

Preparing for the next pandemic is more than responding to a virus. Preparation means working together to create a healthy planet. A healthy interdependent planet will mean a healthier human species. Indigenous people find resilience in our collective cultural values and connectivity to the land. Culture binds us together in collective meaning and strength; the natural world not only sustains people, it also heals as we engage in healthy relationships with others. Pandemic preparation is a process of reclaiming the best aspects of the human creature—of reclaiming our sacred place in Creation as equal members of a sacred system of being. Pandemic preparation is bettering ourselves individually and as a species, becoming physically and spiritually healthy and whole. Pandemic preparation is an opportunity to mature as a species—to part from selfish ways and restore relationships with the Earth that sustains us.

Pandemic preparation also allows us to move on from the colonial era, an era that has been among the most destructive in our collective history. Appropriate pandemic preparation requires that we retire selfish colonial values, that we transform inequitable colonial systems and institutions, that we undo the harm perpetuated upon certain peoples due to cultural lies. Pandemic preparation grants an opportunity to restore, reconcile, and reconstruct just and equitable societies. Pandemic preparation allows us to understand what must be done to transform colonial risks into decolonized resilience. Pandemic preparation generates a more civilized and humane society in which all will be included and respected.

Time cycles and then recycles. Time is optimistic and forgiving that way, allowing for multiple opportunities with similar situations to learn or relearn life lessons, such as overcoming our historical bumbles and missteps. Time is recycling with every pandemic with face, testing us on how well we have learned from previous life lessons. Pandemic preparation can be a time to rejoice together that we are indeed growing collectively from those life lessons, taking advantage of the familiarity of the past in the present, and transforming the present to create a better future as a result. What kind of world will we help to create post-pandemic? Will it be a post-colonial world that reflects our collective sacredness?

References

Becker, T. (1997). *Traditional American Indian leadership: A comparison with U.S. governance*. American Indian Research and Policy Institute. https://www.semanticscholar.org/paper/Traditional-American-Indian-Leadership%3A-A-with-U.S.-Becker/99737b2266bcf9d89913b4291c7788865871d3b8

Blume, A. W. (2022). Global inequity, climate change, and sustainability: An indigenous perspective. In J. L. Chin, Y. E. García, & A. W. Blume (Eds.), *The psychology of inequity: Global concerns*. Praeger.

Blume, A. W. (2020). *A new psychology based on community, equality, and care of the earth: An indigenous American perspective*. ABC-CLIO/Praeger.

Blume, A. W. & Trimble, J. E. (in preparation). "What really matters is that you have a beautiful spirit": Selected Native American Indian traditional leadership styles. In J. L. Chin, J. E. Trimble, & J. Tan, (Eds.). *Building bridges to inclusive leadership through the lens of cultural narratives*. San Diego: Cognella Academic Publishing.

British Medical Association. (2021, 3 May). *Thousands of overworked doctors plan to leave the NHS, BMA finds*. : Author. https://www.bma.org.uk/bma-media-centre/thousands-of-overworked-doctors-plan-to-leave-the-nhs-bma-finds

Bump, J. B., Baum, F., Sakornsin, M., Yates, R., & Hofman, K. (2021). Political economy of Covid-19: Extractive, regressive, competitive. *BMJ, 372*, n73. https://doi.org/10.1136/bmj.n73

Campbell, W. (2021, October 3). *Labor shortages still order of the day*. Vancouver, WA: The Columbian, A1, A12).

Deloria, V. (2003). *God is red: A native view of religion*. Fulcrum Publishing.

Estrich, S. (2021, July 8). *Mask-free*. Hermosa Beach, CA: Creators Syndicate. https://www.creators.com/read/susan-estrich/07/21/mask-free

Facher, L. (2021, September 3). *The white house wants $65 billion for an 'Apollo'-style pandemic preparedness program*. Boston: STAT News. https://www.statnews.com/2021/09/03/biden-wants-65-billion-for-apollo-style-pandemic-preparedness-program/

Fowlkes, A., Gaglani, M., Groover, K., Thiese, M. S., Tyner, H., & Ellingson, K. (2021). Effectiveness of COVID-19 vaccines in preventing SARS-CoV-2 infection among frontline workers before and during B.1.617.2 (delta) variant predominance—eight U.S. locations, December 2020–August 2021. *MMWR, 70*. https://www.cdc.gov/mmwr/volumes/70/wr/mm7034e4

Garber, J., & Brownlee, S. (2021). 'Honoring' health care's bad actors. *National Geographic, 240*(1), 15–18.

Herper, M. (2021, October 1). *Merck's antiviral pill reduces hospitalization of Covid patients, a possible game-changer for treatment*. Boston: STAT News. https://www.statnews.com/2021/10/01/mercks-antiviral-pill-reduces-hospitalization-of-covid-patients-a-possible-game-changer-for-treatment/

Hickel, J. (2019). I it possible to achieve a good life for all within planetary boundaries? *Third World Quarterly, 40*(1), 18–35. https://doi.org/10.1080/01436597.2018.1535895

King, M. W. (2021, May 26). *Why the next stage of capitalism is coming*. London: BBC. https://www.bbc.com/future/article/20210525-why-the-next-stage-of-capitalism-is-coming

Kirzinger, A., Kearney, A., Hamel, L., & Brodie, M. (2021, April 6). *KFF/the Washington Post frontline health workers survey*. : Kaiser Family Foundation . https://www.kff.org/report-section/kff-the-washington-post-frontline-health-care-workers-survey-toll-of-the-pandemic/

Luhby, T. (2021, May 7). *South Carolina and Montana to end all pandemic unemployment benefits for jobless residents*. New York: CNN . https://www.cnn.com/2021/05/06/politics/montana-pandemic-unemployment-benefits/index.html

Mackenzie, D. (2020). *COVID-19: The pandemic that never should have happened and how to stop the next one*. Hachette Books.

McCausland, P. (2021, October 8). *EMS services warn of 'crippling labor shortage' undermining 911 system*. New York: NBC News. https://www.nbcnews.com/news/us-news/ems-services-warn-crippling-labor-shortage-undermining-911-system-rcna2677

Scientific Advisory Group for Emergencies. (2021, July 30). *Long term evolution of SARS-CoV-2, 26 July 2021*. London: Government of the United Kingdom. https://www.gov.uk/government/publications/long-term-evolution-of-sars-cov-2-26-july-2021

Index

A. W. Blume, *Colonialism and the COVID-19 Pandemic*, International and Cultural Psychology, https://doi.org/10.1007/978-3-030-92825-4

The manufacturer's authorised representative in the EU is Springer Nature Customer Service Centre GmbH, Europaplatz 3, 69115 Heidelberg, Germany. If you have any concerns regarding our products, please contact ProductSafety@springernature.com

Printed and bound by CPI Group (UK) Ltd, Croydon, CR0 4YY
30/09/2026
02225293-0005